Sturkie's Avian Physiology

FIFTH EDITION

PEDIATRIC OPTOMETRY

SECOND EDITION

JEROME ROSNER, O.D.

Professor
College of Optometry
University of Houston

JOY ROSNER, O.D.

Associate Professor
College of Optometry
University of Houston

Butterworths
Boston   London   Singapore
Sydney   Toronto   Wellington

To our young patients

Library of Congress Cataloging-in-Publication Data

Rosner, Jerome.
   Pediatric optometry / Jerome Rosner, Joy Rosner.—2nd ed.
     p. cm.
   Includes bibliographies and index.
   ISBN 0-409-90063-X
   1. Vision disorders in children—Diagnosis.   2. Optometry.
I. Rosner, Joy. II. Title.
  [DNLM: 1. Optometry. 2. Vision Disorders—diagnosis.
3. Vision Disorders—in infancy & childhood. WW 600 R822p]
RE48.2.C5R67 1990
618.92'0977—dc20
DNLM/DLC
for Library of Congress   89-9711

British Library Cataloguing in Publication Data
Rosner, Jerome
   Pediatric optometry.—2nd. ed
   1. Children. Eyes. Diagnosis
   I. Title II. Rosner, Joy
   618.92'097715

   ISBN 0-409-90063-X

Butterworth Publishers
80 Montvale Avenue
Stoneham, MA 02180

10 9 8 7 6 5 4 3 2 1

Printed in the United States of America

CONTENTS

INTRODUCTION

It is not that long ago that the optometrist perceived his or her young patients as miniature adults. The main difference in clinical management was often nothing more than a pillow or a telephone book on the examination chair to compensate for their smaller-than-adult size. And, in fact, the optometrist's perceptions were justified. Conventional wisdom supported the notion that children need not visit the optometrist unless or until they displayed reasons for doing so: typically, blurred vision or strabismus.

A marked shift has occurred over the past few decades, for a number of reasons:

First, major discoveries have been achieved in vision-science (e.g., [1,2,3,4]) and major improvements have been made in clinical technology, procedures, and practices (e.g., [5,6]). Vision development is no longer a speculative topic that fosters a host of intuitively determined examination and treatment procedures. It is a phenomenon that is (and continues to be) well documented, and the remarkably insightful and ingenious examination and treatment procedures of previous decades (e.g., [7]) are being modified to reflect that knowledge.

Second, the optometrist has become much more adept at communicating with his patients. The benefit of that with the young patient is obvious. Too often, a child's inability to communicate has been misinterpreted as an inability to perform (8).

Third, the optometrist has become much more knowledgeable about the fundamental principles of instruction and learning, and how these apply within the context of vision testing and therapy (9,10). He now recognizes the remediation of deficient vergence facility, of strabismus, and of perceptual skills disorders to be reeducation processes that, if successful, will improve function and may ultimately affect structure, rather than the other way around. As a result, his procedures and overall clinical management have acquired a focus that yields effective outcomes.

The purpose of this book is to provide a single source of practical information, to synthesize the major advances of the past few decades into a useful form. It speaks to the optometry student and the optometrist conducting a primary-care practice. As such, it is presumed that the reader is already familiar with the basic principles, standard terminology, and clinical procedures of the profession. No space is devoted to these topics except where the redundancy is essential for completeness and clarity.

—■——————————————————————————————————————

SCOPE

The contents of this book emerge from a central question: "What special skills and knowledge should the optometrist in general practice have in order to serve young patients, children age 12 and younger, as competently as he serves adult patients?" Hence, the young patient is the primary concern, but not exclusively. Many adult patients manifest conditions that stem from their childhood; strabismus and/or amblyopia are obvious examples. They, too, fall within the scope of this volume.

—■——————————————————————————————————————

ORGANIZATION

The book is organized into three parts, each one following a structured format.

Part I is concerned with *examination and diagnosis*. The standard pediatric optometric examination is portrayed as a systematic method for posing a set of eight basic questions—probes that, in most cases, are sufficient for generating the information the optometrist needs to provide competent clinical care. These are:

1. Why is the patient seeking professional services (i.e., chief concern[s]?)
2. What other information might be relevant (i.e., history)?
3. How clearly does the patient see (i.e., visual acuity)?
4. Are there signs of pathology and/or structural anomalies (i.e., health assessment)?
5. Is there a significant refractive error (i.e., refractive status)?
6. Does the patient use his two eyes together at all distances (i.e., binocular status)?
7. Can the patient's eyes adapt effectively to reasonably stressful conditions (i.e., vergence and accommodation ranges and facility)?
8. Is the patient's developmental status appropriate for her age (i.e., level of behavioral development, with particular emphasis on visual perceptual skills)?

The first seven questions are very familiar. They pertain to all ages. They constitute the bedrock of the profession. This volume deals with how those standard practices and procedures may be modified in order to accommodate the young patient.

The eighth question signals a significant departure from the standard. It acknowledges the expanding scope of the profession by incorporating a concern for the child's general development—the extent to which the young patient is "on schedule" in achieving the milestone behaviors that exemplify normal development, with special attention devoted to perceptual skills development of elementary school-aged children (11).

Each of the eight questions is addressed in the eight chapters of Part I. Where appropriate, a chapter is then organized into subsections, each focusing on a separate age group. For example, the chapter devoted to assessing visual acuity is organized this way because the best methods for measuring the visual acuity of a 4-month-old differ from the methods appropriate for a 2-year-old, which, in turn, differ from the best methods for 4-year-olds and 6-year-olds. Different age groups present characteristics specific to their respective ages. Each has to be accommodated in a somewhat different way.

Part II focuses on the *postexamination process*—the various actions the optometrist might initiate, given a particular diagnosis. Here the reader will find information regarding the options available in the clinical management of refractive deviations, strabismus, amblyopia, nystagmus, inadequate vergence/accommodation facility, and perceptual skills disorders. Treatment alternatives are identified, along with prototype therapeutic and compensatory regimens; treatments that the primary-care practitioner is equipped to implement and supervise.

Part III comprises the final chapter of this book (Chapter 16). It offers a number of *case reports*. The cases we selected are representative; they describe children who present in all our offices with great regularity. Our reason for including them is not only to illustrate diagnosis and treatment; they are also meant to aid the reader in the process of translating technical knowledge into patient management, adjusting testing and treatment methods for the patient's age. To accomplish this, we include some cases representative of the same clinical condition manifesting in children of different ages.

Following each case report are a number of open-ended questions that are designed to stimulate productive discussion regarding salient aspects of the case. They are intended to aid instructors using this book to initiate discussion.

THE FLOW DIAGRAM

Traditionally, books of this sort contain a large body of information that is organized into major topical units. It is customary for the clinician to use such a book as a reference, going to it when information is needed and deciding, on his own, how and where to apply that information.

This book does not follow that custom. Rather, it follows a basic, problem-oriented design. The information is presented in a way that relates it directly to practical clinical situations.

The basic organizer is the flow diagram, a device that attempts to illustrate the sequence an optometrist follows and the factors he considers as he probes, interprets what he learns, makes decisions, acts, assesses the outcomes of those actions, and modifies his decisions and actions accordingly.

The flow diagrams in this book are neither fail-safe nor essential. Experienced clinicians will be able to use the information presented here without the aid of flow diagrams, but they may find them to be useful nonetheless. Less experienced clinicians will not become master practitioners because of the device, but it will help them also. The point is that the flow diagram is an aid, not a substitute, for competent clinical judgment. It helps organize clinical management into efficient sequences, nothing more. But that in itself is quite a lot.

□ How to Use a Flow Diagram

A properly designed flow diagram is self-explanatory. In essence, it is a road map that defines the most efficient route for getting from one place to another in the face of varying conditions. One simply starts at the beginning and works through it, step by step. Each flow diagram is intended to depict a different aspect of a clinical examination or treatment.

The flow diagrams in this book use two different types of landmarks—"roadsigns"—each identified by a different geometric shape. A rectangle signals a directive, a suggestion for doing something at that point in the sequence. Rectangles have only one exit path. A hexagon identifies a decision point, a fork in the road from which two paths emerge. It always contains a question that requires a "yes" or "no" response, which, in turn, determines the next step in the sequence.

Many of the rectangles and hexagons are marked with a capital letter. The letter indicates that additional, relevant information is contained in the text, where it is identified with the same letter.

■ PRACTICAL SUGGESTIONS

Each chapter of this book contains a Practical Suggestions section that is devoted to bridging the gap that often exists between textbook information and clinical implementation. These are compilations of helpful hints, explanatory illustrations, definitions, questions that are often posed (and proposed answers), and what have you.

■

REFERENCES

1. Hubel DH. Wiesel TN. Receptive fields of single neurones in the cat's striate cortex. J Physiol 1959; 148:574.
2. Wiesel TB, Hubel DH. Effects of visual deprivation on morphology and physiology of cells in the cat's lateral geniculate body. J Neurophys 1963; 26:978.
3. Mitchell DE, Freeman RD, Millodot M, Haegerstrom G. Meridional amblyopia: evidence of modification of the human visual system by early visual experience. Vis Res 1973; 13:535.
4. Fantz RL, Ordy JM, Udelf MS. Maturation of pattern vision in infants during the first six months. J Comp Physiol Psych 1962; 55;907–17.
5. Harter MR, Suitt CD. Visually evoked cortical responses and pattern vision in the infant: a longitudinal study. Psychonom Sci 1970; 18:235–37.
6. Regan D. Evoked potentials in psychology, sensory physiology and clinical medicine. London: Chapman and Hall, 1972.
7. Getman GN. Techniques and diagnostic criteria for the optometric care of children's vision. Duncan, Okla.: Opt. Ext. Program, 1959.
8. Romano RE, Romano JA, Puklin JE. Stereoacuity development in children with normal binocular single vision. Am J Ophthal 1975; 79(6):966–71.
9. Feldman J. Behavior modification in vision training: facilitating prerequisite behaviors and visual skills. JAOA 1976; 52(4):329–40.
10. Cooper J, Feldman J. Operant conditioning and assessment of stereopsis in young children. AJOPO 1978; 55(8):532–42.
11. Rosner J. Screening for perceptual skills dysfunction: an update. JAOA 1979; 55(10):1115–19.

ACKNOWLEDGMENTS

It is impossible to recognize all those who helped us in writing this book. There are simply too many; if we tried to list them, undoubtedly we would omit some unintentionally. We do not want to do that. However, we would be ungrateful to the extreme if we did not acknowledge the very great help supplied by Suzanne Ferrimer, Director of the University of Houston Optometry Library, Rebekah Estrada, her Prime Minister, and the rest of the library staff. All of them were helpful—always. We doubt that we could have written this book without their help.

I

EXAMINATION
AND DIAGNOSIS

1

Question 1
Why Is the Patient/Parent
Seeking Services?

☐

A. DETERMINE CHIEF CONCERN

Clinical examinations are not exhaustive; no single case warrants the use of every test in the optometrist's armamentarium. Clinicians use tests heuristically, in ways that enable them to obtain the information they need as efficiently as possible. They typically employ the strategy of seeking to answer broad-based, pivotal questions first, then the more focused ones, posing their questions in two ways: verbally, in a standard interrogation mode, and by way of objective and subjective clinical test procedures.

There are two fundamental reasons for eliciting a statement of chief concern from the patient or the patient's parent.

1. It identifies an issue that the optometrist must discuss knowledgeably and informatively before the visit ends (i.e., "I, the patient, or the patient's parent, am concerned about this." "Is it serious?" "What, if anything should/can be done about it?").

2. It defines the focal point of the visit, not to the exclusion of all else, but enough so that it influences the scope and sequence of the examination.

On the basis of the patient's/parent's chief concern, and from what he observes firsthand at this point, the optometrist commences the investigative process. He formulates one or more unstated hypothetical explanations for what he is told and what he sees, and then proceeds with the multibranched process of confirming or rejecting his hypotheses. He uses inductive and deductive methods; he infers certain conditions and rules out others on the basis of related pieces of information. He does not simply shrug at contradictory observations and unexplained phenomena. He *keeps them in mind*—a ubiquitous phrase in the flow diagrams, and for good reason—and accepts responsibility for resolving the contradictions and explaining the inexplicable.

The purpose of this section is to describe that first step as it typically pertains to the young patient (see Figure 1.1 flow diagram).

□ Typical Concerns

Ordinarily, children are brought to the optometrist for one or more of the following reasons:

1. The child complains and/or shows signs of substandard visual acuity. This may include sitting close to the television, holding reading material very close to her eyes, squinting, and/or complaining of not being able to see the chalkboard clearly from the back of the room.

2. The child complains and/or shows signs of eye-related discomfort and/or eyestrain and/or pain. This may include headaches and chronic visual fatigue.

3. The child failed a vision screening test. This may include a report of deficient visual acuity, binocular coordination, and/or perceptual skills.

4. The child appears to have a "turned eye" or some other oculomotor difficulty. This may occur sometimes or always, and manifests as an eye that "turns in/turns out" when "she is tired" or "looks at distance" or "looks at something close to her eyes." She may shut one eye when doing close work or when in bright light, she may tilt and/or turn her head in an unusual manner, and/or her eyes may appear to be constantly in motion, "jiggling" from side to side or up and down.

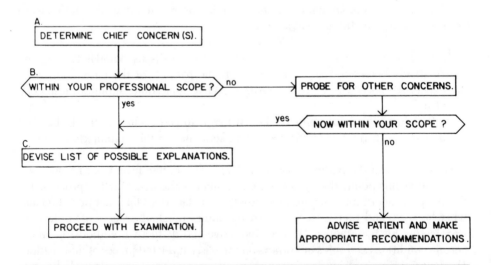

Figure 1.1   Question #1: Why is the patient/parent seeking services?

5. The child's eyes, or the tissue surrounding them, do not look normal in health and/or structure. This may range from "puffy" eyelids to a cloudy cornea, to a "white" pupil.

6. The child is having some/much difficulty in school. This may range from a specific problem (e.g., sloppy paper work, difficulty in copying from the chalkboard and/or from a book, loses place while reading, displays a persistent tendency to reverse certain letters—such as the b and d) to a general achievement problem in reading and/or arithmetic that has been identified as evidence of a learning disability, dyslexia, or an attention deficit disorder, see Practical Suggestions 1-2 and 1-3.

7. The child does not manifest any unusual symptoms or signs. Her parents simply want assurance that her eyes are healthy, normally formed, and performing appropriately for her age. This may have been inspired by a family history of a specific visual or ocular anomaly, but just as often it is the result of a newspaper or magazine article relevant to some aspect of children's vision.

■

B. WITHIN YOUR PROFESSIONAL SCOPE?

There are, of course, instances when the patient's stated chief concern does not fall within the scope of the practitioner. When this occurs, further probing may reveal that the patient has indeed come to the wrong professional or the patient's concerns are within the optometrist's scope, once they have been redefined. In the latter case, the redefinition is essential.

For example, and not an uncommon example at that: suppose the parent's stated chief concern is that the child had been identified as having a "learning disability" or "dyslexia." The purpose of the visit is to determine the validity of that diagnosis: to answer the question, "Does my child have this condition?" Answering that question is beyond the scope of the average optometrist. It requires psychoeducational data that are not usually measured in optometric offices.

Further probing clarifies the situation. The chief concern becomes, "My child has a reading problem. Does he also have a visual problem that might be causing, or contributing to, his school difficulties?"

The investigation may now begin. Both parent and practitioner agree on the purpose of the examination—on what is being sought. Both have reason to believe that the search is worthwhile and that the optometrist is the appropriate person to conduct it. The outcome, insofar as the child's reading problem is concerned, is not predictable. But there is no question about the optometrist's ability to meet the responsibility he accepts. It is well within his professional scope. There are no false expectations, no misrepresentations.

■

C. DEVISE A LIST OF POSSIBLE EXPLANATIONS

Listed below are some of the hypotheses, possible explanations that will occur to the optometrist as he maps out his strategy for managing the case effectively and efficiently. The list is not exhaustive, but it will serve as an advance organizer in many cases.

□ Concern 1: Blurred Vision

POSSIBLE EXPLANATIONS

    1. Ametropia, pseudomyopia (see Chapter 5).

    2. Amblyopia, eccentric fixation, nystagmus (see Chapters 4 and 6).

    3. Trauma: e.g., optic nerve damage, cataract, retinal detachment, corneal scarring, luxation of the lens, vitreous hemorrhage, macular edema (see Chapter 4 and *Nonaccidental trauma*, below.)

    4. Systemic illness: e.g., diabetes, severe anemia, sickle-cell disease (see Chapter 2).

    5. Drug reaction: e.g., sulfa, antihistamines, phenothiazides (see Chapters 2 and 4).

    6. Ocular disease: e.g., acute glaucoma, tumor, keratitis, corneal dystrophies, retinal hemmorhage (see Chapters 2 and 4).

    7. Central nervous system involvement: e.g., optic neuritis, papillitis, tumor, parietal lobe lesion, hydrocephalus, meningitis (see Chapters 2 and 4).

    8. Congenital: e.g., albinism, Best's disease, Stargardt's disease, Coat's disease, Tay-Sachs disease, retinoblastoma (see Chapters 2 and 4).

    9. Malingering (see Chapters 3 and 5).

    10. Nonaccidental trauma (the abused child).

The optometrist must always consider the possibility of child abuse when confronted with a youngster who displays clear signs of trauma. It is not as farfetched a suspicion as was once thought. The prevalence of nonaccidental trauma is astounding and growing: in excess of 34,000 cases were reported in Texas alone in 1975, as compared with 4000 in 1973. The growth factor is explained by the fact that laws now have been passed in every state of the United States requiring that all suspected cases be reported; failure to report a case of suspected child abuse is a crime (1). Hence, there probably has not been a major surge in child abuse; rather, more cases are being identified. Small comfort!

Most cases of nonaccidental trauma involve children younger than 3 years of age. They come from all socioeconomic groups, but they tend to belong to families

Intraocular hemorrhages (retinal, preretinal, vitreous, hyphema)
Periorbital edema/ecchymosis
Detached retina/dialysis
Chorioretinal atrophy
Cataract
Subluxated lens and traumatic mydriasis
Papilledema
Subconjunctival hemorrhage
Esotropia
Corneal opacity and nystagmus
Optic atrophy

Harley RD, Spaeth GL. Ocular manifestations of child abuse. In: Francois J, Maione M, eds. Pediatric Ophthalmology. New York: John Wiley & Sons, 1982.

Table 1.1   Ocular Manifestations in the Child-Abuse Syndrome
(Arranged According to Reported Frequency)

where there is a social dysfunction; e.g., alcoholism, perversion tendencies, marital stress, financial difficulties (2).

The abused child is often socially withdrawn. She may refuse to talk and will be inclined to be wary of physical contact, especially with adults. She is apt to display school learning difficulties (3). The ocular manifestations may or may not be apparent externally; i.e., observable without an ophthalmoscope. Table 1.1 lists these ocular manifestations in their order of frequency.

As already noted, the law in every state of the United States requires that all suspected cases of child abuse be reported. In some states, major units have been organized to receive and follow up on these reports; in others, the standard legal mechanisms come into play. Guidelines for a given state may be obtained from any district attorney's office within that state. They can also advise you of the protection the law provides to the reporters of such cases; most states offer the reporter anonymity and protection from civil liability.

□ Concern 2: Eye-Related Pain/Discomfort

POSSIBLE EXPLANATIONS

1. Ametropia: e.g., hyperopia, astigmatism, anisometropia (see Chapter 5).
2. Unstable binocular status: e.g., intermittent diplopia (see Chapter 6).
3. Inefficient binocular skills: e.g., reduced fusional vergence/accommodation amplitudes; inadequate vergence/accommodation facility (see Chapter 7).
4. Ocular inflammation: e.g., conjunctivitis, keratitis, uveitis, glaucoma, ciliary neuralgia (see Chapter 4).
5. Systemic disease: e.g., sinusitis, hypothyroidism (see Chapter 2).

□ Concern 3: Failed Vision Screening Test

POSSIBLE EXPLANATIONS

1. Reduced visual acuity (see Chapter 5).
2. Binocular dysfunction (see Chapters 6 and 7).
3. Perceptual skills dysfunction (see Chapter 8).
4. Malingering (see Chapters 3 and 5).

VISION SCREENING

Vision screening takes on many different forms, depending upon the sponsoring agent and the target population. The discussion that follows gives an overview of the topic as it pertains to children. We first describe vision screening tests that are frequently used in schools, then the screening of preschool children, and finally, some comments about the optometrist's role in these enterprises.

Vision screening tests are designed to determine the extent to which an individual's performance compares with some predetermined standards (4). Or, said more directly, "Vision screening tests are designed to discover children with vision disorders." (5, p. 333). As such, vision screening tests are not designed to diagnose visual disorders. Rather, their purpose is to identify those children who should be seen by a professional for examination, diagnosis, and subsequent recommendations.

School-Based Vision Screening Programs

Vision screening has become a well-established activity in our schools, primarily because of the obvious connection between clear eyesight and school achievement and secondarily because schools have tended to adopt the role of a public health agency in this domain (6,7,8,9,10).

There are no nationally accepted standards that prescribe when school-based vision screenings should be conducted or the form they should take (4). These decisions, more often than not, rest with the local school boards, although many states in the United States do mandate that screenings be conducted at specified points in a child's school experiences (11).

VISION SCREENING TESTS

Some school-based vision screening tests are very limited, focusing on a single visual ability; others comprise a number of different subtests. Some employ only an acuity test chart and can be administered by any reasonably intelligent person; others require complex optical apparatus and the participation of optometrists or ophthalmologists (4,5,12,13). Some are *true distance tests*, others are *simulated distance tests*. The latter use optical devices to simulate different test distances; the former may also use optical devices, but not for the same purposes. A farpoint assessment with a true distance test requires the patient to fixate at a distant (e.g., 6 meters) target. A simulated distance test will attempt to elicit from the patient the visual responses of farpoint fixation while actually placing the target at some closer position.

True Distance Tests

- The farpoint visual acuity test is the method selected most often for school-based vision screening programs; this despite the fact that those who select it are usually quick to admit its limitations (but not all; see [14,15]). Clearly, its popularity is attributable to its economy. It can be administered by lay volunteers, requires very little time, space, and equipment, and in fact provides relatively reliable information about a very key, albeit single, aspect of vision. Typically, the criterion for "passing" this test is 20/30 acuity or better in each eye.

- The plus 1.75-Diopter lens test entails having the child who has already demonstrated clear farpoint acuity (e.g., 20/20) attempt to read the same size letters through a pair of +1.75-D. sphere lenses. The reasoning is obvious. If the plus lenses do not cause a reduction in acuity, then the child is probably hyperopic to at least that degree in at least one eye. Therefore, being able to read the 20/20 line of print through a pair of +1.75-diopter lenses constitutes a failure, a reason for referral to a professional (see [16,17,18] for a contrary view).

More Comprehensive Screening Protocols

Some schools have adopted more comprehensive screening procedures (19). These range from the use of a commercially produced instrument under the supervision of a school nurse or a trained volunteer to the implementation of a "modified clinical technique" (MCT): a scaled-down version of a professional assessment that requires some professional participation (20).

A representative listing of these appears below. No attempt was made to list all available instruments. Those listed here were selected because of their relative popularity.

- *The Massachusetts Vision Test (MVT)** (21,22) comprises four subtests.

Test 1. Distance visual acuity. Instead of a full-size letter chart, only two lines of letters are presented, one made up of 20/30 letters, the other, 20/20. In application, if the child cannot read the 20/30 line of letters, it is scored as a "fail" and referral is indicated.** If the child cannot read the 20/20 letters but can read the 20/30 ones, then it is a "partial failure" and is recorded as such.

Test 2. Visual acuity with plus lenses. This is the aforementioned plus lens test, used here with the two lines of letters. As already noted, if the child is able to

---

*The MVT, originally marketed by Welch-Allyn, Auburn, N.Y., and American Optical Co., is now out of print. We include it here because many were installed in schools and are probably still in use, because there is virtually nothing to wear out in the instrument.
**Note: A screening procedure is often terminated as soon as one of the critical criterion is failed. There is no need to complete the full battery of tests, since the purpose of the activity is to "screen" rather than diagnose.

read the 20/20 line of letters through the +1.75-D. lenses, it is scored as a "fail" and referral is indicated. If he cannot read the 20/20 line through the plus lenses but can read the 20/30 letters, then it is scored as a "partial fail." (In the MVT, two partial fails constitute a fail.)

Test 3. Distance phoria test. A red Maddox rod is placed before the child's right eye. His left eye is directed to a line drawing of a house, in which there is a line drawing of a window, in which in turn there is a small light. The vertical phoria is measured first, with the acceptable limits being the upper and lower boundaries of the "window." (This is the equivalent of 1 1/4 prism diopters.) Then the lateral phoria is measured, and, once more, the test is failed if the child reports that the red vertical line is located outside the left and right boundaries of the "window." (This is the equivalent of 6 esophoria or 4 exophoria.)

Test 4. Near phoria test. This test is done at a 40-cm viewing distance. The fixation target is a small light that is centered within a drawing of an airplane, which, in turn, is enclosed within a drawn rectangle. Once again, if either the vertical or the horizontal red line produced by the Maddox rod falls beyond the boundaries of the rectangle, then the test is failed. (This is the equivalent of 1 1/4 prism diopters vertically and, horizontally, 6 esophoria or 8 exophoria.)

Simulated Distance Tests

All of the instruments in this category are variations of the Brewster stereoscope. That is, they use convex lenses combined with prisms and appropriately designed stereoscope targets to simulate optical infinity when the actual test distance may, in fact, be only 20 cm. We will describe one of these, the Keystone Visual Skills Screening Test, and then mention the others merely as variations on that theme.

- *The Keystone Visual Skills Screening Test.* This test (Keystone View Division of Mast Development Company, 2312 East 12th Street, Davenport, Iowa 52803) calls for a Telebinocular: a Brewster stereoscope in which orthophoria at optical infinity is achieved by maintaining a 95-mm center-to-center, between-target separation. The battery is made up of a set of ten farpoint tests and five nearpoint tests, each one presented on a separate stereoscope card. (Note: Certain of these tests are deleted in some schools, usually because of the bias of the person administering the test or the opinions of the community optometrists and opthalmologists.)

Farpoint Keystone Visual Skills Screening Tests

Test 1. Simultaneous vision. A drawing of a pig is presented to the left eye; a drawing of a dog to the right eye. The animals are positioned on the card so that if the patient is binocular and both eyes are open, the child will report seeing "a dog jumping over a pig." If only one animal is seen, then the subtest is failed and the obvious inference is that the child does not manifest simultaneous binocular perception.

Test 2. Vertical imbalance. A horizontal green line is presented to the left eye; a vertical row of geometric designs to the right eye. Adjacent to the designs is a vertical column of numerals, ranging from 3 to 0 (in the center) to 3 again. The binocular patient without a vertical phoria will report seeing a horizontal line passing through the center of the middle geometric design, and the "0" alongside it. The patient with a vertical phoria will report in accord with his deviation.

Test 3. Lateral imbalance. The left eye views an arrow, pointing upward. The right eye sees the numerals 1 to 15 arranged in sequence, from left to right (see Figure 1.2). When viewed in the Telebinocular by a binocular individual, the arrow appears to be pointing to a numeral, or between two numerals. Hence, this is a phoria test, wherein wide variance—ranging from high exophoria to orthophoria to high esophoria—may be displayed.

Test 4. Fusion. Two dots—a red one and, below it, a white one—are presented to the right eye. The left eye also sees a white dot but now with a blue one below it. The child displays normal fusion by reporting that he observes three dots: a red, a white, and a blue, aligned vertically. Misalignment—a slanted row of dots or a report of four dots—indicates an instability or a lack of fusion under these viewing conditions.

Test 5. Right eye—usable vision. Each eye is shown a photographed scene containing a series of signposts that recede into the distance along a railroad bridge. Each signpost displays five white diamond-shaped spaces. The right half of the stereoscopic card is designed so that there is a black dot in one of the diamond shapes in each signpost. Hence, when viewed stereoscopically, the individual should see the signposts in three dimensions, each one appearing to be somewhat more distant than the one just preceding it.

The child's task: indicate which diamond in each of the signposts contains the black dot, starting with the nearest one. Thus, this test provides two kinds of information. One, it gives evidence about the child's visual acuity, as illustrated by his ability to discriminate the dots as they, and the signposts, become smaller and appear to recede into the distance. Second, it can reveal a central suppression. If some or all of the dots are not visible to the child unless his left eye is occluded, then the only reasonable explanation is that, when both eyes are open and directed to the same point in space, the right eye manifests a central suppression; hence the invisible dots.

Test 6. Left eye—usable vision. This is exactly like test 5, except that conditions for each eye are reversed. Hence, this test is sensitive to left eye visual acuity and the possibility of a central suppression area in that eye (see Figure 1.2).

Test 7. Both eyes—usable vision. This test is very much like tests 5 and 6, with one important difference. In this test the black dots are presented simultaneously to both eyes. It is not designed to reveal central suppression; rather, it is simply an indicator of binocular visual acuity as measured under these conditions.

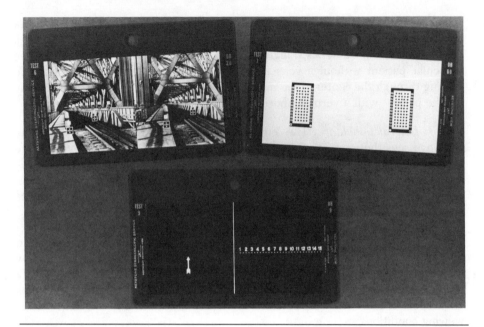

Figure 1.2 Keystone Visual Skills Farpoint Screening Tests #3, 6, and 8.

Test 8. Stereopsis. Matching arrays of geometric designs, organized into twelve horizontal lines, five designs in each line, are presented to both eyes (see Figure 1.2). If the patient is binocular, these will be perceived as a single array. The geometric designs are positioned so that one design in each line appears to "float" forward—seemingly closer than the other designs in that line.* The patient is then asked to identify that design in each of the twelve lines, starting from the top; the discrimination task becomes increasingly more difficult as he works his way down the display.

Test 9 and 10. Color perception. These two are similar. Both are designed in a manner similar to the Ishihara color plates: numerals made up of colored dots embedded in a field of multicolored dots, with all the colors carefully controlled. Test 9 is designed to test for red/green perception; test 10 for blue/violet discrimination.

---

*This is accomplished by decentering the design in each line that is to appear to "float" so that it stimulates noncorresponding retinal points, with the target viewed by the right eye positioned to the left of the target viewed by the left eye; in other words, in a crossed disparity condition. If they were in an uncrossed disparity condition, the effect would be that of placing the image *farther away* rather than closer (see Chapter 6 discussion regarding stereopsis).

Nearpoint Keystone Visual Skills Screening Tests

Test 1. Lateral imbalance. This test is analogous to test 3 in the distance-test group. It is the nearpoint version of the phoria test wherein an arrow, seen by one eye, points to a horizontal row of numerals, visible to the opposite eye.

Test 2. Fusion. This is analogous to test 4 in the distance-test group. Fusion is demonstrated when the patient reports "three balls": a red, a white, and a blue one in vertical alignment.

Test 3, 4, and 5. Usable vision. Like their distance-test counterparts (distance tests 5, 6, and 7), these three tests provide information about visual acuity and central suppression. Test 3 measures the right eye, with the left eye open; test 4 does the opposite; and test 5 presents the same visual stimuli to both eyes simultaneously.

- *Keystone Preschool Vision Test* (Keystone View Division of Mast Development Co., 2312 East 12th St., Davenport, Iowa 52803). This test, too, is designed for the Telebinocular. In fact, the only major difference between this and the Visual Skills Screening Test is in the appearance of the stimuli provided for the various items. This series, called the "Peekaboo" series, contains figures that are intended to be more appealing to young children (see Figure 1.3). For example, instead of an arrow in the phoria test, there is a hand with the index finger pointing upward; instead of a sequence of numerals, there is a row of

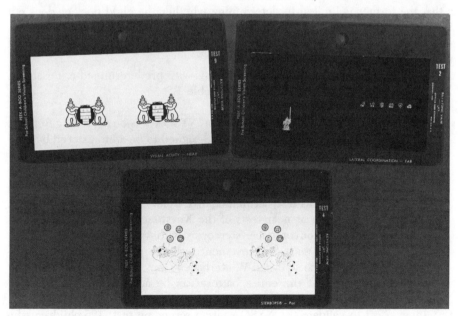

Figure 1.3   Keystone Preschool Vision Screening Tests #2, 4, and 9.

familiar objects; instead of the three colored dots in the test for fusion, there is a rotund clown, and so on. Despite all these, the test is difficult for young children because of its receptive and expressive language demands.

- *Titmus Optical Vision Tester* (Titmus Optical Co., 1312 West 7th Street, Piscataway, N.J., 08854). The T-O Vision Tester is very much like the Telebinocular and the Visual Skills Screening Test. It, too, is built on the principles of a Brewster stereoscope; it, too, uses tests that measure binocular alignment and stereopsis in addition to visual acuity. The main difference: the test items are printed on glass slides that are housed within the device, lighted from behind, and changed by turning a wheel that is situated on the side of the instrument.
- *Ortho-Rater* (Bausch & Lomb, Rochester, N.Y. 14602). The Ortho-Rater is yet another Brewster stereoscope, resembling very closely the T-O Vision Tester both in optical design and in the kinds of tests it contains.
- *MCT*. We have already noted that this method can be characterized as an attenuated professional examination. As the MCT was defined in the landmark Orinda (California) study (20), it screens for four categories of problems:

1. Organic problems—with a hand magnifier and an ophthalmoscope.
2. Visual acuity problems—with an acuity chart.
3. Refractive problems—with a retinoscope.
4. Binocular coordination problems—with cover test and a 5-diopter prism.

The main difference between the MCT and a full-scale professional evaluation is that the former is limited to determining whether the child does or does not display a problem in any one of the aforementioned categories. A screening does not take the second step of establishing the exact nature and appropriate treatment of the problem.

The MCT is administered on a pass/fail basis with predetermined criteria. The criteria for the Orinda study are shown in Table 1.2

- *The New York State Optometric Association (NYSOA) Vision Screening Battery*. The NYSOA vision screening battery was designed to be administered by non-professionals. It comprises a number of different subtests, which, in the aggregate, "screens a child's visual skills as they are needed in the classroom for efficient learning" (23, p. 981). These include visual acuity at distance and near; plus (+) 1.50 diopter lens test; accommodative facility at near; vertical balance, fusion at far and fusion at near tests of the Keystone Visual Skills Tests (see above); near point of convergence; stereopsis with Wirt circles; eye tracking (with the NYSOA K-D saccadic movement test; see p. 320); visual-motor integration as tested by the so-called Winterhaven Copy Forms Test (see p. 305). The authors report that the entire battery can be administered in about 20 minutes by a properly trained person.

In an effort to validate the NYSOA vision screening test, 125 children who had been previously tested with the NYSOA screening battery were given

Characteristic Evaluated	Compilation	Orinda Vision Study
Organic problems	Any	Any
Visual acuity	20/40 or less either eye	20/40 or less either eye
Refractive error		
Hyperopia	+1.75 D.S. or more	+1.50 D.S. or more
Myopia	−0.50 D.S. or more	−0.50 D.S. or more
Astigmatism	±1.00 D.C. or more	±1.00 D.C. or more
Anisometropia	±1.00 D. or more	±1.00 D. or more
Coordination problems		
At distance		
Esophoria	5 Δ or more	5 Δ or more
Exophoria	5 Δ or more	5 Δ or more
Hyperphoria	2 Δ or more	2 Δ or more
Tropia	Any	Any
At near		
Esophoria	6 Δ or more	6 Δ or more
Exophoria	10 Δ or more	10 Δ or more
Hyperphoria	2 Δ or more	2 Δ or more
Tropia	Any	Any
Perceptual problems		
Fusion		
Stereopsis	Must await further investigation; not a cause for referral at present	Not evaluated
Aniseikonia		
Color vision		

Peters HB. Vision screening. In: Hirsch M, Wick R, eds. Vision of children: an optometric symposium. Philadelphia: Chilton Books, 1963.

Table 1.2 Criteria for Referral

complete visual examinations. Sensitivity of the NYSOA test was determined to be 71.7 percent and specificity to be 65 percent. In contrast, the Snellen (visual acuity) test with these same children was found to be 100 percent specific (i.e., no false-positives) but overlooked "75.5 percent of the children found to have vision problems when given a complete visual examination" (24, p. 165).

The NYSOA vision screen test represents a noble undertaking but appears to suffer from the zealousness of its designers. In the process of identifying the behaviors that "represent the visual skills needed in the classroom for efficient learning," many subjective, nonvalidated opinions were exercised; there is little evidence available to substantiate the cause-effect relationships of some of these behaviors to school performance. Hence, the test battery, despite its positive features, lacks the qualities that would justify its implementation. Too many children would fail it on the basis of performance that too few optometrists perceive as "vision problems."

Teacher Judgment

This is the least technical of the screening methods, yet it is used and should be included in this discussion (1). No equipment is employed, other than, in some instances, a printed "checklist" of signs and symptoms that might signal a visual problem. (Figure 1.4 shows one such list.) In many schools, there is no printed checklist; simply a community-sponsored attitude that encourages teachers to stay alert for signs of vision problems among their students, and to mention these observations and/or intuitions to the children's parents when it seems appropriate to do so.

COMPARISON OF SCHOOL-BASED SCREENING METHODS

In comparing vision screening methods, the following three factors have to be kept in mind and in balance:

1. The validity of the test results.*
2. The effectivity of the test results.**
3. Costs: time, personnel, equipment.

Peters (2) provides some relevant data. Table 1.3 compares the following tests: Snellen visual acuity test, MCT, visual skills screening test, Massachusetts Vision Test (MVT), and teacher's judgment. It appears that the MCT had, and continues to have, much to recommend it (20); but one does have to acknowledge that professional participation costs have escalated remarkably since those data were collected, much more than has the cost of equipment. (The Orinda study cites part-time professional costs at $6.00 per hour [25].)

SUMMARY AND FUTURE PROSPECTS

School-sponsored vision screening programs are here to stay. Their worth is well recognized, and it is difficult to find anyone who will argue against them. When disagreement does occur, it tends to be over which tests should be included in a vision screening, not on the basic worth of the enterprise itself. Some would like to see vision screening tests become even more comprehensive than the MCT. Peters (5) discussed the possibility of screening for "perceptual problems" but dismissed this because of lack of "adequate information." More recently, proposals regarding the appropriateness of screening for specific perceptual skills dysfunction have appeared and are gaining acceptance in some sections of the United States (26,27).

Despite the data, the MCT is not growing in popularity. One reason: professionals are not inclined to volunteer their services, and costs are an important factor. Another reason: the professional community itself has not come to grips

*Validity: an index of how well the test measures what it purports to measure; i.e., what is the likelihood that a professional will agree with the referral (2)?
**Effectivity: an index of the likelihood of the test overlooking a problem that a professional would identify (2).

TEACHER:
SCHOOL:

Teacher Observation Checklist

It has been shown that the teacher is frequently the best "screening instrument" for identifying those vision problems that tend to cancel the teacher's efforts in the classroom. The following checklist contains many of the observable clues and symptoms that are often associated with a vision problem. Please read through this list and check those items you have noticed in this case.

( ) Skips words or sentences
( ) Rereads lines or phrases
( ) Reads too slowly
( ) Uses finger or marker to guide eyes
( ) Says words aloud or moves lips
( ) Reverses words or letters
( ) Poor ability to remember what is read
( ) Unusual fatigue or restlessness after maintaining visual concentration
( ) Complains of letters or lines "running together" or "jumping around"
( ) Complains of blur while reading or writing
( ) Comprehension poor as reading continued or loses interest quickly
( ) Poor eye-hand coordination
( ) Unusual awkwardness
( ) Thrusting head forward or backward while looking at distant objects
( ) One eye turns in or out at anytime
( ) Excessive tearing of the eyes
( ) Frequent styes
( ) Reddened eyes or lids
( ) Headaches in forehead or temples
( ) Repeatedly omits "small" words
( ) Writes up or down hill on paper
( ) Complains of seeing double
( ) Misaligns both horizontal and vertical series of numbers
( ) Repeatedly confuses right-left directions

( ) Mistakes words with same or similar beginnings
( ) Blinks excessively
( ) Frowns, scowls, or squints
( ) Holds reading closer than normal
( ) Moves head while reading
( ) Covers or closes one eye
( ) Avoids close work
( ) Short attention span
( ) Daydreaming
( ) Tilts head to one side
( ) Rubs eyes frequently
( ) Rests head on arm when writing
( ) Improper or awkward posture while reading or writing
( ) Confusion of similar words
( ) Fails to recognize same word in next sentence
( ) Fails to recognize same word in different book
( ) Confuses likenesses and minor differences
( ) Makes errors in copying from reference books to notebook
( ) Difficulty copying from the chalkboard
( ) Slowness in all schoolwork
( ) Slowness in copying from the chalkboard
( ) Large pupils in normal light
( ) Excessive squinting from bright light
( ) Difficulty following verbal instructions
( ) Writes crookedly and/or poorly spaced

Figure 1.4   Teacher's observation checklist.

Screening Method	Reliability	Validity	Effectivity	Professional Agreement
Snellen visual acuity	+0.84	+0.71	+0.42	90%
Teachers	+0.72	+0.68		
Nurses	+0.84	+0.71		
Massachusetts vision test	+0.62	+0.68	+0.59	70%
Visual acuity	+0.85	+0.71		
Plus sphere test	+0.71	+0.38		
Lateral phoria at distance	+0.45	+0.41		
Lateral phoria at near	+0.41	+0.37		
Vertical phoria at distance	+0.34	+0.86		
Telebinocular vision skills	+0.53	+0.57	+0.51	55%
Simultaneous vision	+0.57	+0.40		
Vertical phoria at distance	+0.68	+0.63		
Lateral phoria at distance	+0.62	+0.54		
Fusion at distance	+0.43	+0.54		
Visual acuity right	+0.60	+0.61		
Visual acuity left	+0.61	+0.63		
Stereopsis	+0.60	not available		
Lateral phoria at near	+0.57	+0.58		
Fusion at near	+0.41	+0.49		
Modified clinical technique	+0.93	+0.95	+0.95	90%
Visual acuity	+0.93	+0.96		
Skiametry	+0.92	+0.94		
Cover test	+0.92	+0.93		
Organic problems	+0.97	+0.92		

Peters HB. Vision screening. In: Hirsch M, Wick R, eds. Vision of children: an optometric symposium. Philadelphia: Chilton Books, 1963.

Table 1.3 Vision Screening Test Evaluation

with the importance or nonimportance of binocular problems. This is especially true in the case of heterophorias (1). More than one school nurse has stopped making referrals on the basis of a significant heterophoria. School nurses have been embarrassed once too often by eye-care professionals who ignore binocular measures (aside from strabismus), thereby implying that the school nurse was not conducting a valid screening. School nurses in this situation have no recourse but to accept "blame" for making a needless referral, hardly a way to keep them enthusiastic about screening for binocular problems.

On the plus side, however, we know that the possibilities are not yet exhausted. It seems quite probable that new tests will be produced that will not require professional involvement yet will be valid and effective. Recently, for example, the Random-dot E stereotest (28,29) has been found to be very sensitive not only to strabismus, but also to anisometropia and/or acuity deficits, and a layperson can use it with very little pretraining (30).

There is every reason to believe that even better instruments will be produced.

Vision Screening Programs for Preschool (18- to 48-month-old) Children

As noted in our introductory remarks, much has been learned during the past three decades about the development of vision. For example, we now know that certain visual conditions (e.g., amblyopia) respond much better to treatment during the first few years of life than they do if treatment is delayed until, say, age 7 or 8 years. It is not surprising, therefore, that interest is growing in early detection. The first efforts at early detection of visual problems centered on measuring the visual acuity of 3- and 4-year-olds with the Tumbling E test (see p. 48). However, too many children in this age group are unable to respond reliably to that test, for a variety of reasons: the four orientations of the E may present insurmountable perceptual demands, for one; for another, the 6-meter test distance is too great for some children (31). This prompted the use of less sophisticated acuity targets, such as the Allen Picture Card Test and the Broken Wheel Test (see Chapter 3), neither of which causes as much difficulty as the Tumbling E's, but nonetheless are often too demanding for children younger than age 3 years (32).

The search for better testing methods, and an interest in testing more than visual acuity, has generated some innovative approaches. One that has attracted attention is the stereoacuity test. The TNO, the Random-dot E stereotest, and a modified version of the Frisby stereotest (see Chapter 6) all show promise. Young children are able to comprehend them, and they can be administered by lay persons with very little pretraining. Various reports show that the TNO is effective in identifying monocular amblyopia in 3-to 6-year-old children (33) ; the Random-dot E stereotest is applicable with children as young as 30 months and is very sensitive not only to strabismus, but also to anisometropia and/or acuity deficits when it is administered at a 1.5-meter distance (28,29,30); and the Frisby stereotest, when modified to be used as two-item, forced-choice instrument, can be used successfully with children as young as 13 months of age (34).

Vision Screening Programs for (0- to 18-month old) Infants

Efforts are also underway to develop valid, inexpensively administered screening tests for very young (0- to 18-month-old) children. A number of different tests have been devised, but in general, they fall into two categories: tests for measuring visual acuity and tests for determining the refractive status of the eyes. The former typically employ a forced-choice, preferential looking (FPL) approach. It has been shown to be valid with very young infants. (See Chapter 3 and [35] for a fuller description of the method.) The latter involves a procedure that has been labeled "photorefraction." Different versions of this latter procedure have been described (36,37,38,39,40), but, as an example of a relatively typical application, the method involves the use of a 35mm single-lens reflex camera with a narrow ring (flash) light source attached to the outer margin of the lens. This ring also contains a flickering fixation light. If a color photograph is taken at a distance of 0.5 meter from the face of a subject who is accurately fixating and focusing with both eyes on the camera fixation light, the fundus reflex in each pupil will appear to be absent or dark red and the corneal light reflexes will be symmetrical. If one or both eyes are not accurately focused or fixating, the fundus reflex will be brighter and much lighter (yellow or white). One study reports photoscreener photographs of 161 infants and children, some with normal acuity, some with reduced acuity and/or strabismus, who were assessed by independent observers who had no prior knowledge of the subjects' visual conditions. The screening technique obtained a sensitivity of 93 percent and specificity of 82 percent. The authors concluded that "it is a simple method applicable to routine screening of all one year old infants for impediments to normal visual development" (41, p. 43).

Both the FPL and photorefraction tests appear to have excellent potential for accomplishing what they were designed to accomplish—identifying young children with visual conditions that should be treated early in life. Ideally, a visual screening should include both of them. However, if this is not feasible, if only one is to be used, then the latter—early identification of abnormal refractive status with photorefraction—appears to be the more useful of the two. It requires far less time and patient participation than does FPL, and it provides information that is readily translated into clinical implications. Assessment of visual acuity by FPL will, indeed, identify a certain number of vision problems, but not as many as will valid refraction methods, particularly at the age when visual acuity is far from acutely developed (42).

□ Concern 4: Binocular Misalignment, Ocular Motility Disorder, Unusual Head Posture

POSSIBLE EXPLANATIONS

1. Pseudoesotropia, pseudoexotropia, unusually large positive or negative angle kappa (see Chapters 4 and 6).

2. Exophthalmos, hypertelorism, hypotelorism (see Chapter 4).

3. Structural anomaly; e.g., Brown's syndrome, Duane's syndrome, Mobius syndrome, VI nerve palsy, "trapped" extraocular muscle due to fractured orbit (see Chapter 4).

4. Central nervous system involvement; e.g., tumor, myasthenia gravis, meningitis, aneurism, syphilis (see Chapters 2 and 4).

5. Congenital; e.g., cerebral palsy, Marfan's syndrome (see Chapter 2).

□ Concern 5: Eyes Do Not Look Healthy/Normal

POSSIBLE EXPLANATIONS

1. Relation of eyes to orbit; e.g., pseudoproptosis, proptosis, enophthalmos (see Chapters 2 and 4).
2. Eyelids; e.g., pseudoptosis, ptosis, lagophthalmos, blepharospasm, unusual blinking pattern, swollen lids, epicanthus, blepharitis, blepharophimosis, euryblepharon, coloboma, poliosis, trichomegaly, madarosis, distiachisis, synophyrys (see Chapters 2 and 4).
3. Tears/tear glands: e.g., dacryoadenitis, gland enlargement, bloody tears, excessive tears, dry eye (see Chapter 4 and nonaccidental trauma above).
4. "Red" eyes; e.g., dilation of conjunctival vessels, discolored sclera, scleritis, trauma, "bump," or "lump" (see Chapter 4).
5. Pupils; e.g., very large, coloboma, iridoschisis, unequal size, white pupil (see Chapters 2 and 4).
6. Iris; e.g., heterochromia, nevi, atrophy, siderosis (see Chapters 2 and 4).

□ Concern 6: School Difficulties

POSSIBLE EXPLANATIONS

1. Sloppy paper work; uncorrected hyperopia, convergence insufficiency, accommodative insufficiency, substandard visual perceptual skills, insufficient familiarity with the letters and the mechanics of penmanship (see Chapters 5, 7, and 8).
2. Loses place while reading; reduced near visual acuity, uncorrected hyperopia, convergence/accommodation insufficiency, inadequate reading skills (see Chapters 5, 7, and 8).
3. Reverses letters; e.g., confuses the b and d; inadequate visual perceptual skills; practicing a "bad habit" developed when initially taught the letters (see Chapters 8 and 15).
4. Reading problem:
   - *word recognition:* reduced near visual acuity, convergence/accommodation insufficiency, substandard auditory and visual analysis skills, unfamiliar with the printed letters, language deficit.
   - *reading comprehension:* substandard word recognition skills, deficient vocabulary, inadequately familiar with subject matter dealt with in text, uncorrected refractive error, substandard visual analysis skills (see Chapters 5, 7, 8, and 15).
5. Unsatisfactory arithmetic achievement: uncorrected refractive error, convergence/accommodation insufficiency, substandard visual analysis skills, inadequate prerequisite number fact knowledge (see Chapters 5, 7, 8, and 15).

☐ Concern 7: None; Simply Seeks Reassurance

POSSIBLE EXPLANATIONS

Family history of visual/ocular problem (amblyopia, strabismus, glaucoma, retinitis pigmentosa); has been advised that it is wise to rule out deficits before their effects become manifest, i.e., routine precaution (see Chapters 2, 5, 6, 7, and 8).

___■_____

PRACTICAL SUGGESTIONS

1-1. Schedule appointments for young children at the beginning of a major time segment; i.e., the first appointment in the morning, the first after lunch, etc. This reduces the possibility that the child will have to wait very long before being seen.

1-2. When making an appointment for a school-aged child who is experiencing learning problems, ask the parents to bring with them copies of pertinent test records they may have, such as reports of school achievement testing or IQ testing.

1-3. Advise parents of children brought to you because of learning problems that they should feel free to bring along the child's school teacher. Learning problems are not solved in your office. They occur in school and must be addressed there as well. Enlisting the aid of a cooperative teacher will greatly improve the child's chances of overcoming his problem.

1-4. If the patient is very young (e.g., less than 1 year), advise the parent to bring along a nursing bottle. This (or a pacifier) can be very effective in quieting the child during those tests that require the examiner to position himself close to the youngster; e.g., ophthalmoscopy. (Note: Avoid the temptation of suggesting that the child be offered the bottle before it is needed; save it for important circumstances.)

1-5. If, when making the appointment, the parent states that the chief concern is a "crossed eye" or a "droopy lid," ask them to bring with them some baby photographs of the child. Parents often report that the condition "just came on," in their 5-year-old, yet photographs of the youngster when he was two (or younger) may reveal that it was already present then.

1-6. Create a "children's corner" in your waiting room. Furnish it with a table and chairs that are scaled for young children. Provide suitable toys, books, magazines, and pictures. Have paper and crayons available and, if space is no problem, a wall-mounted chalkboard. (Avoid easel-mounted chalkboards; they are apt to topple and cause damage.)

1-7. Have some small give-away trinkets available, such as balloons, plastic toys, etc. Do not be too quick in handing them out; use them judiciously—at the beginning of the visit as an inducement, perhaps; or at the end, as a reward.

1-8. Stay on the lookout for appropriate waiting room reading material that emphasizes the importance of eye examinations for young children.

1-9. Maintain a supply of disposable diapers, just in case. Identify a table or counter top in the office on which a baby's diaper may be changed. Have available, also, a soft, plastic-covered pad to place under the baby.

1-10. Designate an area where a nursing mother may feed her baby in private.

1-11. If the locale of your practice is appropriate, consider establishing a small lending library for your elementary school-aged patients. Encourage them to borrow from it, leaving one of their own books in return, if they so choose.

1-12. When equipping your office, try to purchase an examination chair that can be substantially elevated and has the potential to be adjusted to accommodate a young child; i.e., footrest, adjustable seatback. Bending over for prolonged periods of time is hard on the optometrist's back; sitting in a chair that is much too large is not conducive to obtaining the child's sustained attention.

1-13. Have the following books/articles available for fast reference:

Various pediatric optometry textbooks

A syndrome reference book

Merck's manual

Physician's Desk Reference (PDR)

Copies of figures and tables that pertain to developmental milestones, etc. (These are best stored in a loose-leaf binder.)

1-14. Speak to the child in *your* way; do not try to imitate someone else's style. Children respond well to naturalness, and they tend to be suspicious of artificiality. Avoid "baby talk" or other postures that do not reflect your personality. They do not expect you to be their "pal"; neither do they expect or want you to be their adversary.

1-15. Try to avoid direct confrontations with the child. Do not offer her choices unless you truly intend to honor them. Asking the child: "Do you want to come into the examination room with me?" opens up the opportunity for her to say "No." It is better simply to say "Come with me," in a matter-of-fact, nonthreatening manner.

1-16. Do not try to separate the apprehensive child from his mother, or insist that he sit down. Children feel safest when standing—especially if they are allowed to stand close to their parent. There is no reason why he should not be allowed to do this as you obtain the preliminary information. It also may help to place a toy before the child as you "ignore" him.

1-17. If a child does not respond to a question you pose or a test you present, it does not mean that she cannot do what she is being asked to do. Some children feel safer if they are not required to speak or, for that matter, even to make eye contact with the examiner. With such children, time will solve the problem; and until it is solved, try to limit your queries to the child to those that can be answered with a simple (verbal or nonverbal) *yes* or *no*.

1-18. Avoid referring to your test procedures as "games"; it is better to identify them as "work." Some children, upon hearing the word *game*, or *fun*, immediately adopt an attitude that is counterproductive to reliable data gathering. Most children past the age of 2 years know the meaning of the word *work* and are not intimidated by it. Young children like to "work," and they address it seriously. What they do not like is punishment (real or implied) because they did not meet expectations.

1-19. Whispering sometimes attracts a child's attention better than speaking loudly.

1-20. Avoid touching the child or making any other kind of physical contact until he has overcome some of his initial anxieties.

1-21. Try to overcome your inhibitions about singing and/or otherwise amusing the child. Memorize a few nursery songs and rhymes, and try to develop a repertoire of sounds that will divert him.

1-22. Avoid using the words *left* and *right* with children not yet in second grade. Better to show the child how to express a direction by pointing, touching one shoulder (or elbow) or the other, or identifying landmarks in the room, such as "on my side," "your mom's side," "the window side," etc. (See Practical Suggestion 1-30 for additional discussion regarding this.)

1-23. Avoid using such words as *first, second,* and so on—as when administering a visual or stereoacuity test. Better to identify the stimuli in a line by moving your hand from the child's left knee to his right knee, designating different ordinal positions spatially and, at the same time, with the spoken words, e.g., "circle/letter number 1," "number 2," "number 3," etc.

1-24. Be prepared to alter your standard examination sequence with young children. For example, in some cases, it may be best to begin with items from the Denver Developmental Screening Test (see Chapter 8), or with retinoscopy as he watches a film or videotape cartoon. You will be able to get back to your sequence once the child starts to trust you.

1-25. Keep an eye on the child and her actions as the visit gets underway, watching for relevant clinical information, including her apparent developmental status; i.e., the way she manages herself, enunciates words, responds to social queries, expresses herself verbally, separates from her mother, climbs onto the examination chair, takes notice of things, etc.

1-26. Three- and 4-year-olds, when asked their age, tend to respond by showing the appropriate number of fingers. This is a good icebreaker. Once the child has held up his fingers, ask him "How many is that?" or something similar. Once he has uttered his first words, subsequent ones will be more forthcoming.

1-27. Parents can participate in the examination in a variety of ways, thereby providing the child with some additional reassurance. For example, a parent can hold the occluder, visual acuity cards, the stereotest plate, etc.

1-28. Reports are a very responsible way to advertise the types or services you offer the young patient. Send them. Obtain the names and addresses of all those who should receive a report (e.g., pediatrician, school); it is also wise to obtain a signed release from the parent. (See pp. 355–358 for samples of reports.)

1-29. Use a different recording form for your preschool patients—one that reflects the tests you typically use with that age group. Clearly, there is no need for entering data from such sophisticated, subjective tests as negative and positive relative covergence, and so on. Rather, it should be organized to answer the basic questions of the examination as represented by the titles of Chapters 1 through 8 in this book, with the specific tests being determined in accord with the child's ability to respond appropriately.

1-30. It is not necessary to explain tests in advance of administering them. In fact, it is often undesirable to do that with children; it wastes time, and worse yet, it makes the child uncomfortable because often he cannot remember all you are telling him. For example, if you are going to administer the Tumbling E test, avoid such preparatory remarks as "Look at that screen on the wall. I am now going to show you some letter E's on that screen (or pictures of a three-legged table, or what have you) and you are going to tell me which way they point: up, down, this way, that way." It is better simply to initiate the test, having first made sure that the child has the capacity to respond in a way that will make test outcomes meaningful to you. (See the next item for more discussion regarding this.)

1-31. Before administering a test that requires a behavioral response from the child, make certain that he has that behavior in his repertoire. For example, if he is to read the letters on a Snellen chart, or point to matching letters on a key card, have him first name or print to relatively large letters held close to him— thus not testing acuity but, rather, his ability to understand and respond reliably, *if* he is able to *see* the letters; or, if he is to point to the Random-dot E positioned at 1.5 meters, have him first point to it while you hold it at 40 cm; or if you are attempting to measure nearpoint phoria using the Brock procedure described on p. 212, first have him perform the required behavior *without* the red-green filters, etc.

This will be discussed again, in specific sections, but in general it cautions the examiner to pretest the child in the cognitive aspects of the task he is about to engage in before attempting to measure a threshold with a method that assumes he has those cognitive abilities.

1-32. If the child demonstrates a lack of understanding about how he is to respond to a given test, consider teaching it to him. This is completely appropriate, if it can be done in a relatively brief period of time and if it does not invalidate the test results. For example, if the child is uncertain about what he is to do when asked to "point to" a matching picture, or to the Random-dot E, there is no harm done in teaching him, so long as you make sure that you do it under conditions that do not replicate test conditions. Once the child demonstrates that he has learned, the test may be administered under standard conditions; i.e., increase the test distance, introduce new letters/pictures, etc. (To *teach* in this context means to explain or to model for the child what it means to *point to*, then to reinforce his correct responses with praise or, if indicated, more tangible rewards.)

1-33. If the child is not able to learn how to respond to a given test from brief in-office instruction, consider having the parents teach the child at home. For example, the Allen Picture Cards (and most of the others) may be photocopied and given to the parents with instructions that they teach their child to name the seven objects portrayed on those cards or, in lieu of learning the names, to point to matching pictures. (Indeed, the child need not become familiar with all seven pictures. A very valid test may be conducted while limiting the cards to four or five.) Then repeat the test when the child next presents in your office. The test remains valid; the fact that he was *taught* to identify the pictures does not eliminate the relative difficulty of identifying them from prescribed distance, regardless of testing site, so long as the sequence in which they are shown is not held constant.

1-34. Stay on the lookout for small objects and toys that will serve effectively as fixation targets. Be prepared to give them up on appropriate demand from the child.

1-35. When selecting a test that you believe to be suitable for the young patient, avoid coming to a firm conclusion about what she can and cannot manage without first testing that premise. For example, many 4-year-olds are sufficiently familiar with the capital letters to participate in a standard Snellen visual acuity test. At the other end of the spectrum, some first and even second graders are not secure in their ability to identify the letters of the Snellen chart and will avoid answering rather than risk committing an error. The general rule: select the test you think appropriate, but do not hesitate to scale upward or downward if you get any evidence that such a move is called for; and if you have to scale downward, do not "blame" the child—simply explain it as "I chose the wrong test; my error; let me try again."

1-36. When administering a two-item forced-choice test, you should attempt to rule out "lucky guesses." To do this:

a. Insist that the child look before he responds; i.e., say to him, "First look here," indicating one of the two items, and watch his eyes to make sure that he is doing as directed. Then, "Now look here," doing the same with the second item. Then, "Point to the. . . ."

b. When in doubt, repeat the test.

1-37. Maintain the clinician's prerogative to overrule standardized criteria in any test; trust your own clinical judgment. Some forced-choice tests, for example, impose a "four correct responses in four trials" criterion (e.g., Broken wheel acuity test), some, a "four successive correct responses out of six trials" criterion (Random dot E stereotest as modified by Rosner), and so on. These were devised in order to reduce the probability of lucky guesses—to improve the validity of the test. However, experienced clinicians do not need hard and fast rules in making these judgments. There are many instances when the clinician "knows," after only one trial—and would guarantee—that the child saw what he said he saw. At other times, more than one trial is needed. The important point in this regard: Be suspicious until you are convinced that the child's responses are valid. But once you are convinced, trust your judgment, even if the child ceases to respond reliably. (Many times a child will respond reliably to a test for one or two trials, then—given the capricious nature of some children—start to lose interest and display this by responding in random fashion. The clinician recognizes this and interprets accordingly. We are clinicians, after all, not psychometricians; we know that not being able to elicit a repeated behavior from the patient does not mean they did not perform that behavior initially; and having observed that behavior— whatever "that" is—we can infer relevant clinical information.)

1-38. When eliciting the chief concern from the parent, avoid prolonged discussions unless the child appears to need the extra time to adapt to the surroundings. Obtain enough information to form some impressions about the nature of the problem (if any) and the tests that you will want to administer. There will be time for additional dialogue as the examination proceeds. This is particularly true if the chief concern is a school learning problem. It does the child little good to hear her inadequacies discussed at length at this point in the examination.

1-39. If the parent's chief concern is strabismus, and if the condition is not apparent to you as you observe the child, ask, "Is his eye turned (in/out/up/down) right now?" If the parent says "No," then treat his or her observation powers and concerns with respect (43). Suspect an intermittent strabismus and proceed accordingly. If the parent says, "Yes," then, obviously, you will have to discount, somewhat, his or her reliability as an observer. (But only somewhat; see the case report of Patient Michael, a 3-year-old who did not manifest convergence excess until after partial cyclopegia.)

1-40. Be sensitive to signs of a battered child beyond the ocular ones listed on p. 7. In most states, optometrists are legally obligated to report *all* cases of suspected child abuse, even if the child shows no ocular abnormalities. As noted in the text, information regarding how to proceed may be obtained from your local district attorney's office.

1-41. Encourage early (precautionary) examinations of young children by asking parents about siblings and if and when they have ever been examined. Make it clear that the optimum age for a child's first eye examination is when he is about 4 to 6 months old. Explain that at that age you are not only able to detect and diagnose ametropia and certain binoculars anomalies; you also are often able to initiate a treatment that might remediate or substantially reduce the problem and the negative effects the problem will produce if left unattended until the child reaches school age. Do not think of this as advertising and/or mercenary practice building; rather, think of it as a justifiable and important public health effort.

1-42. Become familiar with the vision screening programs used in the public schools of your region so that you will have some idea about what is tested and the criteria for referral; i.e., what a failure might and might not imply.

1-43. It often is advisable to avoid participating directly in locally sponsored vision screening programs that might place you in the position of referring patients to yourself and make you vulnerable to the types of accusations this could evoke. It is better to work out cooperative arrangements with colleagues from other locales whereby you volunteer your services in their communities and they do the same for you.

1-44. Optometrists are frequently asked to help their local schools design an adequate vision screening program. The optometrist is inclined, of course, to recommend a comprehensive protocol—one that will produce the fewest false-positive and false-negative referrals. This means a modified clinical screening. Unfortunately, such a protocol requires that a professional (optometrist or ophthalmologist) participate. Unless the professional is willing to donate all or part of her services, the costs of a modified clinical vision screening usually are prohibitive.

Consider a less-than-perfect approach, but one that can be implemented by nonprofessionals with a minimum of pretraining: one that will serve effectively to identify most, if not all, children who should be referred for a complete eye examination. Such a screening would consist of (a) a distance visual acuity test, with anything less than 20/30 signalling "failure"; (b) a "plus (+) 1.50 test" (see p. 9); and (c) the Random-dot E stereotest at 1.5 meters (see p. 191 for details). All three of these tests can be reliably administered by nonprofessionals; in combination, they will detect most of the children who should have a thorough assessment. Granted, it may very well overlook the child with (a) a very minimal amount of myopia and/or astigmatism, (b) intermittent strabismus; e.g., convergence or divergence excess. However, it will do a far better job than the distance visual acuity test alone, and at very little extra cost in terms of money, equipment, and time.

1-45. For all practical purposes, there is no difference between *dyslexia, learning disability, attention deficit disorder*, etc. They are descriptors, not diagnoses. Like *reduced visual acuity* they offer no information that can be translated into treatment.

■

REFERENCES

1. McNeese MC, Hebeler JR. The abused child. Clinical Symposium (Ciba) 1977; 29:1–36.
2. Fontana VM et al. The "maltreatment syndrome" in children. N Engl J Med 1963; 269:1389–94.
3. Harley RD, Spaeth GL. Ocular manifestations of child abuse. In: Francois J, Mainoe M, eds. Pediatric ophthalmology. New York: John Wiley & Sons, 1982.
4. Jobe FW. Screening vision in schools. Newark, Del.: International Reading Association, 1976.
5. Peters HB. Vision screening. In: Hirsch M, Wick R, eds. Vision of children: an optometric symposium. Philadelphia: Chilton Books, 1963.
6. Lippmann O. Vision screening of young children. Am J Pub Health 1971; 61(8): 1585–1601.
7. Davens E. The nationwide alert in preschool vision screening. Sightsaving Rev. 1966; 36:13–17.
8. Kelley CR. Visual screening and child development: the North Carolina study. Raleigh: Department of Psychology, North Carolina State College, 1957.
9. Knox GE. Classroom symptoms of visual difficulty. In: Robinson H, ed. Clinical studies in reading. II. Supplementary Ed. Monog 77. Chicago: University of Chicago Press, 1975.
10. North FA Jr. Vision care in Project Head Start. Sightsaving Rev 1967; 37:153–56.
11. Nussenblatt H. Symposium on optometry's obligation in vision screening: opening remarks. AJOPO 1984; 61(6):357–58.
12. Amigo G, McCarthy A. The "Pooh Corner" vision study. AJOPO 1976; 53(2):60–65.
13. Davidson DW. The future of vision screening. JAOA 1977; 48:469–76.
14. Vaugn D, Cook R, Bock R. Eye tests for preschool and school age children. Stockton, CA: Medical Eye Council, 1960.
15. Foote FM. An evaluation of vision screening. Exceptional Children 1954; 20:153–61.
16. Stewart CR. Plus lens visual acuity screening tests. Opt Wkly 1950; 41:615.
17. Stewart CR. Investigation of lens visual acuity screening test. Opt Wkly 1951; 42:9.
18. Kohler L, Stigmar G. Testing for hypermetropia in the school vision screening programme. Acta Ophthal 1981; 59:369–77.
19. Ehrlich MI, Reinecke RD, Simons K. Preschool vision screening for amblyopia and strabismus. Programs, methods, guidelines. Surv Ophthal 1983; 28(3):145–63.
20. Peters HB. Remarks on Orinda. AJOPO 1984; 61(6):361–63.
21. Oaks L. Massachusetts vision test. AJPH 1942; 32:1105–9.
22. Sloane AE. Massachusetts vision test. Arch Ophthal 1940; 24:924–39.
23. Cohen A, Lieberman S, Stolzberg M, Ritty JM. The NYSOA vision screening battery—a total approach. JAOA 1983; 54(11):979–84.
24. Lieberman S, Cohen AH, Stolzberg M, Ritty JM. Validation study of the New York State Optometric Association (NYSOA) vision screening battery. AJOPO 1985; 62(3):165–68.
25. Blum H, Peters H, Bettman JW. Vision screening for elementary schools: the Orinda study. Berkeley: University of California Press, 1959.

26. Rosner J. The rationale and design of a perceptual skills curriculum. Pittsburgh: Learning Research and Development Center, University of Pittsburgh, 1969.
27. Rosner J. Helping children overcome learning difficulties. 2nd ed. New York: Walker Publishing Co, 1979.
28. Reinecke RD, Simons D. A new stereoscopic test for amblyopia. Am J Ophthal 1974; 78(4):714–21.
29. Rosner J. The effectiveness of the random-dot E stereotest as a preschool vision screening instrument. JAOA 1978; 49(10):1121–24.
30. Hammond RS, Schmidt PP. A Random-dot E stereogram for the vision screening of children. Arch Ophthal 1986; 104:54–60.
31. Holland SH. 20/20 vision screening. Ped Nursing 1982; March/April:81–87.
32. Sturner RA, Green JA, Funk SG, Jones CK, Chandler AC. A developmental approach to preschool vision screening. J Ped Ophthal and Strab 1981; 18(2):61–67.
33. Molgaard I, Biering-Sorensen K, Michelsen N, Elmer J, Rydberg A. Amblyopia screening in kindergarten with TNO stereotest. Acta Ophthal 1984; 62:156–62.
34. Gruber J, Dickey P, Rosner J. Comparison of a modified (two-item) Frisby with the standard Frisby and Random-dot E stereotests when used with preschool children. AJOPO 1965; 62:349–51.
35. Fulton AB, Manning KA, Dobson V. A behavioral method for efficient screening of visual acuity in young infants. II. Clinical application. Inves Opththal Vis Sci 1978; 17(12):1151–57.
36. Atkinson J, Braddick O. The use of isotropic photorefraction for vision screening in infants. Acta Opththal 1982; Supplement 157:36–45.
37. Kaakinen K, Tommila V. A clinical study on the detection of strabismus, anisometropia or ametropia of children by simultaneous photography of the corneal and fundus reflexes. Acta Ophthal 1979; 57:600–11.
38. Kaakinen K. A simple method for screening of children with strabismus, anisometropia or ametropia by simultaneous photography of the corneal and the fundus reflexes. Acta Ophthal 1979; 57:161–71.
39. Kaakinen K. Photographic screening for strabismus and high refractive errors of aged 1-4 years. Acta Ophthal 1981; 59:38–84.
40. Kaakinen K. Simultaneous two flash static photoskiascopy. Acta Ophthal 1981; 59:378–86.
41. Molteno ACB, Hoare-Nairne J, Parr JC, Simpson A, Hodgkinson IJ, O'Brien NE, Watts SD. The Otago photoscreener, a method for the mass screening of infants to detect squint and refractive errors. Trans Ophthal Soc N.Z. 1983; 35:43–49.
42. Ingram RM, Holland WW, Walker JM, Wilson PEA, Dally S. Screening for visual defects in preschoolchildren. Br J Ophthalmol 1986; 70:16–21.
43. Rosner J, Rosner J. The accuracy of parents as screeners for strabismus in their own children. J Vis Impaired & Blindness 1988; 82:193–94.

2

Question 2
What Other Information
Might Be Relevant?

☐

■

A. OBTAIN CASE HISTORY

As we have already noted, a clinical examination is a formalized process of asking "questions"—some posed orally, some in the form of clinical tests. The case history portion of the examination comprises, in the main, oral queries.

In presenting her questions to the patient—and, often, to others, as well—the optometrist seeks to obtain information that will (1) provide a more complete and detailed picture of the patient's chief concern: its origin, key characteristics, course, and related events; (2) help her select an appropriate treatment, based on the ultimate diagnosis and the factors in the patient's past and present that might be prognostic (1); (3) help her determine whether there are other conditions that warrant her attention, in addition to those identified by the patient.

☐ The Process

Obtaining a case history involves much more than posing a list of predetermined questions and recording the responses (see flow diagram in Figure 2.1)

Obtaining a case history is an open-ended, multibranched, keep-your-eyes-and-ears-open-for-useful-clues endeavor. Once started—and it starts when the patient first presents—it continues as long as the case is active.

At the outset, the optometrist tends to focus on the patient's chief concern, probing it in some depth. Her array of questions will probably include:

1. When was the problem first noted?
2. Describe some of the associated signs and symptoms.

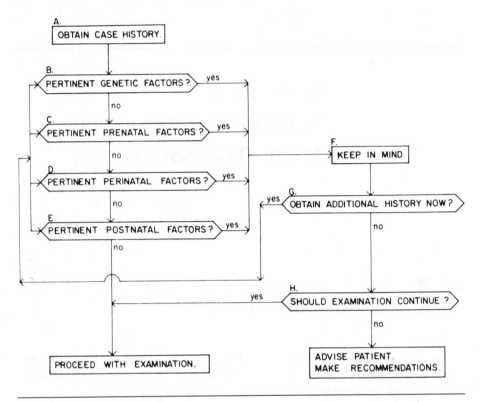

A. OBTAIN CASE HISTORY.

B. PERTINENT GENETIC FACTORS ? — yes / no

C. PERTINENT PRENATAL FACTORS ? — yes / no

D. PERTINENT PERINATAL FACTORS ? — yes / no

E. PERTINENT POSTNATAL FACTORS ? — yes / no

F. KEEP IN MIND.

G. OBTAIN ADDITIONAL HISTORY NOW ? — yes / no

H. SHOULD EXAMINATION CONTINUE ? — yes / no

PROCEED WITH EXAMINATION.

ADVISE PATIENT. MAKE RECOMMENDATIONS.

Figure 2.1   Question #2: What other information might be relevant?

3. How often does it occur?
4. How severe is it?
5. Is it changing? Getting better or worse?
6. Have you sought other opinions, tried any remedies? If so, what?
7. What happened?

In other words, the optometrist seeks information that will enable her to determine "what's wrong" and "what is apt to make it better." But, at the same time, she is committed to not overlooking a problem, or a potential problem, that has not yet become a concern of the patient.

Her process is one of alternately scanning and focusing as the situation requires, narrowing the range as she gets closer to understanding the patient's condition and needs. She asks questions, administers clinical tests, asks more questions, does more tests, and so on, keeping in mind and following up on potential "leads" until she has sufficient information to translate the data into a valid diagnosis and an effective treatment plan.

Almost invariably, her investigations will take her to aspects of the child's background. She will probe (2):

1. Genetic factors
2. Prenatal factors
3. Perinatal factors
4. Postnatal factors

The balance of this chapter is devoted to those topics.

B. GENETIC FACTORS

Genetic factors are investigated in order to answer the following questions: Is there anything in the patient's family background that may contribute to accurate diagnosis and effective prescription? Is there a need for genetic counseling? Is there evidence of something not mentioned as a concern, that should be probed in depth?

As such, the material presented in this section consists of a brief, general overview of the basic principles that govern human genetics and a listing of some of the more common inherited ocular conditions that the optometrist should keep in mind as she compiles the case history.*

□ General Principles

Humans differ from each other in many ways. To a large degree, these differences are the outcome of interactions between unique genetic makeups and the (physical-emotional-cognitive) environments in which the individual lives and has lived; between the characteristics inherited from parents and the circumstances encountered since the moment of conception (3).

Typically, these differences are contained within limits that are called "normal." Occasionally an individual displays a difference that is beyond normal limits. It may be referred to as "unusual" or "abnormal," depending upon the specific nature of the difference and how it is perceived. The seven-feet-tall basketball player is a case in point. He is considered to be unusually tall, nothing more. His height does not warrant professional concern.

Differences are perceived to be abnormal, and to warrant professional concern, when they represent a potential risk to the generations of progeny that may derive from that individual or when they have, or will have, marked impact on the individual's ability to adapt, physiologically and psychologically, to the conditions of a standard environment.

*For a more thorough discussion of this topic, see 4,5,6.

The latter will be discussed subsequently. At this point, we shall consider the first. All somatic cells of the human body contain 23 pairs of chromosomes, which, in turn contain genes, the units of heredity (4,5). Half of the chromosomes, one from each pair, derive from the maternal germ cell: the ovum. The other 23, from the paternal germ cell: the sperm. All but one of the 23 pairs of chromosomes are called autosomes. How they are constituted and organized serves as the determinant, the "blueprint" for most of the individual's inborn characteristics.

The remaining pair of chromosomes is especially unique in that it determines the individual's sex, along with certain other, special characteristics. It is made up of a so-called X chromosome, transmitted from the maternal ovum, and either another X or a Y chromosome, donated from the paternal sperm. When the two chromosomes are the same—that is, XX—then the child is female. When the chromosomes are not the same—that is, XY—then the child is a male.

Among the genetically controlled characteristics transmitted by the other 22 chromosome pairs—the autosomes—some are attributable to *dominant* genes, others to *recessive* genes. When a gene is called dominant, it means that the characteristic related to that gene will be "expressed"—manifested—even if it is the only one of the pair so designed; that is, even if the individual is *heterozygous* for that gene pair. If expression of a particular characteristic depends on both genes of a pair carrying it—on the individual's being *homozygous* for the gene pair—then the characteristic and its respective genes are known as recessive.

Applying these basic principles with some paper and pencil mapping, or by referring to a good text (6), we can determine that in *autosomal dominant* inheritance (a) there is usually a positive family history, with affected individuals presenting in successive generations; (b) in the absence of a family history, an affected individual may represent a new mutation, or the parent may be a carrier in whom the gene is not penetrant; that is, the inherited characteristic is fully expressed *when it is expressed*, but only rarely is it expressed; (c) males and females are affected equally; (d) statistically, each child born to an affected individual has a 50 percent likelihood of being affected.

In *autosomal recessive* inheritance (a) there is usually no related family history; (b) the parents are usually clinically normal heterozygous carriers, but are more apt to be consanguine (an affected individual will have affected children *only* if he/she is mated to someone who is heterozygous, or homozygous for the same gene); (c) males and females are equally affected; (d) each pregnancy carries a 25 percent risk of producing an affected child.

In the case of an *X-linked recessive* disorder (X-linkage refers to the location of the gene on the X chromosome. X-linked genes may be recessive or, less frequently, dominant): (a) the sons of a carrier female face a 50 percent risk of being affected; (b) the daughters of a carrier female face a 50 percent risk of being carriers themselves; (c) all the daughters of a male with an X-linked recessive disorder will be obligate carriers.*

---

*Male-to-male transmission of X-linked disorders does not occur, since a male transmits his Y chromosomes to his sons and his X to his daughters (*except* in those very rare cases in which the son has Klinefelter's syndrome, with the extra X chromosome being inherited from his father [5]).

In the case of an *X-linked dominant* disorder, (a) all the children (male and female) of an affected female face a 50 percent risk of being affected; (b) all the daughters of a male with an X-linked dominant disorder will be affected.

Table 2.1 lists a number of ocular disorders that may be inherited (7). Many of these were also mentioned in the preceding chapter as "possible explanations" for the various chief concerns that accompany a pediatric patient.

C. PRENATAL FACTORS

The term "prenatal factors," interpreted literally, encompasses genetic factors. The two topics are treated separately here, however. In this context, prenatal factors refer to the environment the mother provides from the time of conception until birth, and the extent to which this environment is compatible with the needs of the developing embryo/fetus.

As the optometrist probes for information that might contribute to the diagnosis/prescription processes, he will focus on the following circumstances:

1. Maternal age. The probability of bearing a child with Down's syndrome, for example, increases as a function of the mother's age (8).
2. Radiation. The use of pelvic X-rays during pregnancy has decreased markedly in recent years. This is fortunate. It has been shown to raise significantly the risk of miscarriage and malformation (9). It remains a clinical concern, however, because of the relative recency of this awareness. Many children predate the era of enlightenment.
3. Therapeutic agents. Physicians have become much conservative in recent years, recognizing the marked effects of certain drugs on an embryo/fetus (9). Thalidomide is one unfortunate example.
4. Infection/disease. This factor applies in three ways:
    a. A maternal infection can be transferred to the embryo and—if a miscarriage does not occur—will be well established by the time of birth. Syphilis is an example of this (10).
    b. A maternal infection during pregnancy can impact the development of the organism, resulting in a congenital defect. Rubella during the first trimester of pregnancy is a well-recognized example (11).
    c. Mothers with hemolytic disease (e.g., kernicterus, anemia) are more apt to deliver at-risk children (11).
5. Premature birth. The effects of premature birth can be highly significant (12). All neonates are vulnerable to certain aspects of the extrauterus environment. The premature baby is even more vulnerable (13). A birth is characteristically considered to be premature if (a) it occurs less than 280 days after the first day of the mother's last menstruation and/or (b) the newborn's birth-weight is less than 2500 g (approximately 5 pounds, 8 ounces).

Site	Autosomal Dominant	Autosomal Recessive	X-Linked
Globe	Coloboma/microphthalmos Oculodentodigital dysplasia (microphthalmos)	Anophthalmos	
Eyelids	Blepharophimosis + ptosis + epicanthus inversus		
Extraocular muscles	Familial ophthalmoplegia		Congenital nystagmus External ophthalmoplegia + myopia
Periorbital tissues	Crouzon's craniofacial dysostosis (exophthalmos + hypertelorism + exotropia) Collins' mandibulofacial dysostosis (antimongoloid slant + lower eyelid coloboma) Waardenburg's syndrome (lateral displacement of medial canthi and lacrimal puncta)		
Cornea	Corneal dystrophies—many forms	Corneal dystrophies—several forms	Fabry's disease (corneal dystrophy) Megalocornea
Angle of AC	Aniridia Juvenile glaucoma Rieger's syndrome (angle dysgenesis)	Congenital glaucoma (buphthalmos)	
Lens	Congenital cataract—many forms Ectopia lentis Marfan's syndrome (ectopia lentis) Alport's syndrome (anterior lenticonus)	Congenital cataract—several forms Homocystinuria (ectopia lentis) Werner's syndrome (adolescent cataracts) Marinesco-Sjögren syndrome (congenital cataracts) Rothmund-Thomson syndrome (juvenile cataracts)	Congenital cataract—few forms Lowe's syndrome (congenital cataract)

Table 2.1 Single-Gene Disorders Affecting Vision or Ocular and Periocular Structures in Children and Adolescents*

	Progressive		
Retina	Arthro-ophthalmopathy (myopia + retinal detachment) Wagner's hyaloideo-retinal degeneration Vitelliform macular dystrophy Congenital night blindness Bilateral retinoblastoma Retinitis pigmentosa Spondyloepiphyseal dysplasia (myopia + retinal detachment)	Weill-Marchesani syndrome (spherophakia) Albinism type I (complete) and type II (incomplete) Leber's congenital amaurosis Stargardt's macular dystrophy Gyrate chorioretinal atrophy Favre's hyaloidoretinal tapetoretinal degeneration Pseudoxanthoma elasticum (angioid streaks) Retinitis pigmentosa Complete achromatopsia	Ocular albinism Choroideremia Incomplete achromatopsia Partial color blindness (protan and deutan) Myopia + night blindness Norrie's disease (pseudoglioma) Retinitis pigmentosa Juvenile retinoschisis
Optic nerve	Optic atrophy—congenital and juvenile	Optic atrophy—congenital and infantile	Leber's optic atrophy
CNS & eye	Neurofibromatosis (optic nerve glioma, exophthalmos, glaucoma) Olivopontocerebellar atrophy with retinal degeneration (macular or peripheral) Tuberous sclerosis (retinal astrocytomas) von Hippel-Lindau syndrome (retinal angiomatosis)	Cerebral lipofuscinosis/juvenile amaurotic idiocy (maculocerebral degeneration) Retinitis pigmentosa Laurence-Moon-Bardet-Biedl syndrome (retinitis pigmentosa) Cockayne's syndrome (retinitis pigmentosa) Refsum's syndrome (retinitis pigmentosa) Usher's syndrome (retinitis pigmentosa) Abetalipoproteinemia (retinitis pigmentosa)	

*Where a named syndrome is given, the major ocular feature(s) follow in parentheses.
Crozier G. Genetic counseling and single-gene disorders. *Rev. Optom.* March 1979, p. 45.

6. Malnutrition/drugs. Children born to women with a history of chronic malnutrition that continues into and throughout pregnancy are at risk (14). This is also true of children whose mothers consumed excessive amounts of alcohol, coffee, or other drugs and/or smoked heavily during pregnancy.

D. PERINATAL FACTORS

The circumstances around a child's birth may vary from eventful to uneventful. A birth may be long instead of brief, arduous instead of easy, complicated instead of uncomplicated, traumatic instead of injury-free. Any or all of these factors may have long-term and significant effects on the child or they may not.

As such, the questions that the clinician poses regarding perinatal factors—once the issue of prematurity has been dealt with—should center on the condition of the baby immediately after birth rather than attempting to infer the baby's status on the basis of the delivery itself.

☐ Apgar Score

The condition of the baby immediately after birth is now usually determined and reported to the parents, in the form of an Apgar score (15): an index of the newborn's health status at the age of 1 minute.

The Apgar is a composite index, based on five vital signs: the baby's color, respiration, muscular tone, reflex irritability, and heart rate. Each one is rated on a three-point scale according to quality: 0, 1, or 2, with 2 being the best, and with the maximum score therefore being 10. Table 2.2 lists the criteria used to score the observations.

Most infants will score an 8 or higher at age 1 minute, and even better a few minutes after that, indicating that their basic vital functions were intact at birth. A score of 7 or less indicates that the child's basic life-sustaining systems were

Sign	0	1	2
Heart rate	Absent	Slow (<100)	>100
Respiratory effort	Absent	Weak cry; hypoventilation	Good; strong cry
Muscle tone	Limp	Some flexion of extremeties	Well flexed
Reflex irritability	No response	Some motion	Cry
Color	Blue; pale	Body pink; extremities blue	Completely pink

Table 2.2   Scoring Criteria for Apgar

not functioning as well as they should have been at the time of birth. (A score of 4 or less signals a very depressed infant.) This, in turn, indicates that the child either was born in a weakened condition or that he may have suffered some significant insult during delivery that could produce long-term impairment: hypoxia or anoxia, for example. That information will be useful to the optometrist as he attempts to determine treatment and prognosis for certain conditions that will be discussed later—perceptual skills dysfunction, in particular.

□ Brazelton Neonatal Behavioral Assessment Scale (NBAS)

This test, like the Apgar, attempts to document the infant's physical status shortly after birth. It, too, is relatively new, having initially been published in 1973 (16). For this reason, and because it takes significantly longer than the Apgar to administer, the NBAS is not yet widely used. However, it has captured the interest of many professionals and seems to be gaining broader acceptance. As such, we include it here as a means of informing the optometrist of its existence. We will not describe it in any detail.

In general terms, the scale

. . . attempts to capture the complexity of behavioral responses to social stimuli as the neonate moves from sleep states to crying and to alert states of consciousness.

There are

. . . 20 reflex items that tap neurological integrity and 27 behavioral items to assess the neonate's capacity to respond to the environment

(e.g., orientation to animate visual and auditory stimuli; lability of skin color).

As such, these items' scores become a reflection of the baby's capacity to organize his or her autonomic and central nervous system in order to respond to stimuli (17, p. 13).

E. POSTNATAL FACTORS

The neonate faces a challenge. It is not enough that his basic needs for shelter and nourishment are satisfied and that his vital processes function well enough to sustain life. He also must develop—physically, emotionally, and cognitively.

If he was born intact—with all systems functioning properly, as evidenced by the Apgar, for example—then this is likely to happen, as long as the developmental process is not disrupted/impeded by one or more of the following: trauma, infection/disease; deprivation: nutritional, emotional, cognitive.

Unfortunately, many children do experience one or more of these and often display the long-term effects when they present at the optometrist's office.

The optometrist, knowing this, goes beyond the questions directly related to the chief concern (see Chapter 1) and often inquires about the child's background as a possible contributor to explaining the clinical signs and symptoms his patient presents. His queries take two forms. First, he asks about specific events that may have affected the child's development: traumatic accidents, for example, or disease that might have had a significant impact. Table 2.3 lists various systemic diseases and associated ocular conditions (18).

Second, he asks about the child's general development, the ages at which the prominent motor and cognitive milestones were achieved. Figure 2.2 shows some of these and the ages at which they are ordinarily reached (19). (A description of how to assess the developmental status of the preschool child is presented in Chapter 8.)

Systemic Disease	Ocular Signs/Symptoms
Nutritional deficit	
Avitaminosis A	Xerosis; foamy white triangular areas—Bilot's spots—in interpalpebral area; reduced vision at night
Vitamin B deficiency	Ptosis; extraocular muscle palsy
Vitamin C deficiency	Hemorrhages in lid and/or orbit; possible exophthalmos; retinal hemorrhage; hyphema
Endocrine disease	
Diabetes mellitus	Retinopathy; iritis; rapidly changing refractive error; diabetic cataract
Thyroid disease	Lid lag; nystagmus; poor convergence; lid tremors
Hypertension and nephritis	Narrowing of arteries; hemorrhages; exudates
Syphilis	Keratitis; uveitis; choroiditis with a "salt and pepper" fundus
Viral disease	Conjunctivitis; keratitis; uveitis
Mycotic disease	Orbital cellulitis; blood vessel occlusion
Protozoan disease	Chorioretinitis
Blood dyscrasias	
Anemia	Pale retina and disc; retinal hemorrhage; distended veins
Dermatoses	
Impetigo	Inflamed, edematous lids; thin-walled vesicles, bullae, or pustules; may include acute conjunctivitis
Erysipelas	Red, sharply demarcated lesion; conjunctivitis

Table 2.3 Systemic Diseases and Associated Ocular Conditions

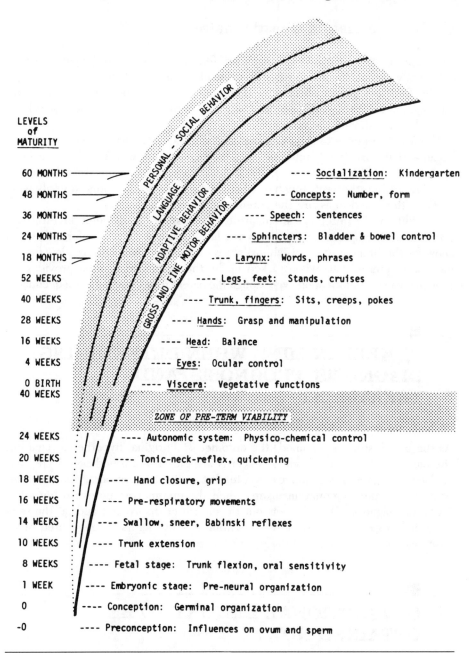

Figure 2.2 The development of behavior in the five major fields (from Gesell AL, Amatruda CS. In: Knoblock H, Pasamanick B, eds. Developmental Diagnosis, 3rd ed. New York: Harper and Row, 1974).

☐ Preexamination Questionnaire

Some optometrists advocate sending a printed questionnaire to the patient's parents in advance of the office visit. The value of this is moot. True, if the questions on the form are posed effectively, then the parent's responses provide useful information about the child. But it is information that could have and would have been obtained during the visit.

The usual response to this comment is that the questionnaire saves office time because that part of the information-gathering process will already have been accomplished. This may be true, but in most cases the optometrist will want to mention, during the visit, much of what the form covered, if only to verify what is stated there and to assure the parent that he read it.

In addition, a printed questionnaire tends to stifle the dynamic investigative process that the optometrist initiates in a face-to-face setting. The form does not allow for the branching that is almost always necessary. Nor does it allow for the incidental remark that, when picked up by the optometrist, often provides exceptionally useful information even though the parent may think it inconsequential.

F. KEEP IN MIND WHEN DETERMINING DIAGNOSIS, PROGNOSIS, AND TREATMENT

As the case history is obtained, the optometrist's original hypotheses regarding the bases for the patient's chief concerns are either confirmed or rejected and replaced by others. The interrogation tends to come to a temporary halt, and the next step in the examination taken, when the optometrist poses (to himself) a tentative diagnosis. He then sets out to confirm or disprove it and, at the same time, investigate further whatever attention-worthy factors he uncovered in the case history, independent of the chief concern.

G. ADDITIONAL HISTORY TO BE OBTAINED NOW?

The critical word in this query is *now*. As already observed, history taking is not a finite enterprise. It continues throughout the examination, diagnosis, and treatment processes.

SHOULD EXAMINATION CONTINUE?

There are occasions when the proper response to this question is *no*. That, when it becomes evident that the patient/parent's concern and clinical history indicate clearly that they would be best served by someone else. For example—a very unlikely one, to be sure—the parent who seeks to obtain contact lenses for a 4-year-old with a mild (e.g., 0.50 D) myopic refractive deviation. Simply stated, there is no justification for prolonging an evaluation when it is evident that the sought-for goals are unreasonable.

PRACTICAL SUGGESTIONS

2-1. When obtaining a case history, avoid making the parent feel anxious and/or guilty by your line of questioning. In other words, do not imply—by words or actions—that they have been neglectful; or worse, that their child's problem is the result of something they did.

2-2. Avoid implying—by words or actions—that there is some genetic factor operating in the case, unless, of course, that is indeed a fact. In other words, try to avoid implying etiology, if you are unsure; by all means, refrain from providing one parent the opportunity to fix blame on the other parent; e.g., "The child gets this from his father's family, not mine!"

2-3. In cases where the chief concern is a school learning problem, it may be useful to inquire about such factors as the stability of:

(a) the child's schooling; i.e., did she attend the same school for kindergarten, first grade, and so on? (All schools strive to teach their students the fundamentals of reading, writing, spelling, and arithmetic by the time they reach the fourth grade; but they often differ in the routes they take to achieve these goals. The child who transfers schools during the primary grades is vulnerable to missing some crucial links in the instructional sequence.)

(b) the teaching staff in the youngster's school; i.e., did she remain with the same teacher throughout the school year, or were there changes due to illness, teacher relocation, etc? A teacher change can bring about changes in instruction that have a detrimental effect on some children.

The purpose of these inquiries is not to identify *the cause* of the child's school difficulties, but it could provide information that would aid in determining some of its roots and subsequent treatment recommendations. (See Chapter 15.)

2-4. As noted in Practical Suggestion 1-5, baby photographs of the child may be very helpful in determining the date of onset of a condition: e.g., strabismus, ptosis.

■

REFERENCES

1. Harvey AM, Barondess JA, Bordley J III. Differential diagnosis. 3rd ed. Philadelphia: Saunders, 1969.
2. Woodruff ME. The visually "at risk" child. JAOA 1973; 44(2):130.
3. Bower TGR. Human development. San Francisco: Freeman, 1979.
4. Porter IH. Principles and examples in ophthalmic genetics. In: Fenman SS, Reinecke RD, eds. Handbook of pediatric ophthalmology. New York: Grune & Stratton, 1978.
5. Punnett HH, Harley RD. Genetics in pediatric ophthalmology. In: Harley R, ed. Pediatric ophthalmology. Philadelphia: Saunders, 1975.
6. Sutton HF. An introduction to human genetics. 2nd ed. Atlanta: Holt, Reinhart and Winston, 1975.
7. Crozier G. Genetic counseling and single-gene disorders. Rev Optom March 1979; 45.
8. Sorsby A. Modern ophthalmology. Vol. 3. Washington, D.C.: Butterworth, 1964.
9. Mann I. The antenatal and postnatal development of the human eye. In: Behrens C, ed. The eye and its disorders. 2nd ed. Philadelphia: Saunders, 1949.
10. Sorsby A. Systemic ophthalmology. St. Louis: Mosby, 1951.
11. Mann I. The development of the human eye. 2nd ed. New York: Grune & Stratton, 1950.
12. Apgar V. Proposals for a new method of evaluation of newborn infants. Anesth & Analg 1953; 32:260.
13. Lubchenco L et al. Sequelae of premature birth. In: Brackhill Y, Thompson GG, eds. Behavior in infancy and early childhood. New York: The Free Press, 1961.
14. Ellerbrock VJ. Developmental, congenital and hereditary anomalies of the eye. In: Hirsch MJ, Wick R, eds. Vision of children. Philadelphia: Chilton Books, 1963.
15. Apgar V. Evaluation of the newborn infant—a second report. JAMA 1958; 168(15):1985.
16. Brazelton TB. Neonatal Behavioral Assessment Scale. Clinics in Developmental Medicine, No. 50. Philadelphia: Lippincott, 1973.
17. Brazelton TB. In Sameroff AJ, ed. Organization and stability of newborn behavior: a commentary on the Brazelton Neonatal Behavior Assessment Scale. Chicago: SRCD Monograph, 177 (5-6), University of Chicago Press, 1978.
18. Gunderson T, Liebman S, Podos SM. Ocular manifestations of pediatric systemic diseases. In: Liebman S, Gellis S, eds. The pediatrician's ophthalmology. St. Louis: Mosby, 1966.
19. Gesell AL, Amatruda CS. In: Knoblock H, Pasamanick B, eds. Developmental diagnosis. 3rd ed. New York: Harper & Row, 1974.

3

Question 3
How Clearly Does
the Patient See?

☐

■

A. MEASURE PATIENT'S
VISUAL ACUITY

Visual acuity is always a central concern. Not only is it of primary interest to the patient, it is also one of the optometrist's principal indices of ocular integrity. Normal acuity may not guarantee a healthy, structurally intact eye that is free of significant refractive error, but it does enable one to rule out, partially or totally, a long list of potential problems. And, just as important, substandard acuity may not signal active pathology, but the possibility must not be ignored. As such, an accurate measure of visual acuity is exceptionally informative and should be accomplished if at all possible (see Figure 3.1).

This chapter addresses two main topics: (1) How to measure visual acuity when standard, adult-appropriate methods are unsuitable, either because the patient is not sufficiently familiar with the letters on the chart and/or because he lacks adequate ability to communicate what he sees. A number of objective and subjective methods are described. (2) What is considered to be normal visual acuity for children below the primary-grade age level, with a linking of those norms to the methods by which they were determined.

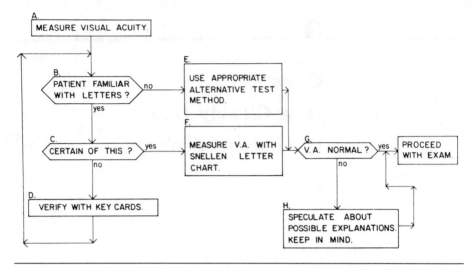

Figure 3.1   Question #3: How clearly does the patient see?

___

B. IS THE PATIENT SUFFICIENTLY FAMILIAR WITH THE LETTERS ON THE STANDARD SNELLEN CHART?

Ordinarily, this question is superfluous with children in the first grade and beyond. But even with this age group it is better to consider the question than to go directly into visual acuity testing with a standard Snellen chart. Some second and even third graders are unsure about certain letters, but not willing to admit it.

___

C. ARE YOU CERTAIN OF THIS?

There are numerous ways to determine whether the child is sufficiently familiar with the letters on the Snellen chart. The simplest: ask the child or the accompanying adult. This is satisfactory most of the time. Nonetheless, it is wise to have a demonstration (or "key") card available to help answer this question.

■
D. VERIFY YOUR JUDGMENT WITH A "KEY" CARD

The key card will probably have to be homemade. It is not difficult to construct. Simply print the Snellen chart letters on an index card. These should be large enough so that when the child is asked to "read" them, it may be assumed that his ability to name the letters is being tested, not his ability to see them. This should be done binocularly. The orientation of the letters should not match the visual acuity chart. This would prefamiliarize the child with the test and reduce some of its validity.

■
E. USE AN APPROPRIATE ALTERNATIVE TESTING METHOD

There are many children's visual acuity tests, and there is a wide diversity of opinion about their relative clinical values (see, e.g., 1,2,3,4,5,6,7). Typically, the tests differ in (a) optotype design (pictures, letters, black and white stripes, etc.); (b) number of optotypes presented in a single display (some present one at a time; others, more than one); (c) presence or absence of contour interaction stimuli (some of the single optotype stimuli are surrounded by contour interaction bars, some are not); (d) acuity range (some do not provide stimuli small enough to document 20/20 acuity; e.g., American Optical Co. picture slide; Allen Picture Cards); (e) test distance (some are designed for a 6-meter distance, some for 3 meters, and some, of course, for nearpoint); (f) response requirements (some tests require the child to name what she sees; some provide key cards that allow the child to point to a matching optotype without necessarily naming it correctly; yet others require only that the child discriminate between two items and identify the selected one by pointing to it; and some—designed for the very young— require nothing from the child other than that she "look at" a visual display as the examiner observes and attempts to infer visual acuity on the basis of the "preferential looking patterns"). (For a comprehensive review of the literature regarding distance visual acuity tests for the preschool child, see [8].)

The procedures described below are organized according to the minimum ages for which they are appropriate. The first ones are applicable with children as young as 5 years, children who are just short of being able to read all of the letters on the Snellen chart. The methods that follow these are for younger children. (In designating age levels, our tendency was to be conservative. Hence, if an age designation is found to be off target, the error is apt to be on the side of under-estimating the child's ability to meet the requirements of the test.)

Start by selecting a test from among those designated as appropriate for the patient's age, but be ready and willing to scale up or down accordingly. (Without doubt, there will be occasions when a child will respond paradoxically, being able to deal with a test that is identified as more difficult than a second test, which, for some reason, confounds him. But this will be the exception.)

In general, the rule to follow is: use the highest level test that does not confuse the child. The benefit of using a higher level test is that the acuity measured with such a method is likely to be closer to a true value than what is obtained from one of the lower level tests. There is no benefit, however, in collecting inaccurate data by confronting the child with a task that demands more from him than he can provide. In those cases, use a lower level test instead.

□ Five-Year-Olds

TUMBLING E TEST

This test has become the standard alternative. It is ubiquitous, being the test method of preference for most mass vision screening efforts that involve preschool children (9).

An inspection of the test reveals its similarity to the Snellen letter test (10). It consists exclusively of E's, oriented in one of four positions: to the right (as an E), to the left, up, or down. The structural components of the E's are single lines that subtend the same visual angles as do the Snellen letters of equivalent acuity value. In other words, this is a Snellen letter test, arranged in exactly the same format, in which only one letter is used—the E—but where the orientation of the letter is varied. It therefore is a very accurate measure of visual acuity, correlating closely with standard Snellen letter chart acuities.

To administer the test, follow the steps listed below:

1. Have on hand a key card similar to the one described for the Snellen letter test, which comprises only four E's, each oriented in one of the four principal directions. The E's should be large; this step is to assess the child's ability to respond, not his visual acuity.

2. Show the E key card to the child and ask him to indicate, either orally or by pointing, which way each of the E's is "pointing." (Some examiners prefer to call the E a "table," with "legs" that point in different directions.) (See Practical Suggestion 3-9.)

3. No response does not necessarily mean that the child cannot see the E's. He may simply be shy, or too intimidated by the situation to respond (see Practical Suggestion 1-17).

4. Some optometrists prefer an alternative response mode: the child is given a fairly large E, made of wood or heavy stock paper, and asked to hold it in the

same orientation as the E on the test chart. (In our opinion, this adds to the complexity of the task for many youngsters.)

5. If the child performs acceptably in the pretest activity, then measure his acuity with the Tumbling E chart. As usual, monocular acuities are measured first, then binocular.

LANDOLT C TEST

This test is similar to the Tumbling E test. It merely substitutes a printed C for the E, with the test chart consisting of open circles of diminishing diameters (11). The break in the circle may occur in any one of the four principal locations, and the size of the break is equal to the width of the line that forms the C. As such, each C compares with equivalent size letters on the Snellen letter chart. The patient's task: identify the location of the breaks in the circle.

The Landolt C test provides a valid measure of visual acuity, but it is not of any unique value with young children. Experience shows that it has no advantages over the Tumbling E test and, in fact, is often more difficult for the child to understand.

□ Four-Year-Olds

SJOGREN HAND TEST

This test (12) closely resembles the Tumbling E test, except that it uses diagrammatic representations (silhouettes) of an open hand (fingers extended) in lieu of the letter E. The child's task: identify the direction in which the fingers of the hand are pointing: to the right, the left, up, down (see Figure 3.2).

Figure 3.2
Sjogren Hand Test.

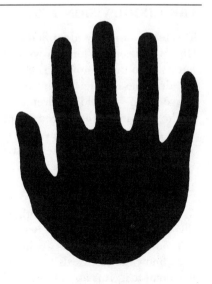

The test has certain faults. First, Snellen standards can be applied to the fingers only, and even there only loosely. Second, because the palm of the hand is large, it is easy to distinguish. Identifying its position aids in determining the location of the fingers, even when the fingers themselves are not at all clear. Hence, the test outcomes are less valid than desired. Finally, young children who are confused by the response requirements of the Tumbling E test are likely to be equally perplexed by the response requirements of the Sjogren test.

BLACKBIRD VISION SCREENING TEST

This test is very much like the Sjogren Hand test. The child is asked to indicate the orientation of a schematic "bird" (it could also be called an "airplane"), and, as a means of indoctrinating the child to the response requirements of the test, a story is provided about a blackbird that flies in different directions (13).

BROKEN WHEEL ACUITY TEST

This is a two-alternative, forced-choice, nonverbal test. Seven pairs of 5 × 7-inch posterboard cards are provided for presentation at a test distance of 10 feet. Each of these displays a black and white drawing of a car. Within each pair, the wheels of the car on one card are Landolt C's (called "broken wheels" by the tester), while on the other card they are unbroken circles. The stimuli range in size from 20/20 to 20/100 (when viewed from 10 feet). To administer the test, the examiner displays a pair of cards of equivalent size and asks the child to indicate ("point to," "show me," etc.) the car with the broken wheels. To reduce the risk of correct guessing, a four-correct-out-of-four-trials criterion is suggested (14) (see Practical Suggestion 1-37).

PRESCHOOL VISION TEST

This test, commonly identified by its author's name as the Allen Picture Card test (15), was designed for use with children who cannot—or will not—respond to letters or to the Tumbling E chart. The test is made up of seven black and white line drawings of objects that were selected because they are within the experience of average 3-year-old children (5). These are shown in Figures 3.3A and 3.3B.

The drawings are printed on plastic 4 × 4-inch white cards. There are four cards in all, a drawing appearing on each side of each card, except for the eighth side, which contains the test instructions.

To administer the preschool vision test, perform the following steps:

1. First, prepare a key by arranging the test cards into two clusters—four cards in one cluster, three in the other—and photocopying them. You may not need this but, on the other hand, you may (see below). (An alternative to this is to use a second set of test cards as the key.)
2. Show the test cards to the child and ask him to name each of the objects as you point to it. It is not important that the child name the objects correctly, simply

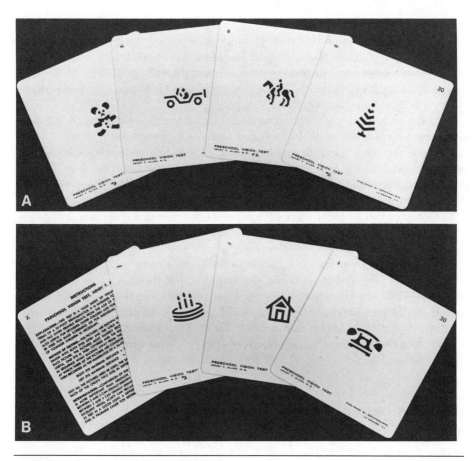

Figure 3.3 Preschool Vision Test.

that he have a specific and consistent verbal label for each one. For example, many youngster will call the drawing of the birthday cake simply "birthday." This is acceptable; it does not invalidate the acuity measure. In other words, do not turn the test into a vocabulary lesson (see Practical Suggestion 1-33).

3. If the child fails to respond orally, take a different tack. Show the child one of the test cards—still held at a close viewing distance—and say to him, "This is mine." "Show me one just like it on yours." "Yours," of course, refers to the key cards. This mode of testing relieves the child from speaking; he need only point to a matching picture.

4. If the child responds appropriately—that is, if he either names or points accurately when the pictures are held close to him—then proceed with measuring his visual acuity. (Note: A helper is needed with this test, if only to hold the occluder. Also, if the child is to respond by pointing to the matching picture on the key rather than by naming the object, then the helper will have to hold the key card and assess the accuracy of the child's responses.)

5. With the room fully illuminated, and one of the patient's eyes occluded, present the pictures, one at a time in random sequence, from a 15-foot testing distance. (Allen suggests that a 75-watt bulb in a gooseneck lamp, located 5 feet from the test cards, will provide suitable illumination [5, p. 1097].) Make sure that no hints are given to the child about the accuracy of his responses, and remove the test picture immediately after he responds.

6. If the child does not respond accurately, shorten the test distance in 5-foot increments (i.e., move up to 10 feet) and repeat the procedure.

7. If, on the other hand, the child responds accurately and with relative ease, move back in 5-foot increments until the test distance is about 30 feet—if that much leeway is available. If not, then move back as far as possible, and take note of the distance.

8. Consider three to four successive correct responses at a specific test distance to be evidence that the child can see the drawings from that distance (see also Practical Suggestion 1-37).

9. Record acuities as fractions, wherein the denominator is 30 (the maximum test distance, measured in feet) and the numerator is the maximum distance at which the child could accurately identify the test pictures. For example, if the maximum distance at which the child could accurately identify three successive test drawings is 15 feet, then his acuity is 15/30. This fraction may be converted directly into the standard Snellen fraction: 15/30 translates to 20/40, 30/30 to 20/20, and so on.

AMERICAN OPTICAL COMPANY PICTURE SLIDE

This test is designed for use with the A.O. Projecto-chart. The slide contains three types of targets: Tumbling E's, Landolt C's, and line drawings of familiar objects. The latter are very similar to those that appear on the aforementioned Allen cards. Specifically, the slide contains the same drawings of the birthday cake, telephone, horseman, and automobile along with two novel figures: a bird and a hand with fingers extended upward.

The drawings are organized in the format characteristic of distance visual acuity charts. They present an array of sizes representative of 20/200 to 20/30 acuity when viewed from the designated testing distance.

To administer this test, follow this procedure:

1. Prepare a key card and proceed as described for the Preschool Vision Test procedure above. When indoctrinating the child, move her closer to the screen—within arm's reach—thereby assuring that her ability to identify the drawings is being assessed rather than her ability to see them clearly (see Practical Suggestion 1-31).

2. Once she has displayed an ability to communicate reliably regarding what she sees, proceed with the test itself.

SHERIDAN LETTER TEST

This test was originally published as part of the Screening Test for Young Children and Retardates (STYCAR) (16). The other STYCAR subtests are less complicated than this one; they will be mentioned subsequently.

The test comprises seven letters, obviously selected on the basis of their symmetry; they appear the same when perceived as reversed. These are the H, O, T, V, X, U, and A. The letters range in size from 6/6 to 6/60 when shown at 6 meters and are shown one at a time, each one printed on a separate 5 × 5-inch card. The test also includes a key card.

To administer the test:

1. Show the child some of the larger letters from a near viewing distance and determine whether he can name the letters in the set or, if not, whether he is able (and willing) to point to matching letters on the key card. If he responds appropriately, proceed to measure his acuity from the proper distance.

2. If he does not respond appropriately, then you may want to attempt to teach the child how to use the key card. Obviously, if this is too difficult for the child, then select a less confusing test.

H-O-T-V TEST

This test, produced by Lippman (17) is a slight modification and simpler version of the Sheridan test. It uses only four opto-types: the letters H, O, T and V, and is designed for a 10-foot testing distance. The child responds by naming the letters or pointing to a matching letter on a key card.

□ Three-Year-Olds

NEW YORK LIGHTHOUSE FLASHCARD TEST

This test was originally designed for use with "low-vision" children: children with poor acuity that cannot be improved in the customary ways (18,19). It resembles, but is less complicated than, the previously described Allen cards test in that it is based on the use of three picture symbol flash cards: line drawings of an open umbrella, an apple, and a house (see Figure 3.4). These are printed, one drawing per card, in seven different sizes, ranging from a 20/200 size down to a 20/10 size. Thus another difference from the Allen cards: the test is designed to be administered from a single fixed distance. (This is not always done, nor need it be.)

To administer the New York Lighthouse Flashcard Test, the Preschool Vision test (Allen cards) procedure is generally appropriate.

FFOOKS SYMBOL TEST

Like most of the test already described, Ffooks (20) designed his test as a less-confusing alternative for the Snellen and Tumbling E tests. His solution: use

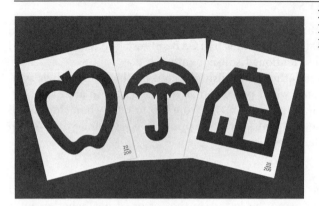

Figure 3.4
New York Lighthouse
Flashcard Test.

familiar geometric designs as test targets rather than E's or hands, both of which require a more sophisticated understanding of spatial orientation than many pre-school children are able to display. He originally prepared wooden cubes on which circles, squares, and triangles of different sizes were presented to the child for identification. More recently, the test has been redesigned, and now the geometric forms are displayed in a printed chart format. But the basic principle remains the same.

To administer, the Preschool Vision test (Allen cards) procedure is appropriate.

PARSONS VISUAL ACUITY TEST

The Parsons Visual Acuity Test (PVAT) is a nonverbal picture test that was spe-cifically designed for difficult-to-test patients including preschool children (21). Testing is administered at 13 inches using a stereoscope-like device in which a 20-foot viewing distance is simulated by introducing +3.00D lenses. The test employs three pictures: the hand, bird, and cake targets from the Allen Card series. The patient's task is to identify the hand when presented with these three. The test has been compared with the standard Snellen with normal 6- to 30-year-olds, and has been found to be invalid as a measure of distance visual acuity. However, the investigators did acknowledge that "the PVAT has clinical value in testing (near) vision of those patients who are unable to perform on the other more efficient acuity tests" (22, p. 18).

□ Two-Year-Olds

The tests described in this section, with the exception of the Dot Visual Acuity and the Bailey-Hall Cereal Tests, fall under the general heading of "miscellaneous informal measures of acuity." Their principal value is in providing a way for comparing the monocular acuity of the two eyes when the patient is too young to be tested in the standard ways. These informal probes have merit and should not be ignored.

THE DOT VISUAL ACUITY TEST

This test resembles the Candy Bead Test (see below) but attempts to obtain more exact information. It is designed to measure one's detection threshold for a black dot on a white background. The child is asked to touch a black dot that is situated somewhere on a white circular field. The dots range in size from 40 minute arc (20/800) to 1 minute arc (20/20) when viewed from 25 cm. Its authors report that the test produces visual acuity measures that are not significantly different from those obtained from the Tumbling E test (23,24).

BAILEY-HALL CEREAL TEST

This test uses a two-alternative, forced-choice approach wherein pairs of stimuli are presented to the patient. One of these is a drawing of a "cheerio" (a doughnut-shaped breakfast cereal product); the other is a rectangle of the same dimensions and color. The patient is asked simply to identify one from the other and is reinforced with cheerios. The test comprises six pairs of different sized targets and, according to its authors, Snellen fraction acuities may be derived on the basis of the maximum distance from which the patient is able to discriminate between a given pair (25). To date, there is very little validation data by which to assess the clinical usefulness of the test.

MINIATURE TOY TEST

This is another component of the previously cited STYCAR test (16,26). Its original purpose was for use with "severely handicapped children; in particular, those with low intelligence and those whose opportunities to learn from experiences had been so limited that they were not only unable to match single letters but were also unable to name or match colored pictures of common objects pasted singly on cards" (27, p. 453).

As the name indicates, the test uses pairs of miniature objects (toys) and requires the child to name them or select from an assortment of similar toys the one that matches the one shown by the examiner. The toys include pairs of the following: automobiles (2 inches long), airplanes (2 inches), dolls (2 inches), chairs (2 inches × 1 inch), knives, forks, and spoons (each 3 1/4 inches long; fork prongs 8/10 inches, spoon bowls 1 inch), and smaller knives, forks, and spoons (each 2 inches long; fork prongs 1/2 inch long; spoon bowls 7/10 inches long). (See Figure 3.5.)

To administer the test:

1. Orient the child to the task. Start off by determining his ability to name or at least find a matching toy, when the toys are shown to him one at a time.
2. If this is too difficult for him, then spend some time attempting to teach the response behavior. (Note: It is often helpful, when one knows in advance that the child might have difficulty with this activity, to have his parents teach the response behavior at home, before his visit. They can use standard-sized utensils for this.)
3. If the task remains unmastered, then scale down to a less demanding task.

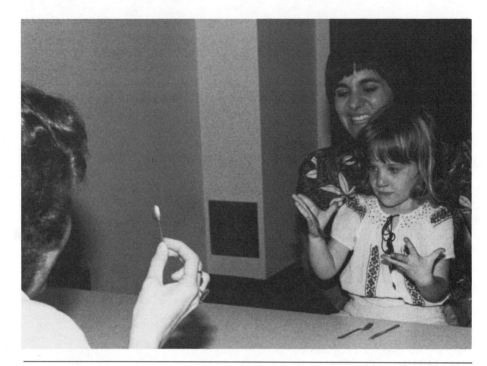

Figure 3.5 Visual acuity testing with STYCAR utensils.

4. If the child comprehends the task, then assess his ability to discriminate the various test objects when they are displayed from a distance of 10 feet.

5. Although strict standards have not been established for this test, its author states that being able to discriminate between the large toy fork and spoon from a distance of 10 feet is equivalent to 20/30 acuity; the smaller ones, 20/20. She suggests also that there is reason for considering acuity significantly substandard if the child cannot distinguish all of the seven larger toys from the 10-foot distance.

COIN TESTS, ETC.

Both Watchurst (28) and, before him, Young (29) described simple ways to use common coins as acuity targets. The former suggested using an English King George VI 3d. piece, asking the child to distinguish between the two faces of the coin; i.e., to indicate whether he sees the "daddy" or the "flower," as the coin is moved farther and farther away from him.

Young suggested using coins of different denominations—dimes, nickels, and quarters, for example—as the test distance was increased. Brock (30) proposed a variation, recommending the use of pairs of fine screws, washers, and other items of this sort, as targets to be picked up after they are scattered randomly on a sheet of paper. He urged a game format and an avoidance of language confusion by playing the game of "Do as I do" with the child.

□ One-Year-Olds

Once more it is obvious that the tests described here are informal and inexact measures of acuity.

BOCK CANDY TEST

The chief value of this test (31) is its appropriateness for children as young as 1 year, or even younger. The visual stimuli are unique in that they are edible and tasty: small candy beads such as those used for candy and cake decorations (see Figure 3.6). It would be erroneous, of course, to view test outcomes as analogous to responses on a Snellen letter test, but reasonably refined qualitative judgments are, in fact, possible (32).

To administer the test:

1. Place a number of the beads on a sheet of clean paper, or in the palm of your hand.
2. Guide the child's hand to a bead. Place one of his fingers on a bead; make sure that the bead adheres to the finger. Then guide the child's finger to his mouth. This single experience is usually sufficient to convince the child that the activity is worth repeating.
3. Occlude one eye, then the other, and observe differences, if there are any, between the two.

IVORY BALL TEST

Worth (33) designed this method for assessing the visual acuity of preverbal children. He proposed the use of five ivory balls, ranging in size from 1/2 inch to 1 1/2 inches in diameter. With one eye occluded, the child is asked to retrieve each ball after it has been rolled on the floor to a distance of about 20 feet. The child is to observe the ball being rolled; the examiner is urged to spin the ball as he rolls it.

Worth attributed an acuity value of 20/200 to the 1 1/2-inch ball when it is viewed from a 20-foot distance, and the 3/4-inch ball as 20/80. In practical terms, of course, the Ivory Ball test is out of date. But there is no reason why other objects (brightly colored marbles or beads, for example) could not be used as substitutes.

GRADUATED SIZE BALLS TEST

Sheridan, author of the STYCAR, developed a test similar to the Ivory Ball test (34). It uses Styrofoam spheres of graduated sizes that are rolled in front of the child along a black cloth strip with variations in the speed, distance of roll, and side from which the ball was cast. The examiner assesses the quality of the youngster's fixations in relation to the size of the sphere being presented. It has been subsequently reported that a black background is not desirable for this test because

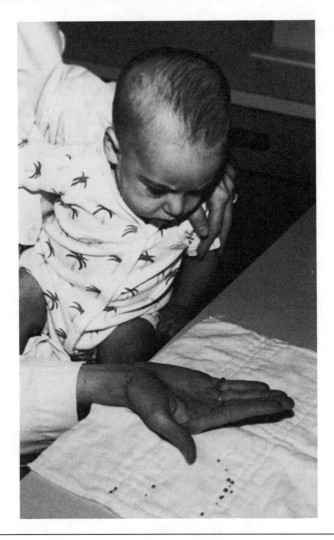

Figure 3.6 Visual acuity testing with candy beads.

increasing blur makes the white ball easier, rather than more difficult, to identify; hence a neutral background would be more appropriate for this procedure (35).

RELATIVE MONOCULAR BEHAVIORAL DIFFERENCES IN RESPONSE TO OCCLUDING ONE EYE

As the name suggests, it may be helpful simply to observe how a child responds to having his right eye occluded as compared with when his left eye is covered. If the child fusses more under one circumstance than the other, then it is reasonable to infer that the acuity of the one eye is significantly worse than the other (36).

□ Neonates

All of the visual acuity tests presented thus far have been based on subject-response tasks. That is, they depend on the child being willing and able to engage in visually guided tasks that range from naming different letters positioned 20 feet away to locating small objects at varying distances. Not surprisingly, these methods become increasingly less satisfactory as the age of the patient decreases.

Over the past four decades or so, new measurement methods have been developed. Most of these exploit the young child's apparently innate tendency to fixate on "interesting" visual stimuli presented in distractor-free contexts (37). Acuity is inferred by observing the child's instinctive behavioral response. For example, conditions that evoke *pendular eye movements or the optokinetic nystagmus reflex (OKN)* or the phenomenon of *preferential looking (PL)*. A few are based on measures of unobservable, central nervous system responses; i.e., *visually evoked potentials (VEP)*.

All of these procedures have been used in enough different settings by enough different investigators to be accepted as reasonably valid, albeit context-specific, procedures (i.e., the outcomes of the different tests cannot be interpreted as equivalent; not yet, at any rate). Some have been used clinically; some have not, but probably soon will be. As such, they warrant the clinician's interest. A brief description of each follows.

The tests are discussed more or less in the sequence in which they were developed and reported. First, the various categories of behavioral tests; then the electrophysiological procedures.

PENDULAR EYE MOVEMENTS

Very young children are inclined to fixate on an interesting visual stimulus, if they can see it and especially when no distractors are present. Recognizing this, Goldmann (38) reasoned that one could measure a young child's visual acuity by presenting oscillating visual stimuli of different sizes and determining the smallest stimulus that elicits pendular—"following"—eye movements. He used a small (38 x 15-cm) board containing a vertically oriented stripe (6.2cm wide) of black and white squares (each 1.15cm) centered in a field of smaller (0.36cm) black and white squares.

The board was initially presented at a 30-cm distance, and moved from side to side (each excursion = 18.5cm) at the rate of 40 times per minute. While this was going on, an observer watched the patient's eyes for movements, by viewing the conjunctival vessels through the 20D lens of an opthalmoscope. When eye movements were detected, the board was gradually moved farther away from the patient until that point where eye movements were no longer observed. Visual acuity measures were then calculated on the basis of the visual angle subtended by the larger squares from that threshold viewing distance.

Schwarting (39) modified this technique by adapting a metronome to accommodate interchangeable steel wires of different diameters, ranging from thick (20mm) to very thin (0.15mm).

The metronome, illuminated by a built-in light source, was presented in a darkened room at a distance of 1m. The examiner watched the patient's eyes as the device was activated, and visual acuity was inferred on the basis of the thinnest wire that elicited pendular eye movements. The author reported effective application with young children.

Bouman and associates (40), Popkowski and Markiewicz (41), and Millodot and Harper (42), among others, described variations on this method, but none of these investigators worked very much, if at all, with children.

Catford and Oliver (43) produced a motorized oscillating drum that displayed dots of various sizes, ranging from a 15-mm diameter down to 0.5-mm diameter. The device allows the examiner to control which one of the dots is visible at any given time and the rate at which the drum—and, hence, the dot—oscillates (see Figure 3.7).

When viewed from a distance of 2 feet, the dots are purported to represent stimuli comparable to Snellen acuities ranging from 20/600 to 20/20. The patient is instructed to watch the dot as it moves and, while this occurs, the examiner watches the patient's eyes for "following" movements. If these are observed, the dot is replaced by a smaller one and the test repeated. This continues until no oscillating eye movements are evident. Visual acuity is inferred from the smallest dot that evokes following movements. The device was designed for use with adults and children.

In one of their early reports (43), the authors of the test cited data from two groups of children. One group consisted of children with strabismus and varying degrees of amblyopia. Good correlations were found between acuities measured in the standard way and with the Catford apparatus. The second group of children were younger and not known to have visual disorders. Their visual acuities were measured with the Catford apparatus only. From these data, the authors concluded that normal children have 20/600 visual acuity at age 6 weeks and adult acuity by age 3 years.

Other investigators have found fault with the Catford apparatus. One team (44, pp. 2090-91) noted that

> . . . the subject must consciously fixate and follow the moving target across the visual field, rendering a part of this testing a subjective phenomenon requiring the subject's full cooperation. It is not exclusively an involuntary reflex and may be easily suppressed. . . . It would seem to have questionable value as a screening test with individuals where subjective acuity is unreliable or unobtainable.

A second group compared visual acuities as measured by the Catford apparatus to those obtained from the Landolt C acuity test and found that the Catford drum significantly overestimated visual acuity (45).

Figure 3.7
Catford Vision Testing
Apparatus.

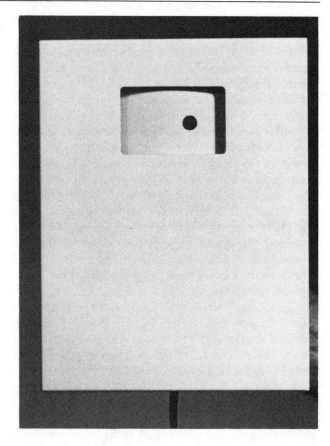

SUMMARY

Interest in this method of measuring visual acuity (i.e., by monitoring pendular eye movements) appears to be waning as investigators turn their attention to more promising methods. At this time, there is not enough evidence to argue strongly to the contrary.

OPTOKINETIC NYSTAGMUS

Optokinetic nystagmus (OKN) is defined as an "involuntary rhythmic oscillation of the eyes produced by a repetitive stimulus passing in front of the visual field. There is a slow phase as the eyes follow one target and then a correction fast phase as they shift to pick up the next target coming into view. The phenomenon has sometimes been called 'railroad train nystagmus' because it resembles the eye movements of a passenger on a moving train who is watching passing telephone poles" (46, p. 324).

Barany (47), while seeking a method for assessing the peripheral fields of infants, recognized the possibility of testing central visual function by way of the opto-kinetic nystagmus reflex.

McGinnis (48) followed up on Barany's observations by demonstrating that the optokinetic response could be elicited from infants as young as 75 minutes after birth—this by holding before the child's eyes a vertically oriented, slowly spinning drum on which black and white stripes had been drawn. He observed that if the stripes are visible as the dum rotates, the child will fixate upon a line and follow it until it goes out of view, then refixate on another line, and repeat the behavior.

McGinnis noted further that the speed at which the drum is rotated has effects. If it spins too rapidly, one cannot identify a single line upon which to fixate; hence, nystagmus is not evoked. If it moves too slowly. fixation is apt to be given up by the impact of competing distractors. (Borish [49] reports that if an object moves faster than 1 to 5 degrees per second, the slow, smooth following movements of the OKN response will become saccadic [p. 395]). When an appropriate speed is obtained, the nystagmus response is observed, if the child can resolve the separate vertical lines on the drum. Hence, inference of the child's visual acuity may be drawn on the basis of the minimum width of the black and white stripes that elicit the OKN response.

Gorman and associates (50) used a striped paper scroll draped over a transparent plastic canopy apparatus to test the visual resolution abilities of 100 infants, all under 6 days of age. The canopy was mounted so that it arched over the infant's head. The striped scroll was attached to rollers at each end, thereby making it possible to move the stripes either to the left or the right. The OKN responses were observed directly while the rollers were activated and the stripe widths were gradually reduced or increased depending upon the procedure followed on that particular trial. Here, again, an estimate of the infant visual acuity was made on the basis of the thinnest stripes that elicited the OKN response.

Later, using a device similar to Gorman's, Dayton and colleagues (51) introduced a different and more precise method for monitoring OKN eye movements: re-cording them with electo-oculogram tracings (EOG) and confirming these with direct observations.

Kornblatt and Saferstein (52) and Harcourt (53) described interesting procedural variations. The former reported a technique that involved presenting a vertically striped drum that was spinning too rapidly to elicit nystagmus and allowing the drum to slow down until the OKN response was finally elicited. They recorded the RPM that produced this effect and reported that the lower the patient's visual acuity, the slower the drum had to rotate before the phenomenon was observed.

Harcourt described a somewhat different device—a motor-driven drum, ori-ented horizontally, displaying a continuous wrap-around stripe: a helix. As the roller was turned, the stripe appeared to move horizontally along the roller. Harcourt went on to suggest a similar but simpler device that could be constructed by winding black tape of different thicknesses around a horizontally held paint roller.

SUMMARY

There now appears to be a declining interest in using the OKN response to measure visual acuity. This, for at least two reasons: (1) newer, more promising procedures are being reported; (2) not everyone accepts as fact that this method provides a valid measure of visual acuity. Fantz and Ordy (54) argue that it ". . . involves peripheral as well as central vision, it is reflex in nature, and it probably can be mediated by subcortical visual centers" (p. 161). Reinicke and Cogan (55) disagree, but do not refute the argument convincingly enough to remove a reasonable doubt.

ARRESTING THE OKN RESPONSE

Ohm's work (56) helps to resolve one of the criticisms of the OKN response as a measure of visual acuity. He designed a procedure that measures the size of the smallest visual fixation stimulus that would disrupt an ongoing OKN response. In brief, once nystagmus has been evoked, a stimulus is introduced into the patient's central visual field. If the patient sees this stimulus and fixates it, the nystagmus stops. Thus, the size of the smallest target that stops the nystagmus action may be translated into a visual acuity measure.

Wolin and Dillman (57) improved on Ohm's method by incorporating electro-oculography to monitor the eye movements. Voipio and Hyvarinen (58) introduced a variation by using horizontal stripes of varying thickness as the arresting stimulus for a drum containing vertical stripes. They stated that by using stripes instead of a spot, they were measuring "minimum separable" rather than "minimum visible" and were thereby closer to a valid assessment of visual acuity.

Once again, very little of this research involved children and, for now at least, it does not appear to hold promise as a useful procedure for the young patient.

PREFERENTIAL LOOKING

A few decades ago, Fantz (37) reported that when two objects are presented simultaneously in a distractor-free environment to an infant age 6 months or younger, the child is apt to look at the more "interesting" of the two. All else being equal in the two stimuli—e.g., luminance, color, size—an important "interesting" feature to Fantz's subjects was the internal composition of the visual stimulus. In other words, the infants he studied typically spent more time looking at a circle containing black and white checkerboard patterns than at a blank gray circle of equal size and luminance (59). This observation opened up a new avenue for measuring the visual acuity of very young children.

These early studies documented the percentage of time, within each 30-second test exposure, the child attended to one target as compared with the other. Thus, by reducing the size of the squares in the checkerboard pattern, and later on in a pattern of vertical stripes (60) a threshold for fine detail could be inferred, *if*, in fact, the child ceased to look more at one of the paired set when the stripes became too thin to be differentiated from the plain gray field. Fantz defined acuity on the basis of the narrowest stripes that attracted 75 percent or more of the infants of that age, when the stimuli were shown alongside a gray, homogeneous field of equal size and luminance.

Modifications of this technique have been developed. Teller and associates (61), using a similar apparatus, devised a forced-choice preferential looking technique (FPL) which has since been modified (62) and applied clinically (63).

In this clinical procedure (see Figure 3.8), the infant is seated on someone's lap before a screen containing two 9-cm circular apertures, separated horizontally and equidistant from a centrally located 4-mm peephole. The distance from the child's forehead to each of the two circular apertures is 36 cm. An eyeshield projects from the screen in such a way as to prevent the person holding the infant from seeing the two apertures, and thereby perhaps consciously or subconsciously prompting the infant.

A striped grating is placed in one of the two apertures, a plain (homogeneous) gray card of equal luminance in the other, and observations of the child's looking behaviors are noted. As the test stimuli are changed (i.e., stripes of different widths), they are shifted randomly from one aperture to the other, the opposite aperture always then displaying a homogeneously gray target of equivalent luminance.

The stripe widths vary from wide to narrow—from 20/800 (stripes that subtend a visual angle of 40 minutes from the 36-cm distance), the starting point for infants up to the age of 7 weeks; 20/600 (or 27 minutes) for infants ages 8 through 11 weeks; and 20/400 (or 20 minutes) for 12-through 16-week-old infants. There were chosen on the basis of normative studies carried out with the same apparatus.

Three adults are required for the activity. One acts as an *observer* and is located behind the screen, watching the infant through the center peephole. The observer's task: predict which of the two apertures contains the stripes—this on the basis of the infant's behavior and the assumption that the infant will choose to look at the stripes, as long as he is able to resolve them. The second participant: a *holder*, who holds the infant, but cannot see the two apertures. The third, an *experimenter*, who controls the stimuli, records the observer's judgments, determines their accuracy, and reports trial-by-trial results to the observer.

In the clinical validation study (64), each trial was allowed a maximum of 2 minutes, but the investigators report that this amount of time was rarely needed. The entire FPL test usually required between 5 and 10 minutes—and it is worth noting that in about half of these cases (total N = 121), the observers were the children's mothers, who, after being positioned behind the screen, were simply asked, "Which side does your baby like to look at more, the left or the right?" They were given no other information.

The study was supportive in that infants with identifiable ocular deficits that would cause substandard visual acuity were readily identified by the FPL procedure. In the conclusion of their report, the investigators state that their "observations, to date, indicate that the FPL screening test effectively identifies infants with binocular visual problems" (63, p. 1156). They were not yet ready to claim that it measures Snellen equivalent visual acuities, but they expressed no

Figure 3.8
Schematic drawings of OPL apparatus with animal reinforcer (from Mayer DL, Dobson V. Assessment of vision in young children: a new operant approach yields estimates of acuity. Inv Ophthal 1980; 19 [15]:556).

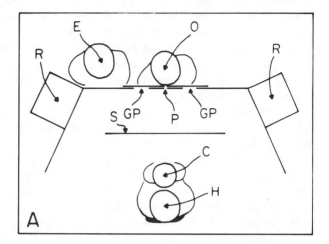

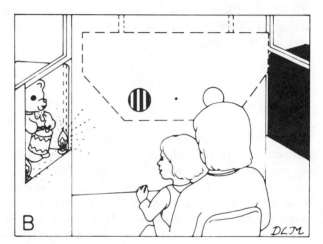

reservations about the test's ability to identify clinically important differences between an infant's monocular acuities.

Another group (64) has varied this procedure somewhat, measuring differences in preferential looking as a function of stripe orientation.

Later, Mayer (65) reported a modification of the procedure that makes it more effective with children older than 6 months; this by using an operant conditioning paradigm in lieu of depending upon the child simply being attracted to the stripes because they are more interesting than the nondetailed field. The child is entertained ("reinforced") for looking at the stripes by a motorized, drum-beating toy bear. Figure 3.8 shows two schematic drawings of the apparatus.

Many advances have been made during the past few years in the clinical application of this procedure, both in simplifying the apparatus and in speeding up the testing time. Manny, after doing some initial investigations with Boltz, wherein it was shown that blur produced by lenses placed before young children was reflected in their visual acuity as measured by the FPL method (66), has gone on to adapt the method for use on a computer (67). Other investigators have altered the original FPL apparatus by reducing it to a series of "Acuity Cards"—gray rectangular cardboard cards that contain grating targets of various spatial frequencies. The examiner holds the cards before the infant and watches his eye movement patterns. On the basis of these, the examiner infers whether or not the infant can see the gratings. Visual acuity is estimated as the highest spatial frequency that the infant is believed to be able to see. Time estimates for completing this procedure range from 3 to 5 minutes per eye (68,69,70,71,72).

Although not everyone has been able to document a direct link between a child's FPL visual acuity and his refractive status, there seems to be little doubt that the procedure has merit and is likely to become a standard method in optometric offices (73). Two commercially produced devices are presently available (Teller Acuity Cards, Visitech Consultants, Inc., 1327 N. Fairfield Rd., Dayton, OH 45432; Pl 20/20 Vision Tester, American Optical Co., 14 Mechanic St., Southbridge, MA 01550), and there is every reason to believe that, in time, additional ones will be produced.

VISUALLY EVOKED POTENTIALS

The phenomenon of VEP is a relative novelty to clinicians. It is not all that new, however. The basis for it was described over 100 years ago, when Caton (74) pointed out that the brain generates electrical impulses that occur in several distinctive rhythmic patterns, or "waves." The well-publicized alpha rhythm is an example of such a pattern. In essence, alpha is the name given to that intrinsic stream of electrical impulses emitted by the brain that peaks and ebbs at the rate of about 10 cycles per second—at 10 Hz. Most persons produce such a signal under the same set of conditions. Hence, it is a predictable phenomenon, and extreme variations from the norm have diagnostic value. From this, of course, comes the basis for the development of electroencephalography (EEG) in clinical neurology.

Caton also reported the presence of evoked potentials: the electrical activity that results from some specific external stimulus and disappears when the stimulus is removed.

Visually evoked potential is one of these. Simply stated, it is the change in the emitted electrical pattern detected by (scalp) surface electrodes monitoring the occipital cortex following light stimulation of the retina. The phenomenon has been called a number of things over the years: for example, visually evoked response (VER), evoked potential (EP), and visually evoked cortical response (VECP). All of these refer to the same thing and simply illustrate the dynamics of a developing language. It now appears that VEP will be the official, universally accepted identifier.

In operational terms, obtaining a VEP involves introducing a stimulus to the eye(s) and measuring the response from the occipital cortex. This provides data from which one may infer the conditions that the stimulus-generated signal encountered in between the two events. It is not quite so simple, however, because of the great number of variations possible from different stimulus conditions and the sensitivity of the VEP to those different conditions.

This is not the place for an in-depth description of the electronics or neurophysiology of the VEP procedure, but a very brief discussion of the fundamentals would be useful. First, some of the underlying neurophysiology that makes the VEP procedure possible; then a nontechnical description of the procedure itself, with some elaboration on the parameters of the stimulus conditions and the different effects these have on the measurements one obtains (75).

About half of the occipital cortex is devoted to representing 5 degrees or so of the central retina. This remarkable allocation of central nervous system capacity is, of course, what equips the human eye to see as clearly as it does, *when the stimulus falls on macula*, as opposed to peripheral retina.

As such, electrical impulses generated by occipital cortex tend to reflect macular function rather than peripheral. This sponsors the assumption that the impulses will differ according to the nature of the external stimulus, the impact of the ocular media on that stimulus as it travels through the eye to the macula, the ability of the macula to resolve the stimulus, the integrity of the optic tract that transports the signal back to occipital cortex, and the cortex itself. And the assumption appears to be correct.

The VEP Apparatus and Procedure

Four components are characteristic in most VEP setups: (a) a stimulus generator, situated a fixed distance from the patient's eyes; (b) three scalp electrodes; one attached to the back of the skull, slightly above the inion; another, serving as a reference, attached to one ear lobe; and the third, serving as a ground, attached to the other ear lobe (in some installations children are fitted with a strap helmet to which the electrodes are attached); (c) an amplifier and a computer that make the evoked signal apparent by separating it from the background activity; and (d) a recording device to store the output data.

Assume a patient is "wired up" and awaiting the introduction of a visual stimulus. If one monitors the occipital cortex at this moment with a VEP apparatus, potential is recorded—there is a lot of activity—but it tends to be random, intrinsic "noise." When a visual stimulus is introduced—a flash of light, say, patterned or unpatterned (more about this in a moment)—a specific response is generated from the occipital cortex. But it is not a very strong signal and will therefore be buried in the ongoing aforementioned noise. In order to make the signal useful, something has to be done to separate it from the noise. An amplifier is used to enhance the VEP signal, and a computer to translate the ongoing noise into a baseline component and to make the VEP response a unique and apparent event that is time-linked with the stimulus in a cause-effect fashion.

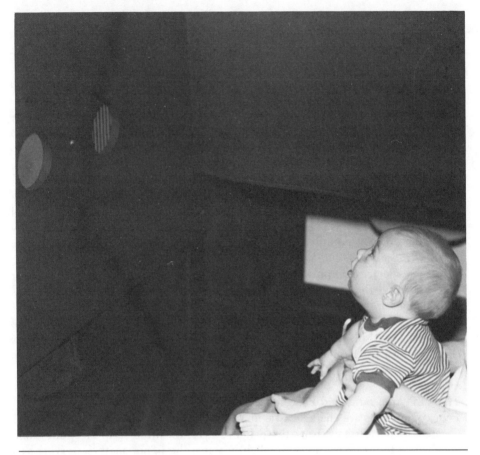

Figure 3.9 Preferential looking. (Photo courtesy of R. Manny and R. Boltz.)

Considering all of this, it is easy to recognize the strong influence of the stimulus conditions on the response signal. Variations in the former have an immediate and direct effect on the latter and, because of this, the procedure has clinical value. By altering stimulus conditions in a controlled manner, and noting the change in the response, the examiner can infer the impact of what happened in between these two events—i.e., what happened as the stimulus passed through the eye and the neural system to the occipital cortex and, ultimately, the electrode at the back of the skull.

Stimulus Conditions
Stimuli may be patterned or unpatterned light. Inasmuch as the topic here is visual acuity, the former is more pertinent than the latter. An unpatterned light stimulus is more apt to be used when the eye is incapable of resolving patterns, such as when a cataract obstructs a view of the retina.

Variations in Patterns

Patterned stimuli may differ in appearance. They may be checkerboardlike, with the checks ranging from large to small, or they may be contrasting stripes (black and white, multicolored, etc.) oriented in a specific meridian and/or ranging from narrow to wide. They may also be dots on a contrasting background that vary in size and density, or they may be something less geometric. Patterns may also vary widely in luminance and contrast.

Variations in the Rate of Pattern Presentation

Stimuli may be presented at various rates. Two basic presentation modes have been developed. One involves making an abrupt, unique alteration in stimulus conditions (such as a flash), then repeating this at a relatively slow rate (e.g., one per second). The other involves a very rapid rate of stimulation that tends to obscure the separateness of each presentation, blending them into an ongoing, continuous pattern. The former condition produces what is called a "transient VEP," where each stimulus input generates a separate VEP output. The latter condition, in contrast, produces a "steady-state VEP," where a continuous wave-like output is obtained.

Given all these variables, it begins to become evident why there are so many reports in the VEP literature that appear to contradict each other. The VEP is so responsive to variations in conditions that slight alterations will produce marked differences, and major alterations will generate something well beyond that. But it is reasonable to assume that, as the research is continued, some optimum set of conditions will be defined and validated. In the meantime, it is also reasonable for the optometrist to assume a wait-and-see attitude. The day for installing a VEP measuring system in the standard optometric office has not yet arrived, but it is surely on the way.

Two landmark studies signal this very clearly. Both addressed the question. "How soon following birth does a child achieve the visual resolution abilities of the adult?"

Marg and colleagues (76) offer evidence suggesting that human infants are able to resolve squares subtending 1 minute of arc (organized in a checkerboard format)—the equivalent of 20/20—at the age of 6 months. Their procedure: children were tested regularly from the time they entered the study (some as young as 1 month) until they were 6 months old. At each testing session, the child was linked up with a VEP apparatus and shown, first a blank gray luminous field. This was then replaced, tachistoscopically, by a 40-msec exposure of a checkerboard, made up of squares measuring 1 minute of arc along each dimension. The gray field was then restored at the end of the 40-msec flash, thereby producing a transient VEP. (The luminance of both displays was equivalent.)

Evidence of the patient's ability to resolve the small squares was based on a change in the VEP that occurred coincident with the 40-msec flash. If the flash brought about no change in the VEP, the assumption was that the child could not resolve the individual squares, that his eyes detected no change in the visual stimulus during the tachistoscopic exposure of the checkerboard pattern. The children in this study showed VEP responses to the 1 minute of arc squares when they were approximately 6 months old, and to larger squares prior to that time.

Sokol and Dobson (77) took a somewhat different approach. They based their study on knowledge that adults respond best (i.e., show the highest amplitude) in a steady-state VEP to a stimulus that is made up of checkerboard squares that subtend 10 to 20 minutes of arc. (The steady-state VEP was achieved by alternating the checks, from black to white and from white to black, at the rate of 6 cycles per second, while holding luminance and contrast unchanged.) Larger and smaller squares caused an attentuation of the VEP amplitude. They found that infants respond similarly by age 6 months. The authors go on to acknowledge that they are inferring a great deal when they reason that, because of this, one can conclude that infants at this stage are able to see as well as adults with 20/20 visual acuity, but their data are noteworthy.

Sweep VEP

One of the impediments to the use of VEP acuity assessment with infants has been the amount of time required to carry out the procedure. This problem appears to have been solved by the development of a procedure known as "sweep VEP," wherein vertical black and white stripes of different spatial frequencies are presented in very rapid sequence; e.g., a different spatial frequency each 0.5 seconds (78). One recent study used it with young (1- to 53-week-old) infants and showed that by age 8 months, VEP grating resolution was not significantly different from adult levels with the same apparatus. In other words, 8-month-olds appear to see as well, on average, as do adults (79).

VISUAL BEHAVIORS OF THE NEONATE

There are times when conditions prevent implementation of standardized tests; this is particularly true with very young infants. In those situations, it behooves the optometrist to be familiar with the visual behaviors—listed below—that are characteristic of the normal neonate so that atypical behaviors can be recognized.

At birth, infants display the following characteristics:

1. Eye position appears homodirectional with head-neck-hand (i.e., "fencing position" or tonic neck reflex [TNR]).
2. Blinking reflex usually present unless delivery was very premature.
3. Occasional nystagmus, but this soon disappears.
4. Passive raising of the head and of the trunk often causes the eyelids to open.
5. Eyes are apt to open as child sucks.
6. Pupils constricted but somewhat reactive to light.
7. May react to loud sounds, or stimulation of nose or eyelids, usually by inhibiting actions; e.g., stops movements.
8. Doll's eyes reflex may be present; i.e., when infant's head is rotated laterally, the eyes are pulled synergistically in the opposite direction, then return to the middle of the palpebral fissure.

9. Eye openings and excursions are sporadic and brief. Child fixates momentarily on a bright object that is held directly in its line of vision.

By the end of the second week, the following traits are noticed in the infant:

1. More alertness, wider excursions (same plane of TNR), more sustained gaze, as if staring.
2. Push away reflex—infant pushes away hands of person who attempts to force eyelids open.
3. Provoked nystagmus (rotatory or caloric); absent during the first month of prematurity.

By the end of the infant's fourth week, we note the following characteristics:

1. Eyes move approximately 90 degrees in the horizontal plane and about 20 degrees downward. Eye coordination and symmetry is much improved, often accompanied by associated head movements.
2. Defense reflex, i.e., lids close when attempt is made to force them open, associated with bilateral limbal movements and head disengagement.
3. Eyes fixate on a light source.
4. Fixation is more sustained for close, but not too close, objects (10 to 30 inches).
5. Supine position and TNR are still preferred, but the infant also begins to stare more at his surroundings; child starts to show evidence of an emerging symmetrotonic posture (STR) (80, 81).

■

G. IS THE VISUAL ACUITY NORMAL?

There is no debate about the criterion for normal visual acuity in the adult; 20/20 is uniformly accepted. But, this single index cannot be applied to young children. With them, one has to take into account specific ages and, in recent years, the measurement method that was used to gather the normative data.

As recently as 1939, it was generally accepted that children did not acquire 20/20 acuity until about age 5 years (50). With the advent of innovative measurement procedures, this statistic has been questioned strongly and now appears to belong to the category of "quaint notions held in the olden days"; it can no longer be taken seriously.

What, then, is normal acuity for young children, recognizing that measurement methods have to be included in the consideration? Table 3.1 shows the outcomes of a number of studies where different methods were used and relates visual acuity with age and with method.

Age (months)	Tumbling[a] E	Pendular[b] Eye Movements	OKN[c]	PL[d]	VEP[e]
1			20/300	20/400	20/300
2			20/150	20/300	20/200
3			20/150	20/200	20/60
4			20/150	20/200	20/50
5			20/60	20/150	20/40
6		20/400			20/20
12	20/140	20/200	20/40		
24	20/48	20/100	20/30		
36	20/46	20/50	20/20		
48	20/40				
60	20/33				

[a]Slataper.
[b]Schwarting.
[c]Allen; Catford.
[d]Allen.
[e]Sokol; Marg; Harter.

Table 3.1   Changes in Visual Acuity as a Function of Age and Measurement Method

The data shown there reveal two basic facts: one, young children acquire the ability to see clearly far earlier in life than had once been thought; second, a great deal more normative data are needed from all of these methods, in greater depth and across broader age ranges, before a firm position is taken on what is and what is not normal visual acuity for children between the ages of 1 day and 3 years. There are too many blank spaces in the table, leaving too much to speculation. But what there is helps the clinician far more than what was available only a decade ago.

■

H. SPECULATE ABOUT POSSIBLE EXPLANATIONS FOR THE LOWERED ACUITY

Substandard visual acuity may be the result of a number of different conditions. With the young patient, four general categories of possibilities stand out. These are as follows:

1. Refractive deviations
2. Pathology and/or structural anomalies
3. Binocular anomalies
4. Malingering

The first three are discussed in other sections (see Chapters 4, 5, and 6). Only malingering will be discussed here.

□ Malingering

As a general rule, preschool children do not malinger, at least not with sufficient conviction to make it a clinical problem. Typically, the preschool child who decides to complain about his eyes and/or eyesight, in the hopes of achieving some special goal (e.g., a pair of glasses or some other special attention), will not sustain at the mission long enough to cause real concern.

School-aged children are another matter, however. One does encounter malingering with this age group, and it is often accomplished with sufficient conviction to become a clinical problem.

CLINICAL SIGNS OF MALINGERING

The critical diagnostic indicator of malingering is evidence that the patient is consciously feigning poor visual acuity and/or whatever other difficulties he reports. Clearly, the optometrist cannot act on a hunch, regardless of how strong. Substandard acuity must either be explained on the basis of reliable data or, at the least, every other conceivable, clinically significant explanation must be ruled out. In other words, the only way to be certain that the patient is malingering is to acquire proof that the patient does not suffer from what he claims to suffer.

METHODS FOR DIAGNOSING MALINGERING

Interrogation. The malingerer will often overstate his case by claiming such poor visual acuity that one can legitimately question how he finds his way about his house, the optometrist's office, etc. If this appears to be the case, ask the child to explain the paradox, and ask it in serious tones. This often sets the stage for more valid responses.

Measure visual acuity at different viewing distances. Many young patients do not recognize the direct relationship between letter size and viewing distance. The malingerer, for example, will sometimes display 20/100 acuity and then insist that the rest of the chart remains too blurred to read (or improves but one line) even when the viewing distance is reduced by half.

Place into a trial frame lens combinations that add up to plano, or thereabouts. Determine whether this "improves" acuity (e.g., O.U. + 2.00 = −2.00D. spheres).

Present the child with a forced-choice condition in acuity testing. For example, show him a series of two (20/60, say) letters that he previously claimed to be unable to see, and ask him to try to identify which of the two is the _____ (examiner names one of the letters). The malingerer is apt to select the wrong one consistently, a pattern that random guessing would rarely produce.

Measure visual acuity on a vectographic chart. Using Polaroid filters intermittently, make it difficult for the child to "figure out" how to answer your questions. Do not allow any extra time as this is being done.

Have the child hold his hands in front of him and simply look at them. The malingerer is likely to avoid looking at his hands even though his proprioceptive reflexes rather than his eyesight will make this possible. Or have him—with eyes open—stretch his arms out to his sides and then either touch his nose with one index finger or bring the two index fingers together in front of him, fingertip to fingertip. Again, proprioception, independent of eyesight, makes these actions possible. Hence, the child should have no difficulty with these activities unless, of course, some underlying neurological deficit is affecting his behavior.

If only one eye is involved, introduce a reading bar between the child and some printed matter while he is reading it. The bar should have a detrimental effect on the child's ability to read that portion of the text that can be seen only by the involved eye.

Place a variety of informal assessment stimuli about the room. For example, use pictures containing specific details on the walls, small figures and/or toys on bookshelves and cabinets across the room. Identify details that require acuity of 20/50 or better in order to distinguish. Talk casually to the child about one or more of these, attempting to elicit evidence of his being able to see them. (It may be useful to do this while conducting an ophthalmoscopic or retinoscopic procedure in that there is nothing about those that hints at acuity assessment.)

MALINGERING, HYSTERICAL AMBLYOPIA, AND THE NONMALINGERING SYNDROME

The optometrist is sometimes confronted with the dilemma of distinguishing between malingering, hysterical amblyopia, and a condition that has been labeled the nonmalingering syndrome (82). Most often, the distinction between the first two is based upon certain behavioral signs: Hysterical amblyopes tends to display (a) no difficulty in orientation (the malingerer frequently exhibits exaggerated difficulty); (b) tubular fields, usually sharp-edged and circular in shape, that remain the same size regardless of test distance (83). One report also mentions diminished corneal sensitivity (84). The distinction between malingering and the nonmalingering syndrome: The latter patient (a) tends to hold reading matter far closer to his eyes than is normal; and (b) displays unstable bell and book retinoscopic reflexes (85).

The three conditions (presumably) stem from different etiologies. The origins of hysterical amblyopia are, by definition, psychogenic; the non-malingering syndrome is purported to stem from nearpoint focusing (accommodation/convergence) difficulties, and the malingerer is simply keen on obtaining glasses. As such, the three call for different treatments.

This concerns us. We have no quarrel with the notion that some children who feign poor visual acuity do so because of psychological difficulties. However, we are inclined to reject the idea that their visual behaviors are guided subconsciously. In the many years we have practiced, we recall no child who did not admit better sight once she was convinced that we knew her claim of reduced acuity was false. We suggest, therefore, that it does the child a disservice to label her as an hysterical amblyope. True, if psychological problems exist, they should be attended to; but that does not justify applying the label "hysterical" on the basis of a very limited set of visual behaviors. (It is interesting to note that in one of the reports cited above [84], ten of the eleven patients discussed initially manifested their visual difficulties after reaching adulthood; the eleventh case initially presented at age 10 years and

> completely recovered shortly thereafter. Fields were still normal when she reported for refraction five years later. . . . She has not been seen since, but her father reported 8 years after her last visit that she had recently committed herself to a mental institution, after having various sex problems, the nature of which was not revealed.

The authors then go on to comment that "this suggests a bad psychoneurotic prognosis for children with hysterical amblyopia, even when cured" [p. 1112].)

Neither do we deny the possibility that some nearpoint focusing problems may cause reduced distance and near visual acuity, and that plus lenses for near work could be helpful. But, again in our combined experiences, we have seen very few cases where this has been true.

In our opinion, the labels *malingering, hysterical amblyopia,* and *nonmalingering syndrome* all refer to a single condition in which the patient is seeking to obtain special attention. In some of these instances, the motivation is probably an effort to find some justification for doing poorly in school; in some instances, it is probably attributable to the professional bias of the diagnostician; and, obviously, in some cases, it is the product of a capricious child. (We are ignoring the malingerer who seeks financial reward from an insurance company, etc. These are rarely, if ever, children.)

POSTDIAGNOSIS MANAGEMENT OF THE MALINGERER

The clinical management of the malingering child poses a dilemma: expose the child and leave it at that, or cover up for him? Neither is desirable. The first will embarrass the child and may sponsor parental anger toward him. On the other hand, if the malingering is diagnosed but not revealed to the parent, (a) the child may very well continue the pretense, thereby raising parental anxieties and doubts about his well-being and the optometrist's professional competence; or (b) the child may give up the pretense but not the underlying motivation for it. Neglect of that underlying motive may not be best for the youngster.

Clearly then, one treatment approach will not satisfy each situation. The optometrist will have to exercise the "art" of his profession as he addresses the problem. Hence, each practitioner will differ somewhat in how he manages a case. But, regardless of approach, the goal is the same: Leave the child free of lingering guilt and, if possible, the factor(s) that sponsored his malingering behavior, and his parents free of feeling anger toward him and anxiety regarding his "condition." There is no one perfect way to achieve this, but there are ways, and they should be tried. It is not a trivial matter (86). (See discussion of reassurance therapy, Chapter 9.)

☐ Delayed Visual Maturation

Some otherwise apparently normal infants fail to show normal visual function during early infancy, yet ultimately do display it. During the first few months of life, they do not respond to visual stimuli in an expected manner (see list above); by 4 to 8 months of age, they start to behave normally (87, 88, 89). Obviously, such children cause great anxiety and concern during those early months, and deservedly so. Careful examination is warranted.

The mechanism of delayed visual maturation is not understood. Typically, pupillary reflexes are normal; media is clear; and retina, macula, vessels, and discs appear normal. The key (and often, only) discriminator is electrophysiological testing: ERG responses are normal, VEP responses are not. (One researcher also notes that such children do not manifest the pendular nystagmus movements often observed in blind children by age 3 to 4 months [90].) Later, normal visual behaviors start to appear and VEP responses become normal. Speculation about the causes of this condition includes delayed maturation of the macular photoreceptors, delayed myelination of the visual pathways, and delayed dendritic formation and synaptic development in the occipital cortex. Children with delayed visual maturation are at risk for developing permanent neurological sequelae. They should be seen as early as possible and their condition documented as thoroughly as is practical.

■
_____

PRACTICAL SUGGESTIONS

3-1. The examiner, not the child, should hold the occluder when monocular visual acuity is measured.

3-2. Occlude the child's eye by resting the hand that is holding the occluder on the child's forehead. This enables you to stabilize her head as you occlude the eye.

3-3. Some very young children object to an occluder or, for that matter, anything that touches them. For such children, try placing your palm, your thumb, a thick pencil, a toy, a high plus (e.g., $+8.00D$) lens, or what have you, before the eye to be occluded. (Also keep in mind that with some very young children, the only indicator of reduced visual acuity may be "resistance to occlusion" before one eye but not the other.)

3-4. A very useful and economical projector screen can be constructed with non-depolarizing, washable vinyl (available from Bernell Manufacturing Corp.) mounted on plywood or canvas stretchers, such as artists use. It is far less vulnerable to damage than is a painted screen.

3-5. Most visual acuity tests can be made simpler by administering them in a two-item, forced-choice format. For example, project a pair of Snellen letters (by using the mask built into the projector) while simultaneously showing the child one of these letters drawn on a sheet of paper that is held at nearpoint. Ask her, "Which of the letters out there, on the chart, looks like this one?" Or the reverse: project a single letter and present her at nearpoint with two letters and the request, "Show me which of these looks just like the one out there." The same general modifications can be applied to all of the tests described in Chapter 3.

Remember, however, that you should use the most *informative* test available. A two-item, forced choice format might be necessary for a given child. If it is, then use it, of course. But, if it is not—if the child can respond reliably to a more demanding test—then by all means use the latter, regardless of the child's age. (See also Practical Suggestion 1-35.) Conversely, if the youngster, because of a cognitive deficit, requires a test simpler than her chronological age would suggest, administer it. Do not succumb to the conclusion that, because you "see nothing else wrong," that her apparently reduced visual acuity, measured with the Snellen test, is attributable to a lack of understanding and nothing else. Test her with a simpler test.

3-6. It often is necessary to start off determining a young child's visual acuity with single optotype displays; i.e., by showing one letter/picture at a time. More complex displays can be more than the child can manage. Granted, doing this avoids contour interaction effects; hence, single optotype displays might not yield precisely accurate visual acuities, especially if the child has an amblyopic eye. But, if nothing else is possible, then settle for what you can get, until you can get more.

3-7. The first letters a child usually learns to identify are those in his first name. Hence, in lieu of anything better, perhaps selected letters on the Snellen chart will provide some information about the child's visual acuity.

3-8. Some children who do not yet know the names of the letters are able to "draw them in the air" with their finger. Obviously, if this is attempted, letters should be selected that are easily identified when drawn in the air, such as the T, V, X, O, L, H, J, etc, and the child should be encouraged to "draw them" large so that you can interpret them accurately.

3-9. The Tumbling E visual acuity test often causes difficulty because of the child's inabilility to indicate accurately the right/left orientations of the E. If you suspect this to be the case, limit the test to E's that are oriented vertically (i.e., to those that "point" up and down only), or use all of the orientations but instruct the child to report whether the E's point "up," "down," or "sideways," ignoring the distinction between left and right. (See also Practical Suggestion 1-22 regarding the use of various examination room landmarks to facilitate directional responses.)

3-10. When recording visual acuity thresholds derived from a test in which the standard testing distance was not used, record the test distance as the numerator and the designated stimulus size as the denominator. For example, if the patient's visual acuity threshold was the "20/30"-size Lighthouse Card patterns when held at 10 feet, then visual acuity should be recorded as 10/30. If this system is used routinely, it simplifies interpretation when the records are examined at a later date. (It is also desirable to record which test was used.)

3-11. If the child achieves maximum visual acuity on a test that does not provide optotypes as small as 20/20, indicate in your records that threshold might not have been measured. For example, if the child is able to identify the smallest pictures on the AO Picture Slide, record his acuity as 20/30+, thereby indicating that he might very well have achieved better acuity if smaller stimuli were used.

3-12. Start off Snellen letter visual acuity testing by presenting a single, vertical line of letters, with the largest letter being about a 20/50 size. This will yield an array of letters that ranges from 20/50 down to about 20/20, depending upon which visual acuity slide you use. This enables you to determine quickly the patient's approximate visual acuity, thereby giving you an entering point into the measurement process. In other words, if the patient correctly identifies the 20/50 and 20/40 letter in the vertical line of letters, but not the 20/30 one, then you know that you should probably start to test "line acuity" at about the 20/40 level. (Obviously, if the patient is unable to see the 20/50 letter, then larger ones will have to be presented.)

3-13. Near visual acuity testing of children is awkward and time-consuming, and it rarely provides the optometrist with any unique information. True, it may reveal hyperopia not made evident by distance acuity testing; but surely retinoscopy is a far better way to accomplish this. It might also be useful in determining when cycloplegia has been achieved; but rarely is this needed—reaction time tends to be very predictable. A third possibility: a near visual acuity measure might reveal a significantly reduced amplitude of accommodation; but that condition is exceptionally rare in young children, and when it does exist, it is usually evident in a number of other ways. Hence, although near visual acuity measures will be needed in these cases, there is no need to conduct the test with all children at the outset of an eye examination, unless, of course, state law mandates it.

■

REFERENCES

1. Brant JC, Nowotny M. Testing of visual acuity in young children: an evaluation of some commonly used methods. Develop Med Child Neurol 1976; 18:568–76.
2. DeYoung-Smith MA, Baker JD. A comparative study of visual acuity tests. Am J Orthoptics 1986; 36:160–64.
3. Rosenbaum AL, Kirschen DG. A survey of visual acuity testing in the infant and preverbal child. Am Orthop J 1984; 34:13–21.
4. Greenwald MJ. Visual development in infancy and childhood. Symp Ped Ophthal, Pediatr Clin N Am 1983; 30(6):977–93.
5. Livanes A, Greaves D, Bevan J. Pre-school visual acuity tests. Clin Exper Optom 1986; 69(4):145–48.
6. Simons K. Visual acuity norms in young children. Surv Ophthal 1983; 26(2):84–92.
7. Kastenbaum SM, Kepford KL, Holmstrom ET. Comparison of the STYCAR and Lighthouse acuity tests. AJOPO 1977; 54(7):458–63.
8. Fern KD, Manny R. Visual acuity of the preschool child: a review. AJOPO 1986; 63(5):319–45.
9. Hatfield EM. Methods and standards for screening preschool children. Sightsaving Rev Summer 1979:74.
10. Snellen H. Methods of determining acuity of vision. In: Systems of diseases of the eye. Norris WE, Oliver CA, eds. Vol. 2. Philadelphia, 1897.
11. Landolt A. Bull Soc Franc Opthal 1888; 6:213.
12. Sjogren H. A new series of test cards for determining visual acuity in children. Acta Ophthal 1939; 17:67.
13. Viacrucis KS. Preschool vision screening: a new method fills a need. J Sch Health 1976; 46:480–81.
14. Richman JE, Petito GT, Cron MT. Broken wheel acuity test: a new and valid test for preschool and exceptional children. JAOA 1984; 55(8):561–65.
15. Allen HF. A new picture series for preschool testing. Am J Ophthal 1957; 44(1):38.
16. Pugmire GE, Sheridan MD. Revised vision screening chart for very young or retarded children. Medical Officer 1957; 100:53.
17. Lippman O. Vision screening of young children. AJPH 1971; 61(8):1586–1601.

18. A flash card vision test for children. New York: Low Vision Lens Service, N.Y. Assn. for the Blind, 1966.

19. Faye EE. A new visual acuity test for partially sighted non-readers. J Ped Ophthal 1968; 5(4):210–12.

20. Ffooks O. Vision test for children. Br J Ophthal 1965; 49:312.

21. Cress PJ, Johnson JL, Shores RE. The development of a visual acuity test for persons with severe handicaps. J Spec Educ Technol 1983; 5(3):11–19.

22. Richman JE, Cron MT. Evaluation of the Parsons visual acuity test in screening exceptional children. JAOA 1987; 58(1):18.

23. Kirschen DG, Rosenbaum AL, Ballard EA. The dot visual acuity test—a new acuity test for children. JAOA 1983; 54:1055–59.

24. Kirschen DG, Goochey K, Salomon B. Performance of the dot visual acuity test with uncorrected ametropia resulting in target blur. AJOPO 1986; 63(12):962–65.

25. Bailey IL, Hall AP. New visual acuity tests for children. *AJOPO* 1984; 61:86P.

26. Sheridan MD. Diagnosis of visual deficits in early childhood. Br Orthop J 1963; 20:29–36.

27. Sheridan MD. Vision screening of very young or handicapped children. Br Med J 1960; 2:453.

28. Watchurst GR. Refraction and squint in children. Optician 1963; 145:533.

29. Young JH. Amblyopia exanopsia in children. Br J Ophthal 1940; 24:297.

30. Brock FW. A plea for orthoptic reorientation. Br J Phys Opt 1959; 16:175.

31. Bock RH. Ambylopia detection in the practice of pediatrics. Arch Pediatr 1960; 17:335.

32. Richman JE, Garzia RP. The bead test: a critical appraisal. AJOPO 1983; 60(3):199–203.

33. Worth C. Squint, its causes, pathology and treatment. 5th ed. Philadelphia: Blakiston's, 1921.

34. Sheridan MD. Vision screening procedures for very young and handicapped children. In: Gardner MD, MacKeith V, Smith T (eds). Aspects of developmental and pediatric ophthalmology. London: Spastic Internation Medical Publication 39, 1969.

35. Press LJ. STYCAR Ball acuity in relation to contrast and blur. AJOPO 1982; 59(2):128–34.

36. Woodruff ME. A systems examination of the infant's visual function. JAOA 1973; 45(3):410–15.

37. Fantz RL. Pattern vision in young infants. Psych Rev 1958; 8(2):43–47.

38. Goldmann H. Objektive sehscharfenbestimming. Ophthalmologica 1943; 105:240.

39. Schwarting BH. Testing infants' vision: an apparatus for estimating the visual acuity of infants and young children. Am J Ophthal 1954; 38(5):714.

40. Bouman MA et al. A modification of Goldmann's apparatus for the objective determination of visual acuity. Ophthalmologica 1951; 122:368–74.

41. Popkowski J, Markiewicz B. Klin *Oczna* 1975; 27:520.

42. Millodot M, Harper P. Measure of visual acuity by means of eye movements. AAAO 1969; 46:938–45.

43. Catford GV, Oliver A. Development of visual acuity. Arch Disabled Child 1973; 48:47.

44. Kahn SG et al. Subjective and objective visual acuity testing techniques. Arch Ophthal 1976; 94:2086.

45. Atkinson J, Braddick O, Pimm-Smith E, Ayling L, Sawyer R. Does the Catford drum give an accurate assessment of acuity? Brit J Ophthal 1981; 65:652–56.

46. Keltner J. Neuro-ophthalmology for the pediatrician. Pedi Annals 1977; 6(2):610–20.

47. Barany R. The clinical aspects and theory of train nystagmus. Arch Augenheilk 1921; 88:139–42.

48. McGinnis JM. Eye movements and optic nystagmus in early infancy. Genet Psych Monog 1930; 8:321.
49. Borish I. Clinical refraction. Chicago: Professional Press, 1970.
50. Gorman JJ et al. An apparatus for grading the visual acuity of infants on the basis of optokinetic nystagmus. *Pediatrics* 1957; 19:1088.
51. Dayton G Jr, Jones M, Aiu P, Rawson R, Steele B, Rose M. Developmental study of coordinated eye movements in the human infant. Arch Ophthal 1964; 71:865.
52. Kornblatt S, Saferstein D. An objective measure of visual acuity. AAAO 1963; 40:205.
53. Harcourt RB. The objective assessment of visual function. Br J Orthop 1969; 26:1.
54. Fantz RL, Ordy SM. A visual acuity test for infants under six months of age. Psych Record 1959; 9:159.
55. Reinecke RD, Cogan DG. Standardization of objective visual acuity measurements: Optokinetic nystagmus versus Snellen acuity. Arch Ophthal 1958; 60(3):418.
56. Ohm J. Objektive prufung der schleistungen mit helfe der optokinetischen augen-beivegungen. Stutgart: Enke, 1953.
57. Wolin LR, Dillman A. Objective measurements of visual acuity using optokinetic nystagmus and electro-oculography. Arch Ophthal 1964; 71:822.
58. Voipio H, Hyvarinen L. Objective measurements of visual acuity by arrestovisography. Arch Ophthal 1966; 75:799.
59. Fantz RL. The origin of form perception. Scientific American 1961; 204(5):66.
60. Fantz RL et al. Maturation of pattern vision in infants during the first six months. J Comp Phys Psych 1962; 55(6):907.
61. Teller DY et al. Visual acuity for vertical and diagonal gratings in human infants. Vis Res 1975; 14(7):1433.
62. Dobson V et al. A behavioral method for efficient screening of visual acuity in young infants. I: preliminary laboratory development. Inv Ophthal 1978; 17(12):1142.
63. Fulton AB et al. A behavioral method for efficient screening of visual acuity in young infants. II: clinical application. Inv Ophthal 1978; 17(12):1151.
64. Gwaizda J et al. New methods for testing infant vision. Sightsaving Rev Summer 1979:61.
65. Mayer DL, Dobson V. Assessment of vision in young children: a new operant approach yields estimates of acuity. Inv Ophthal 1980; 19(5):566.
66. Boltz RL, Manny RE, Katz BJ. Effects of induced blur on infant visual acuity. AJOPO 1963; 60(2):100–105.
67. Manny RE. Clinical assessment of visual acuity in human infants. AJOPO 1983; 60(6):464–71.
68. McDonald MA, Dobson V, Sebris SL, Baitch L, Varner KD, Teller DY. The acuity card procedure: a rapid test of infant acuity. Inv Ophthal Vis Sci 1985; 26(8):1158–62.
69. Dobson V, McDonald MA, Kohl P, Stern N, Samek M, Preston K. Visual acuity screening of infants and young children with the acuity card procedure. JAOA 1986; 57(4):284–89.
70. McDonald MA, Ankrum C, Preston K, Sebris SL. Monocular and binocular acuity estimation in 18- to 36- month old acuity card results. AJOPO 1986; 63(3):181–86.
71. McDonald MA, Sebris SL. Monocular acuity in normal infants: the acuity card procedure. AJOPO 1986; 63(2):127–34.
72. Brown AM, Yamamoto M. Visual acuity in newborn and preterm infants measured with grating acuity cards. Am J Ophthal 1986; 102:245–53.
73. Kohl P, Rolen RD, Bedford AK, Samek K, Stern N. Refractive error and preferential looking visual acuity in human infants: A pilot study. JAOA 1986; 57(4):290–96.
74. Catton R. The electrical currents of the brain. Br Med J August 8, 1975:278.

75. Sherman J. Visual evoked potential (VEP): basic concepts and clinical application. JAOA 1979; 50(1):19.
76. Marg E et al. Visual acuity development in human infants. Inv Ophthal 1976; 15(1):150–53.
77. Sokol S, Dobson V. Pattern reversal visually evoked potentials in infants. Inv Ophthal 1976; 15(1):58–61.
78. Tyler CW, Apkarian PA, Levi D, Nakayama K. Rapid assessment of visual funciton: an electronic sweep technique for the pattern VEP. Invest Ophthal Vis Sci 1979; 18:703–13.
79. Norcia AM, Tyler CW. Spatial frequency sweep VEP: visual acuity during the first year of life. Vis Res 1985; 25(10):1399–1408.
80. Esente I, Nardi M. Visual behaviour of the neonatal period. In Francois J, Maione M, eds. Pediatric ophthalmology. New York: J Wiley & Sons, 1982.
81. Mohindra I. Developmental inventory for infants and young children. Optom Wkly 1979; July:505–509.
82. Maino JH. Ocular hysteria and malingering. In Amos J, ed. Diagnosis and management in vision care. Boston: Butterworths, 1987.
83. Borish I. Clinical refraction, 3rd ed. Chicago: Professional Press, 1975.
84. Friesen H, Mann WA. Follow-up study of hysterical amblyopia. Am J Ophthal 1966; 62(6):1106–15.
85. Streff JW. Preliminary observations on a non-malingering syndrome. Optom Wkly 1962; 53:536–37.
86. Korsch BM, Negrete VF. Doctor-patient communication. Sci Am August 1972; 66–74.
87. Mellor DH, Fielder AR. Dissociated visual development: electrodiagnostic studies in infants who are 'slow to see.' Develop Med Child Neurol 1980; 22:327–35.
88. Hoyt CS, Jastrzebski G, Marg E. Delayed visual maturation in infancy. Br J Ophthal 1983; 67:127–30.
89. Fielder AR, Russell-Eggitt IR, Dodd KL, Mellor DH. Delayed visual maturation. Trans Ophthalmol Soc UK 1985; 104:653–61.
90. Illingworth RS. Delayed visual maturation. Arch Dis Child 1961; 36:407–409.

4

Question 4

Are the Eyes Healthy and Normally Formed?

☐

The eyes of a newborn are different than the eyes of an adult. Describing what these differences are and how they diminish as a child matures is one of the goals of this chapter.

Ocular growth and development do not commence at the time of birth. (The terms growth and development have distinctly different meanings. Interpret growth to mean cell proliferation; development, cell differentiation [1, p. 80].) They begin some 280 days before birth, at the time of conception. What we observe when we look at the eyes of a newborn is simply a point along a continuum, a continuum that will not achieve terminal status for a number of years.

Ocular growth and development are very rapid in the embryo. By the end of the first month of the pregnancy, the optic cup has begun to form and the fundamental structures of the vitreous, the lens, and the blood vessels have been laid down. At the completion of the first trimester these have been joined by the uveal and fibrous coats of the eye: the choroid and cornea/sclera (2, p. 83).

As the second trimester of pregnancy comes to an end, basic ocular anatomical development is almost complete. Everything but the macula and the pupillary dilator muscles are in place and presumably ready to function. Thus, many of the final prenatal development changes are *reduction* processes, such as atrophy of the pupillary membrane, the hyaloid artery, and the connective tissue in the angle between the iris and the cornea. These are typically completed by the time of delivery. What remains to be accomplished in postnatal life is the development of precise function and maximum physical growth (3).

The optometrist keeps this in mind as she assesses the health and structural integrity of her young patient's eyes. By means of various procedures, she attempts to determine:

1. The normalcy of the growth and development that has occurred
2. The health status of the existing ocular structures
3. The functional status of the existing ocular structures

To do this, she will look at the components of the eyes in a systematic fashion (4). Sometimes, however, she will alter her customary sequence, influenced by some compelling factor discovered during an earlier part of the visit—while determining the patient's chief concern and case history, perhaps, or while measuring visual acuity. She is, after all, a clinician, primarily devoted to solving patient's problems, not collecting information for its own sake (see Figure 4.1).

This brings up a topic directly related to clinical assessment: *relative intensity,* the extent to which the clinician attaches extra importance to some aspects of an examination protocol; the extent to which she will switch to a slower-paced, finer-grade, in-depth analysis mode during certain parts of her examination.

We noted earlier that the optometrist's characteristic style is not (a) collect all available date; (b) then analyze the data; (c) then diagnose. Rather, her usual approach is, from the onset, to formulate hypothetical explanations for what she hears and sees, and then to test these by way of clinical investigation, rejecting, or altering, or even posing new hypotheses as evidence is accumulated and juxtaposed with what she has already learned about the patient. (The experienced

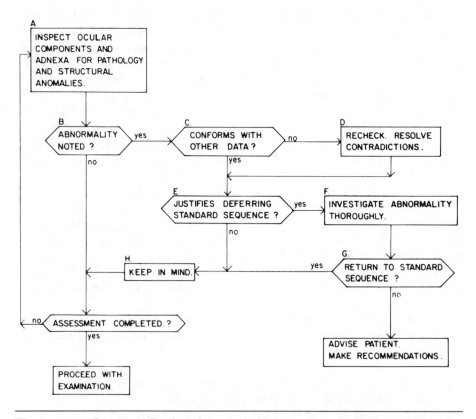

Figure 4.1   Question #4: Are the eyes healthy and normally formed?

clinician does not simply record contradicting information without questioning it and/or trying to explain it.)

The process commences when the child first comes to her attention—either by way of professional report from a school counselor or referring colleague or anxious inquiries from a concerned parent or direct observations of the child himself. It continues while she obtains preliminary information and observes the child. It goes on as she determines the parent's chief concerns and starts to elicit a case history. It is maintained as visual acuity is measured.

During all of this, certain hypotheses fall by the wayside, no longer plausible in the light of the data. Sometimes, a new hypothesis is introduced, triggered by something observed during a clinical test. In short, the process is one of accumulating and filtering, wherein, through successive approximations, the clinician narrows her scope, homing in on a decreasing number of possible explanations (diagnoses) for what she knows about her patient and her patient's clinical problem(s) (5).

The process is carried over to that portion of the examination that is characterized by the working question, "Are the patient's eyes healthy and normally formed?" In fact, the process actually influences how this question will be addressed: the degree to which extra attention may be devoted to some aspects of the clinical picture and not to others.

Suppose, for example, that Patient A's chief concerns are "red eye," "slightly blurred vision," and "some ocular pain." Patient B's chief concern is simply preventive. His parents want to know, "Are his eyes ready for school?" Patient B has no ocular complaints, and his parents have not observed any unusual signs. Suppose further that Patient A's case history reveals that he was treated for keratitis a year ago. Patient B's history is uneventful.

Their visual acuities are found to be different. Patient A's farpoint acuity is 20/40 in each eye. Patient B's farpoint acuity is better than 20/20 in each eye.

How will this affect the assessment of these patient's respective ocular health statuses? It certainly will not give one license, nor would a responsible clinician even think to ignore Patient B's ocular health. A thorough examination of his eyes and adnexa will be conducted, but *not as thorough* as with Patient A, and particularly not when it comes to slit lamp assessment of the corneas.

What does this mean? That clinicians exercise at least two levels of concentration when conducting an examination: one, a standard level; the other, high-intensity and fine-grained. The standard level is characterized by completeness, but no single portion of the eye is studied more completely than is customary, and with good reason. It would be abusive to the patient in many ways; it would be unjustified.

The high-intensity level is employed when a particular problem is suspected. Patient A warrants a high-intensity level of investigation. Patient B does not, at least not on the basis of existing evidence.

The point? Some patients require more in-depth work ups than do other, and the basis for deciding who and when is (a) What is already known about the case? and (b) What questions remain to be answered?

A. INSPECT OCULAR COMPONENTS FOR PATHOLOGY AND STRUCTURAL ABNORMALITIES

The balance of this chapter is organized into twelve sections, each devoted to a major ocular component (see below). An heuristic approach is taken. Within each of these sections, key diagnostic sites and signs are identified—the structural and functional landmarks of that ocular component that the clinician should examine when assessing ocular health. Each of these key diagnostic sites and signs segments is, in turn, organized into three subsections, as follows:

1. The normal clinical picture that should be seen at this site (Prerequisite to being able to identify an abnormal ocular condition is being able to identify a normal condition.)
2. Procedures appropriate for examining this site
3. Potential abnormalities and their possible causes

The twelve major ocular components and their respective diagnostic sites and signs are as follows:

1. The orbit
   a. Relative size, shape, and position of the outer orbital margins
   b. Apparent fit of the globe within the orbit
   c. Physical appearance and relative comfort of the lids and anterior segment of the globe
2. The eyelids
   a. Size and shape of the palpebral fissures
   b. Mobility patterns
   c. Physical appearance of lid tissues
3. The lacrimal system
   a. Appearance and volume of tears accumulated within the palpebral fissure
   b. Appearance and relative tenderness of the tissues in the region of the lacrimal gland
   c. Appearance and relative tenderness of the tissues in the region of the nasolacrimal duct
4. The conjunctiva
   a. Color and transparency
   b. Degree of vascular dilation
5. The cornea
   a. Size and shape
   b. Appearance of the cornea and circumcorneal regions

6. The sclera
   a. Color
   b. Degree of vascular dilation
7. The anterior chamber
   a. Depth
   b. Clarity
8. The iris and pupils
   a. Pigmentation
   b. Anatomical structure/physiological status
   c. Status of adjacent components
9. The crystalline lens
   a. Size
   b. Shape
   c. Position
   d. Transparency
10. The vitreous body
    a. Clarity
11. The fundus
    a. Optic disc
    b. Blood vessels of the fundus
    c. Peripheral (extramacular) fundus
    d. Macula
12. The oculomotor system
    a. Fixation accuracy
    b. Fixation stability
    c. Motilities

□ The Orbit

RELATIVE SIZE, SHAPE, AND POSITION OF THE OUTER ORBITAL MARGINS

Normal Clinical Picture

The shape of the orbit is often compared to a pear or a quadrilateratal pyramid, where the base is directed forward and laterally, and the apex backward, upward, and inward. Fully developed, the orbit is about 45 mm in depth with the apex containing the optic foramen and the superior orbital fissure (2, p. 412).

The orbit of a full-term newborn occupies much more of the face, relatively speaking, than it will when he achieves adulthood. At birth, the height of the outer orbital margin is about half of the baby's total face; at adulthood it will occupy approximately one third of the space (6).

At birth, the outer orbital opening tends to be circular (about 20 mm in diameter) or approximately so; by age 6 years, it is larger and more rectangular (about 30 × 33 mm in the male; slightly smaller in the female), and at adulthood it measures approximately 33 × 40 mm (2, p. 309).

The interorbital distance is usually about 49 mm in the newborn; it will increase to about 64 mm by the time adulthood is reached (6).

In infancy, the orbital margins are quite sharp and are located fairly close to the globe, particularly in the region near the equator of the eye. As the child matures, the margins commence to flatten; they become rolled, losing their sharpness (6).

Examination Procedures

Face the child and compare the two orbital openings for size, shape, and position symmetry. It may be useful to measure these dimensions with a ruler and compare them with the norms cited above, recognizing that there will be normal variance. It may also be useful to compare current measurements to those made at an earlier date, if these are available.

Use your fingertips to probe the orbital margins and the relative snugness of fit between the orbital wall and the globe. Compare the one eye with the other, and both to what you have established, from experience, as normal.

Abnormalities and Their Possible Causes

Developmental Anomalies. As a rule, abnormal size, shape, and/or position of the outer orbital margins stem from an anatomical deviation that is developmentally derived. It suggests that other bone structures of the skull will also display unusual characteristics (7). Some of the more common developmental anomalies of the orbit are discussed below.

Craniostenosis, a deformity of the skull, is caused by premature closure of one or more cranial sutures; it consequently causes a cessation of skull growth. It is often accompanied by exotropia, diplopia, papilledema, optic atrophy, seizures, and mental retardation.

Dysostosis (defective ossification) of cranial bones presents as a combination of cranial and facial abnormalities; e.g., strabismus, exophthalmos, parrot-beaked nose, hypoplastic maxilla. It manifests in Crouzon's disease, Franceschetti's syndrome, and Treacher-Collins syndrome.

When meningoceles and encephaloceles exist, part of the cranial contents protrudes through a defect in the skull. If only the membrane protrudes, it is known as a meningocele; when some of the cerebral substance also protrudes, it is an encephalocele (8).

Oculoauricular dysplasia (Goldenhar's syndrome) includes epibulbar dermoids or fibrodermoids (subconjunctival near the limbus), malformations of the pinna of the ear, and lid coloboma.

Hypotelorism is characterized by an abnormally reduced distance between the two orbits. It occurs in such developmental anomalies as Apert's syndrome, Lowe's syndrome, Conradi's syndrome, cri du chat syndrome, Crouzon's disease, and Hurler's syndrome.

Hypertelorism is characterized by an abnormally increased distance between the two orbits. It occurs in such developmental disorders as ocular-dental-digital dysplasia, trisomy 13-15, Cockayne's syndrome, trisomy 21, and Marchesani's syndrome.

APPARENT FIT OF THE GLOBE WITHIN THE ORBIT

Normal Clinical Picture

There should be space in the orbit for the globe and a variety of other tissue, including fat, connective tissue, muscles, peripheral nerves and ganglia, blood vessels, and glandular tissue. The eye should appear to "fit"; it should not be sunken backward into the orbit (enophthalmos) nor bulge forward (proptosis) (7).

Examination Procedures

Face the child and compare the two palpebral fissures. If one is larger than the other, if more globe is apparent within one fissure than the other, then suspect a proptosis of one eye or enophthalmos of the other. Usually it is not too difficult to make the distinction; select the eye that most nearly approximates a normal appearance and use it as the standard against which to compare the other; also exercise the rule-of-thumb that if sclera is apparent above the cornea when the eye is in its primary position of gaze, suspect proptosis.

Have the patient close his eyes in a normal manner. If one lid fails to cover the globe completely, suspect that eye of proptosis.

While the patient's eyes are closed, place a vertically oriented ruler on the center of the upper and lower orbital margins and note the proximity of the straightedge to the closed lid (8). In most instances, the straightedge will just touch the closed lid. If the lid protrudes so that the straightedge causes an indentation, suspect proptosis. If, instead, there is a significant space between the straightedge and the lid, suspect enophthalmos.

Stand behind and above the patient, so that you can look down on his eyebrows. Elevate the patient's lids so that you can see the two corneal apices from above. They should appear to protrude about equally from the frontal plane of the forehead. Continuing on, slowly tip the patient's head forward and down, observing when the two corneal apices disappear from view. If they are similarly positioned in their respective orbits, they should disappear at the same time (8).

If there appears to be reason, measure the position of each corneal apex in relation to the anterior margin of its respective lateral orbital wall with an exophthalmometer. Consider a between-eye difference of more than 2 mm to be significant (9).

Compare the resilience of the orbital contents of the two eyes by palpation—pressing inward on the closed eyes. The two should be equally (and normally) resistant and the maneuver should not generate pain.

If indicated, make arrangements for visualizing intraorbital tissue, using one or more of the following procedures:

1. A-scan ultrasonography. This procedure provides information about the size of an orbital mass and an indication of tissue type.
2. B-scan ultrasonography. This procedure provides an outline of the shape, and details some of the characteristics, of the orbital contents.
3. Films of the skull (including tomograms). These may reveal defects of the bony orbit and size differences between the two orbits and the two optic canals.

4. Computerized axial tomography. This procedure provides information about the shape and the location of orbital lesions.

5. Orbital venography. Use this procedure to detect changes in the configuration and course of the superior ophthalmic vein (and thereby, perhaps, evidence of a mass lesion in the orbit) by x-ray studies of the orbit after a radiopaque substance has been injected into the frontal vein.

Abnormalities and Their Possible Causes

Proptosis.   When there is no indication of a developmental bone anomaly and/or lid inflammation, the following information is needed to identify cause (9;p.332):

What is the history of the proptosis? What was the age of onset? (Congenital tumors are more likely in younger children.) Has the proptosis developed slowly or rapidly? (Benign tumors usually grow more slowly than malignant tumors.) Does the proptosis vary? (Intermittent conditions might be due to congenital or acquired orbital varices or vascular tumors.) Has there been trauma? (A positive response implies bone fracture.)

What is the child's general health? Exophthalmos may be due to endocrine anomaly; e.g., Graves' diseases. (Look for *Graefe's sign:* upper lid lags behind globe on downgaze; *Dalrymple's sign:* upper lid retracted to the extent that sclera is visible above the cornea; *Stellwag's sign:* decreased and incomplete blinking—"lid stare"; *Mobius sign:* decreased ability to keep the eyeballs converged due to insufficiency of the internal recti muscles; *Rosenbach's sign:* inability to close the eyes immediately upon command, closed lids are tremulous; *Gifford's sign:* difficult to evert upper lid; *Joffroy's sign:* absence of forehead wrinkling when eyes are suddenly turned upward.)

Is the condition monocular or binocular? Monocular conditions are less likely to stem from systemic involvements. One of the most common causes of unilateral proptosis is dermoid cyst.

What is the direction of displacement? A straight-ahead displacement suggests a mass within the muscle cone; e.g., a hematoma, a hemangioma, or glioma of the optic nerve. An eccentric displacement indicates a major orbital mass outside the muscle cone, located opposite to the direction of the displacement (10).

What is the result of palpation? Hard masses tend to be malignant and inflammatory. If highly sensitive to touch, suspect a fracture or a neoplasm involving the infraorbital canal.

Is vision affected? Gliomas of optic nerve affect vision rapidly. Tumors near the optic nerve may exert sufficient pressure to produce field changes and optic atrophy. Mechanical obstruction of circulation can result in retinal hemorrhage or edema. Changes in the axial length of the globe will alter refractive status.

Are ocular motilities affected? Reduced motilities suggest pressure on, or invasion of, muscles or motor nerves.

Are there changes in the fundus? Optic nerve pallor, papilledema, venous congestion, and retinal striae in the region of the posterior pole are all indicative of a proximal intruding mass (11).

Enophthalmos.   This condition indicates an increase in the available orbital volume; it may be due to any of the following:

1. an orbital bone fracture; this should be accompanied by (visible and/or reported) evidence of trauma
2. a decrease in volume or orbital soft tissue, such as from fibrosis or atrophy that is related to an inflammatory disease of the orbit.
3. Horner's syndrome (sympathetic dysfunction); usually unilateral, it includes miosis, ptosis, and enophthalmos; also heterochromia if the onset occurred in infancy.

PHYSICAL APPEARANCE AND RELATIVE COMFORT OF THE LIDS AND ANTERIOR SEGMENT OF THE GLOBE

Normal Clinical Picture
The eyelids should be free of redness, edema, echymosis, and tenderness to touch.

Examination Procedures
Inspect lids and anterior segment with the naked eye, with a hand-held magnifier, and/or with a slit lamp.

Abnormalities and Their Possible Causes
Inflamed eyelids might be a consequence of inflamed orbit. Etiology typically is one of the following:

1. Reactive edema of the orbit resulting from an inflammation in a neighboring region (e.g., sinusitis, dacryocystitis, chalazion);
2. Direct infection of the orbit (e.g., from a penetration wound);
3. Infection in the orbit arising from surrounding tissue (e.g., ethmoidal sinusitis, abscessed tooth, lacrimal sac infection, cavernous sinus thrombosis).

□ The Eyelids

SIZE AND SHAPE OF PALPEBRAL FISSURES

Normal Clinical Picture
Width.   The horizontal dimension of the palpebral aperture of the average male newborn is 18 mm; in females, about 16 mm. By age four, it will have grown to 23 mm in the male and 21 mm in the female; by age 12, to about 27 mm, and ultimately to almost 30 mm.

Height.   The average vertical dimension of the palpebral opening of the neonate is about 9 mm. This does not increase very much as the child grows: about 1 mm, with the height-to-width ratio gradually changing from 1:2 to 1:3. The upper lid margins should cover about 1 to 1.5 mm of the upper limbus when the eye is in the primary position of gaze; anything in excess of that signals a possible ptosis; if sclera is visible above cornea, suspect lid retraction.

Symmetry. The two apertures should not differ more than 0.5 mm in the vertical dimension.

Examination Procedures

Compare one eye to the other, and both to normative data. Measure with a ruler where indicated.

Assess levator function: Hold the patient's head firmly against a headrest by placing your hand on her brow so as to inhibit frontalis muscle action. Ask the patient to look down, then up. Compare the upper lid movements of the two eyes as she does this. Normally, both upper lids will move upward a distance of from 12 to 17 mm. In congenital ptosis, there is almost always dystrophic changes in the levator aponeurosis; i.e., there will be reduced levator function on upgaze and a shortened upper lid on downgaze (12).

Abnormalities and Their Possible Causes (12)

Blepharoptosis. There are many varieties of ptosis and many etiologies. In some instances, the ptosis is an isolated phenomenon that has a slight effect on the patient's appearance but nothing else. At the other end of the spectrum, ptosis may signal an active neurological disease that requires immediate attention. Therefore, having identified a ptosis, the optometrist must then attempt to differentiate among the possible origins of the condition, commencing by addressing the question: congenital or acquired? The following information will aid in determining this:

What is the history of the condition? What was the age of onset? (Infant photographs may be informative.) Was there trauma? (A positive response implies that the condition was acquired.)

What is the child's general health? Acquired ptosis is often associated with sympathetic dysfunction (e.g., Horner's syndrome) and tumors affecting the hypothalmic region, medulla, or spinal cord.

Does it vary? Ptosis that varies is apt to be caused by a myoneural transmission defect, such as in myasthenia gravis. It tends to look worse when the patient is fatigued and improves when he is rested, or after the administration of a cholinesterase inhibitor, such as Prostigmin. In addition, the patient has difficulty in sustaining lid elevation in upgaze and often manifests a lid twitch sign—a momentary upward twitch or overshoot when bringing the eyes from downgaze to the primary position (12).

Is the condition unilateral or bilateral? Congenital ptosis is usually bilateral; acquired ptosis tends to be unilateral. (Marcus Gunn's, or jaw-winking, syndrome is a notable exception.)

Are extraocular muscle functions impaired? Congenital ptosis is often accompanied by paralysis of the superior rectus or all the muscles supplied by the III nerve.

Is levator function impaired? Reduced levator function suggests that ptosis is congenital; see Examination Procedures section, above.

Are there any other hereditary defects? When ptosis is inherited, it usually presents with other hereditary defects, such as epicanthus and blepharophimosis.

Often, the final diagnosis of a congenital ptosis is made by the process of elimination. If the ptosis was apparent very early in the child's life, and if there is no reason to suspect a familial or genetic disorder, birth trauma, or significant illness during infancy, then the logical conclusion is that the condition is idiopathic and congenital.

Lid Retraction. The first goal is to differentiate between a physiological and pathological condition.

Newborns normally exhibit lid retraction.

Beyond infancy, the phenomenon, if manifested, is usually temporary and voluntary, such as when the child is exaggerating attentiveness or surprise.

Pathological causes include the following:

Congestive dysthyroid disease or excessive stimulation of levator muscles from nerve fibers of the superior rectus; lid retraction is apparent only with upward eye movement.

Noncongestive type of dysthyroid exophthalmos (as in Graefe's sign), or an aberrant regeneration of III nerve of the inferior rectus to the levator, where the lid retracts only when the eye moves downward.

Duane's retraction syndrome or an underacting lateral rectus muscle that spills over to the levator; manifests only when abduction is attempted.

Supranuclear lesions (e.g., tumors on midbrain, hydrocephalus, syphilis).

Neuromuscular diseases (e.g., peripheral VII nerve paresis with loss of obicularis oculi muscle tone).

Epicanthus. Epicanthus may be due to one of the following:

1. Immaturity, in which event it will disappear by the time the child reaches his sixth or seventh birthday.
2. Inherited racial characteristic.
3. Genetic abnormality. This, chiefly among whites. Often it is one of the signs of a developmental anomaly syndrome.

Other Eyelid Size/Shape Deviations. Although typically congenital, these may be of genetic origin and include the following:

1. Inverse epicanthus. Often accompanied by blepharophimosis and ptosis.
2. Epiblepharon. A condition in which a fold of skin stretches along the border of the lower lid and presses the lashes against the globe. Usually genetic.
3. Oblique lid fissures. May present as a mongoloid or an antimongoloid slant. Usually genetic.
4. Ectropion/entropion. May be congenital or acquired.
5. Anklyoblepharon. Adhesion of the margins of the upper and lower lids by filamentous bands. Usually congenital.
6. Blepharophimosis. Abnormal narrowness of the palpebral fissures in the horizontal direction, caused by lateral displacement of the inner canthi.
7. Symblepharon. An adhesion between the tarsal conjunctiva and the bulbar conjunctiva. Usually due to burns, trauma, diphtheria, trachoma.
8. Coloboma. May be congenital or acquired.

MOBILITY PATTERNS

Normal Clinical Picture
Blinking Rate.   Under normal circumstances, a child will blink involuntarily between two to seven times per minute. A significant increase or decrease in blink rate that appears to be independent of a local, temporary factor is worthy of attention.

Lid-globe Movements.   The lids and the globe should move in harmony in the vertical axis. Horizontal movements of the eyes should elicit no changes in lid elevation.

Lid Closure.   The globes should be completely covered by the lids when the eyes are closed.

Examination Procedures
Engage the patient in conversation and count her blinks. Also keep a lookout for involuntary tics and lid spasms. Have the patient shift her gaze from straight ahead, to up, to down, to the right, etc. Be alert for signs of unusual lid reponses. Ask the patient to close her eyes in a normal fashion, as if going to sleep. Take note of the completeness of the lid closure.

Abnormalities and Their Possible Causes (12)
Lid Spasms.   The patient may present with a myoclonic tic (intermittent) or a reflex blepharospasm (continuous). In both instances, the observed behavior is a spasmodic, uncontrolled closure of the lids, which may be due to a cramp of the obicularis oculi muscle, psychological factors, pain, photophobia, or may be idiopathic.

Inability to Close Eyelids Voluntarily.   This is typically caused by paralysis of the obicularis oculi muscle, stemming from birth injury, congenital factors, or a myogenic/neurogenic disease.

Lid Lag.   May be neuorgenic, neuromuscular, or myopathic.

Lagophthalmos.   May be due to facial nerve paralysis or congenital anatomical anomaly.

PHYSICAL APPEARANCE OF LID TISSUES (11)

Normal Clinical Picture
Tissues should be free of inflammation, edema, echymosis, lesions, and growths.

Examination Procedures
Conduct a direct inspection with a hand-held magnifier and/or a slit lamp.

Abnormalities and Their Possible Causes
Hyperemia.   There are two general classifications: active hyperemia and passive hyperemia. The latter is characterized by a less acute, less red appearance. Active hyperemia is usually accompanied by a localized lesion, such as a stye, chalazion, furuncle, erysipelas, etc. Passive hyperemia is ordinarily associated with systemic or adnexal diseases.

Puffy (edematous) Eyelids.   The patient may present with or without signs of inflammation. Most often, both lids appear to be swollen, but not to the point where lid mobility is significantly impaired.
   Edematous eyelids may stem from general systemic involvements (e.g., allergy), localized conditions (e.g., antigenic, foreign protein such as parasites), or congenital anomalies (13).

Unusual Pigmentation.   The patient may present with hyperpigmentation or hypopigmentation; either condition may be limited and circumscribed, or pervasive. If hypopigmentation exists, look for indications of associated albinism (inherited) and vitiligo (acquired). If hyperpigmentation is present, attempt to differentiate between the following:

Congenital melanosis (usually associated with endocrine dysfunction)

Acanthosis nigricans; caused by endocrine dysfunction; presents as gray-black discoloration along skin folds and the neck as well as lids and eyebrows.

Peutz-Jeghers syndrome (freckles on the face, lids, extremities, and around the mouth, typically connected with a genetic disorder)

Nevus of Ota (an inherited blue-gray melanosis in the area of the first and second trigeminal nerve branches, including the skin, sclera, iris, uvea, conjunctiva, and even the optic disc)

Xanthelasma.   The most common form of xanthoma is xanthelasma (lipid deposits), characterized by soft yellowish spots or plaques on the eyelids. It may signal hyperlipemia, but it also may be idiopathic or familial.

Edema.   Typically, edema derives from general or local disease.

Hemorrhage.   Hemorrhage may occur as a small ecchymosis. If large, it may spread across the bridge of the nose into the opposite lid and even into the orbit or the adjacent tissue of the face. It may be caused by trauma or blood dyscrasias (e.g., leukemia, purpura).

Emphysema.   This is a pathological accumulation of air in the lid tissue, usually due to trauma in the orbital region, combined with nose blowing that forces air into lid tissue.

Eczema.   Eczema is characterized by red skin with superimposed vesicles, cracks, and excoriations. The vesicles may develop into pustules or break and leave raw, bleeding, or weeping surfaces. This condition may be caused by toxin-producing infectious agents of the conjunctiva; e.g., staphylococci. It is sometimes evoked by contact sensitivity-producing agents such as certain antibiotics, cosmetics, and food.

Impetigo.   This is a contagious, pyogenic infection of the skin. Lesions are characterized by thin-walled vesicles, bullae, or pustules, which, upon rupture, form superficial crusts. The condition is often caused by streptococcus or staphylococcus aureus.

Furuncle.   A furuncle is a painful nodule, formed in the skin by circumscribed inflammation of the corium and subcutaneous tissue, enclosed in a central "slough" or core. It can be attributed to staphylococci that enter the skin through the hair follicles.

Erysipelas.   This acute infection of the skin is characterized by a precisely demarcated red lesion accompanied by malaise and fever and, in most cases, conjunctival infection. It is caused by hemolytic streptococci.

Molluscum Contagiosum.   This condition is characterized by a mildly infectious papillomatous lesion of the skin. The papule is usually about 2 to 3 mm in diameter with an umbilicated surface. The condition is caused by virus.

Cysts.   These are very tiny, transparent blebs that are typically situated close to the lid margins, behind the lashes. Cysts are caused by occlusion of the ducts in the glands of Moll, or of the mouth of the meibomian gland.

Hordeolum.   This is found at the lid margin. A localized, pyogenic inflammation with abscess formation in a gland of Zeis, it is usually called a stye. The hordeolum is frequently the outcome of a staphylococcus infection. It may also be caused by any factor responsible for generating hyperemia of the lid margin, or any condition that produces general debility, such as anemia or diabetes (14).

Meibomianitis.   Meibomianitis is an acute or chronic staphylococcus infection of the meibomian glands. If acute, the patient complains of pain in the lid and tenderness over part of the lid. Upon everting the lid, a yellow line is seen extending vertically across the tarsus. If the infection is chronic, a low-grade inflammation of most of the meibomian glands exists. No pain, but some sandy sensation in the eyes is experienced, usually accompanied by chronic conjunctivitis.

Neoplasms.   These may present as basal cell epithelioma. They may be no different in color from the surrounding area, or they may be red, circumscribed, lobulated growths involving the lid margin, or they may have an umbilicated center.

Chronic Blepharitis.   This condition may present as any of the following:

1. *Seborrheic:* lid margin covered with small white or gray scales; aggravated by chemical fumes, smoke, and fog. Tends to be associated with seborrheic dermatitis of the scalp.
2. *Ulcerative-suppurative:* inflammation of the follicles of the lashes and associated glands of Zeis and Moll. Usually caused by staphylococcus or herpes simplex.
3. *Angular:* inflammation of the angles of the lids. Usually associated with angular conjunctivitis, it may also be caused by mites or pubic lice.

Poliosis.   Poliosis is evidenced by whitening of the hair of the eyebrows and eyelashes. It is associated with albinism and vitiligo.

Trichomegaly.   Trichomegaly, or unusually long lashes, may reflect a familial trait or may be a sign of a severe congenital anomaly; e.g., Rubinstein-Taybi syndrome.

Madarosis.   The loss of eyelashes, this condition may reflect local inflammation or infection, or it may be related to some pervasive systemic condition, such as chronic dermatitis, endocrine disease, or sickle-cell anemia.

Distichiasis.   The presence of an extra row of lashes growing from openings of the meibomian gland, or distichiasis, is usually attributed to heredity.

Coarse Eyebrows.   This sign is encountered in a number of congenital anomalies, including Hurler's and Rubinstein-Taybi syndromes. However, it may simply be a normal variation.

Synophrys.   Confluent eyebrows that extend to the midline may be a normal variation or a sign of one of a number of syndromes resulting from a significant congenital anomaly; e.g., Waardenburg's syndrome, trisomy 13 syndrome.

□ The Lacrimal System

APPEARANCE AND VOLUME OF TEARS ACCUMULATED WITHIN THE PALPEBRAL FISSURE

Normal Clinical Picture

The lacrimal system is not fully developed at birth. The lacrimal gland will continue to grow and develop until the child is about 3 to 4 years old.

The nasolacrimal duct is usually functional at the time of birth. Sometimes, however, a membrane separates the lower end of the nasolacrimal duct from the nasal mucosa for the first month or two following birth, thus preventing canalization. Once lysis occurs, effective tear drainage is possible (15,16).

The lacrimal lake should be comfortably full at all times; there should always be enough tear fluid accumulated within the palpebral fissure to meet ocular needs, but not so much that it overflows onto the cheeks.

The tears should be free of foreign matter.

There are two types of weeping: reflex and psychic. Each is stimulated in different ways. *Reflex weeping* is generated by environmental irritants: foreign matter coming into contact with the eye, cold air, wind, trauma, and corneal and conjunctival inflammations. It is usually observed during the first week or so after birth. *Psychic* weeping is typically the outcome of pain and/or emotion. It is always bilateral and is rarely observed in children younger than 2 months.

Examination Procedures

Perform direct visual inspection with good illumination and magnification. (For signs of foreign matter, look particularly at the corneal epithelium and the lid margins.)

Abnormalities and Their Possible Causes

Epiphora.   An abnormal overflow of tears, epiphora can be caused by a hypersecretion of tears or a dysfunction of the drainage system. To differentiate, instill one drop of 2% fluorescein solution and have the patient keep her eyes open (in normal manner) for about 1 minute. Adequate draining is demonstrated if the fluorescein is no longer apparent in the palpebral fissure and/or if there is evidence of fluorescein in the nose. Obviously, if drainage is adequate, the epiphora must be attributed to hypersecretion of tears rather than to inadequate drainage.

Hypersecretion.   This condition can be *primary*, due to disturbance of the lacrimal gland itself; *central or psychic*, stemming from pain or hysteria; or *neurogenic*, provoked by cold, wind, conjunctivitis, ametropia, glaucoma, Horner's syndrome, etc.

Hyposecretion.   Dry eye is caused by local tissue changes (e.g., keratitis, conjunctivitis). To document hyposecretion, use the Schirmer test (17, p. 175):

1. Instill one drop of topical anesthetic in each eye.
2. Place a strip of filter paper over the lateral third of the lower lid margin and allow it to remain there for 5 minutes.
3. Less than 10 mm of moistened filter paper within the five minute period is presumptive evidence of hyposecretion.

Inadequate Lacrimal Drainage. This condition may be caused by any of the following:

1. Congenital anomalies of the lacrimal apparatus (e.g., unformed puncta, obstruction of the canaliculi)
2. Dacryocystitis
3. Eversion of lower lacrimal punctum due to ectropion, tumor obstruction, drugs

Bloody Tears. These may be caused by conjunctival fibroma, malignant melanoma, hemophilia, pannus, and other vascular complications.

APPEARANCE AND RELATIVE TENDERNESS OF THE TISSUES IN THE REGION OF THE LACRIMAL GLAND

Normal Clinical Picture
There should be no evidence of pain, tenderness, or swelling beneath the upper temporal margin of the orbit.

Examination Procedures
Visually inspect and palpate the tissues in the region of the lacrimal gland.

Abnormalities and Their Possible Causes (11,12,15,16)
Dacryoadenitis. This condition may be acute or chronic. In rare instances of acute dacryoadenitis, a catarrhal inflammation of the lacrimal gland exists; it is caused by systemic disease; e.g., mumps, measles, influenza, scarlet fever, erysipelas, typhoid fever.

Chronic dacryoadenitis is characterized by proliferative inflammation of the lacrimal gland; it may be caused by a specific granulomatous disease; e.g., Mikulicz's syndrome, Heerfordt's disease, syphilis, pseudotumor, Boeck's sarcoid.

Enlargement of Lacrimal Gland. The enlargement may be painless or painful. If painless, suspect leukemia or mumps. If painful, consider lymphomatous disease, an orbital pseudotumor, or a lacrimal gland neoplasm.

APPEARANCE AND RELATIVE TENDERNESS OF THE TISSUES IN THE REGION OF THE NASOLACRIMAL DUCT

Normal Clinical Picture
Normally, there is evidence of pain, redness, induration, or swelling of the tissues in the medial portion of the lower lid and sides of the nose. The regional lymph

nodes are neither palpable nor tender. There is no evidence of mucous in the conjunctival sac.

Examination Procedures
Visually inspect the region and palpate. Exert pressure over the region of the sac and watch puncta for regurgitation of mucopurulent material.

Abnormalities and Their Possible Causes (11,12,15,16)
Dacryocystitis. An inflammation of the lacrimal sac and surrounding tissues, dacryocystitis may be acute or chronic.

If acute, it is accompanied by pain, tenderness, induration, and swelling of the tissues of the medial portion of the lower lid and side of the nose. Regional lymph nodes are usually palpable and tender. Generally, it is caused by an infection (staphylococcus, pneumococcus, streptococcus) that stems from a congenital obstruction of the nasolacrimal duct.

If chronic, the inflammation is accompanied by epiphora and regurgitation of mucous into the conjunctival sac, chronic conjunctivitis, and some swelling. It is usually due to infection.

☐ The Conjunctiva

COLOR AND TRANSPARENCY

Normal Clinical Picture
The conjunctiva should appear as a thin, transparent, colorless mucous membrane. The conjunctiva varies in thickness. It is thickest (and looser fitting) in the fornices, somewhat thinner (and tightly fitting to the underlying tarsal plate) in the palpebral zone, and thinnest (and most transparent) in the bulbar region (18).

Examination Procedures
Visually inspect the conjunctiva, including a slit lamp examination. Review the patient's history for evidence regarding systemic involvements and localized trauma.

Abnormalities and Their Possible Causes (11,12,18)
Subconjunctival Hemorrhage. This may be idiopathic or due to trauma, sudden violent cough, strain, or blood disease.

Chemosis of Conjunctiva. Chemosis may be associated with eyelid edema and/or caused by any condition that impairs lymph or blood circulation, including such general conditions as Grave's disease.

Benign Tumors. There are a number of different types, including the following:

1. *Nevi:* slightly elevated lesions; usually salmon color, but may be deep brown.
2. *Dermoid cysts* and *dermolipoma:* elevated, smooth, round, often straddle the limbus in the upper, outer quadrant.

3. *Hemangioma:* congregation of dilated blood vessels; may or may not be elevated.

4. *Pterygium:* connective tissue overgrowth; triangular shaped, usually located in the exposed portion of the bulbar conjunctiva with the apex of the thickened mass pointing to, and sometimes advancing on, the cornea.

Spots. These may manifest as any of the following:

1. *Nevi:* pink to brown.
2. *Pinguecula:* elastic and hyaline degenerative changes of the cornea that manifests as a yellowish-white, slightly elevated, benign lesion on the bulbar conjunctiva.
3. *Pigmentations:* yellow (may stem from bilirubinemia, picric acid, leptospirosis, brucellosis); gray-black (argyrosis); brown (conjunctival melanosis, ocular melanocytosis—nevus of Ota).
4. *Lithiasis:* yellow spots (conjunctival secretions) on the palpebral conjunctiva produced by degenerative changes in the glands of Henle.

DEGREE OF VASCULAR DILATION

Normal Clinical Picture
The conjunctiva is richly vascularized, connecting with the circulatory subsystems of the ciliary body and iris. Ordinarily, however, few of these vessels are apparent. (The picture changes with the onset of disease. Then, hyperemia, discharge, and edema occur in varying degrees) (19) (20, p. 256)

Examination Procedures
The following steps are advised:

1. Visually inspect the conjunctiva, with and without a slit lamp.
2. Use fluorescein staining of the conjunctiva to rule out presence of a foreign body; look for denuded conjunctival epithelium.
3. Investigate the lacrimal drainage system to rule out obstruction of the canaliculus or lacrimal punctum.
4. Rule out glaucoma: measure intraocular pressure, assess size and luster of cornea.
5. Review the case history for evidence of acuity variations, discharge, systemic diseases, seasonal variations, sensitivity to allergens.

Abnormalities and Their Possible Causes
Hyperemia. Hyperemia is evidenced by diffuse redness of the conjunctiva; injection is most intense at the periphery of the bulbar conjunctiva and in the fornix. Vessels appear bright red. There may be some petechial hemorrhages. The patient generally feels irritation, itching, foreign body sensation. May be acute, chronic, recurring. Hyperemia can be due to environmental irritants (e.g., fumes, wind, bright light), ametropia, allergies.

Deep Ciliary Injection of Conjunctiva. Redness is most intense at limbus. Darker red conjunctiva moves easily over limbal vessels and may affect visual acuity. This condition is usually caused by corneal or anterior segment inflammation.

Conjunctivitis. Superficial conjunctival hyperemia is evidenced by redness that is deepest in the fornix, least at the limbus; it may invade the cornea and anterior chamber. Conjunctivitis is accompanied by chemosis, dull pain, exudation of cells and fluid ("sticky lids" after sleeping), and foreign body sensation. It may be infectious or noninfectious, acute or chronic. Possible causes include staphylococcus, streptococcus, gonococcus, virus, allergens, mechanical and chemical trauma.

☐ The Cornea

SIZE AND SHAPE

Normal Clinical Picture
Embryologically, the structure of the cornea is established in the fetus by the third month of gestation. The only significant changes that occur from that time are in corneal size and shape (6).

At birth, the average cornea measures about 10 mm in diameter. By age 1 year, it will have achieved almost fullgrown status: about 11 mm in the vertical dimension and 12 mm in the horizontal (2, p. 306).

The shape of the cornea changes also. It is reported to be relatively spherical at birth, tending to become less so as the child grows, but not to any remarkable degree. It is also flatter at birth than it will be a year or two later, particularly in the central region (2, pp. 306-307). (Note: We recognize that this appears to conflict with what has been reported regarding the prevalence of astigmatism in young children; see Chapter 5. We have no explanation for this paradox.)

The cornea of the newborn is slightly thinner (average thickness, 0.8 mm) than it will be when the child achieves full-growth status (average thickness, 0.9 mm) (2).

Examination Procedures
Visually inspect the cornea. Measure its horizontal diameter. (The corneal-scleral junction is more clearly defined in this region than in the vertical zones.) Also, inspect the curvature of the cornea in profile.

Use the placido disc, the illuminated keratoscope (see Figure 4.2), or the ophthalmometer to obtain direct evidence about the front surface of the cornea (21).

Abnormalities and Their Possible Causes (11,12,22,23,24)
Megalocornea (or macrocornea). This is a developmental anomaly characterized by unusually large (bilateral) corneas—diameter greater than 13 mm at birth, sometimes reaching an ultimate diameter of 18 mm. Normal intraocular pressure,

limbus, anterior chamber angle and pupil exist. The condition is congenital and is probably inherited.

Buphthalmos (or hydrophthalmos).   This is a form of glaucoma characterized by marked enlargement and distension of the fibrous coats of the eye. Corneal diameter is greater than 13 mm. Buphthalmos is usually congenital.

Microcornea.   This is a (usually bilateral) developmental anomaly in which the corneas are exceptionally small (less than 11 mm at age one year). Microcornea is due to an arrest of prenatal development; it may be associated with other ocular abnormalities, such as microphthalmia, hydrophthalmia, multiple defects of the anterior chamber, cataract, and glaucoma. The condition is inherited.

Keratoconus.   This condition does not ordinarily manifest in young (prepuberty-aged) children. It appears to be inherited, but it also has been associated with corneal dystrophies, glaucoma, and aniridia. It occurs in about 6 percent of Down's syndrome cases and in some cases of Marfan's syndrome.

Keratoglobus.   A bulging forward of the entire cornea, this condition is accompanied by a marked thinning of the stroma. Globe size and intraocular pressure remain normal. It is presumably a genetic anomaly.

APPEARANCE OF THE CORNEA AND CIRCUMCORNEAL REGIONS

Normal Clinical Picture
The cornea is an avascular continuation of the conjunctiva and sclera. Its epithelial layer links with the epithelial layer of the conjunctiva; its stromal layer with the sclera.

A normal cornea is pain-free, shiny, and transparent, except perhaps in infants younger than 1 week of age; the corneas of a newborn may be slightly hazy (22).

Examination procedures
Visually inspect the cornea and circumcorneal regions, paying special attention to the following:

1. *The circumcorneal areas and related symptoms.* The cornea's vascular needs are furnished by subconjunctival and scleral vessels that also supply the ciliary body and iris. Hence, long-term corneal lesions are usually accompanied by circumcorneal injection and photophobia.

2. *The nature of corneal reflections.* This provides clues about the status of the various corneal layers and, if a lesion does exist, to the nature of that lesion. To assess, project a light pattern onto the front surface of the cornea.

Also conduct slit-lamp examination of the corneal tissue, including the use of fluorescein to stain possible breaks in epithelium.

Abnormalities and Their Possible Causes (11,12,23)
Congenital Opacities.   These have well-defined borders with no indication of active inflammation; they may be of developmental or inflammatory origin. If the origin is *developmental* the opacities may be associated with leukomas, melanosis corneae, Krukenberg's spindles, and embryotoxon; i.e., arcus juvenilis. If the origin is *inflammatory*, the opacities are generally due to intrauterine infection of the cornea, usually caused by virus or syphilis.

Active Corneal Inflammation.   This will vary from superficial to deep and present in a variety of clinical pictures, depending on etiology.
    Possible causes (22,23,24) include bacterial or viral infection; trauma followed by contaminating agents; and herpes simplex.

□ The Sclera

COLOR

Normal Clinical Picture
The neonate's sclera, composed of dense, whitish bands of collagen, is thinner than it will be a few months later. (Full-grown thickness is about 1 mm at the posterior pole, 0.5 mm at the equator, and 0.9 mm at the limbus.) As a result, the infant's sclera is more translucent than the sclera of an older child. This allows the underlying uveal melanin to be more visible, thereby giving the sclera a bluish cast.
    During the first postnatal year, the scleral fibers thicken, the sclera becomes whiter and more opaque, with discoloration being evident in the normal eye only at those sites where the blood vessels and nerves surface: about 6 mm or so from the limbus. At these points, uveal (bluish-brown) pigment collars may be noted, especially in darker-pigmented children.

Examination Procedures
Direct inspection with the naked eye, hand-held magnifier, and/or slit lamp is sufficient.

Abnormalities and Their Possible Causes (11,12)
Scleral Melanosis.   This condition is evidenced by brown, irregular patches of pigment that may remain unchanged over long periods of time or may become larger. Scleral melanosis is usually attributable to heredity.

Blue Sclera.   Scleral tissue takes on an overall blue cast. This has been attributed to colloidal chemical changes rather than to a thinning of tissue, and it has been explained as stemming from an embryonic arrest in the development of scleral collagen fibers.
    Blue sclera is probably due to heredity. It appears in a variety of syndromes; e.g., Crouzon's, Albright's hereditary osteodystrophy.

Ectasia. This localized thinning of the sclera may be caused by high myopia, inflammation, glaucoma, or trauma.

DEGREE OF VASCULAR DILATION

Normal Clinical Picture
Ordinarily, there is very little vascularization apparent in the sclera despite the fact that it is richly supplied. The scleral coat should appear to glisten, be free of hyperemia and edema, and display no extra-thin or extra-thick areas (22).

Examination Procedures
Perform direct inspection with the naked eye and/or the slit lamp.

Abnormalities and Their Possible Causes (22)
Episcleritis. Episcleritis produces pain, sensitivity to pressure, and localized inflammation. It is mildly recurrent, but it typically heals completely within a few weeks. The engorged blood vessels are deeper than in conjuctivitis. Episcleritis is caused by allergy, toxin, infection, etc. Sometimes it is associated with leptosperosis and Reiter's syndrome.

Scleritis. This condition is characterized by diffuse inflammation involving *all* visible sclera. Deep ciliary injection often lasts for months and heals as a slate gray, transparent, sometimes thin ectatic staphyloma or scar. It is often associated with peripheral choroiditis, iridocyclitis, and secondary glaucoma. Scleritis may be caused by syphilis, erythema nodosum, and rheumatoid disorders.

□ The Anterior Chamber

DEPTH

Normal Clinical Picture
At birth, the anterior chamber is relatively deep—about 3.5 mm. As the lens grows and the cornea flattens, it becomes a bit shallower, ultimately achieving a depth of about 3 mm.

The aqueous drainage channel is usually operational by the time of birth, when little or no connective tissue remains and the aqueous can move readily to Schlemm's canal (2).

Examination Procedures
The following procedures are recommended:

1. Penlight method. Hold a penlight at the temporal side of the eye, directing the beam across the plane of the iris. If the chamber is shallow, a portion of the iris (nasal) is apt to remain unlighted—in a shadow.
2. Slit-lamp method for grading angle width (25).
3. Gonioscopy.

Abnormalities and Their Possible Causes (11,12)
Unusually Shallow Chamber.   Possible causes include angle closure glaucoma, lenticular swelling, anterior luxation or subluxation of the lens, and choroidal detachment.

Unusually Deep Chamber.   This may be caused by posterior subluxation of the lens, aphakia, iridocyclitis, or choroidal detachment.

CLARITY

Normal Clinical Picture.
The aqueous fluid should be completely clear: transparent and free of foreign matter (2).

Examination Procedures
Visually inspect the chamber with the naked eye, a hand-held magnifier, an ophthalmoscope, or a slit lamp.

Abnormalities and Their Possible Causes
Cell-free Opalescence.   This condition occurs with iritis, after blunt trauma, and/ or with vitreous loss.

Opalescence with Cells, Leucocytes, Lymphocytes, Macrophages, etc.   A possible cause is fibrinous iritis.

Hypopyon.   This is probably due to ulcus serpens, hypopyon iritis, and endophthalmitis.

Hyphema.   The possible causes of hyphema include trauma, rubeosis iridis, and hemorrhagic glaucoma. Spontaneous anterior chamber hemorrhage in children occurs with juvenile xanthogranulomatosis, leukemia, and retinoblastoma.

Tumor Cells.   Possible causes include retinoblastoma, metastatic carcinoma, and lymphosarcoma. Tumor cells may be associated with pseudouveitis and hypopyon formation.

☐ The Iris and Pupils

PIGMENTATION

Normal Clinical Picture
Iris color is inherited in Mendelian fashion; brown is dominant to blue; blue is recessive.
   The iris of a white newborn is likely to be blue because the stroma contains very little pigment at this early stage of life. However, the condition changes

during the first six months. Pigment is formed and the color of the iris deepens, with the irides that are eventually going to be brown changing from dark blue to greenish-blue, to greenish-gray, to greenish-brown, en route (27).

Ordinarily, of course, both eyes display and the same color patterns. About half of all white people have pigment flecks—benign melanomas—on the surface of the iris.

Examination Procedures
Visually inspect the iris and pupils.

Abnormalities and Their Possible Causes (11,12,26)
Albinism. Total lack of pigment—complete albinism—is rare. In the case of incomplete albinism, the irides are blue or yellowish green, the fundus is lightly pigmented, and there often is hypoplasia of the macula.

Albinism is inherited and presents in a number os syndromes; e.g., Chediak-Higashi; Waardenburg's.

Heterochromia. This phenomenon presents in the following two forms:

1. *Heterochromia simplex* (hypochromia): an abnormal eye with an iris that is a lighter color than the partner (normal) eye. Possible causes include sympathetic damage in infancy (e.g., Horner's syndrome) and heredity.

2. *Hyperchromic heterochromia:* an abnormal eye with an iris that is a darker color than that of the partner (normal) eye. It is usually accompanied by a hyperplastic iris. Possible causes include congenital tumors and trauma (e.g., retention of an intraocular iron foreign body—siderosis).

Pigmented Lesions. These may be benign or malignant. The latter often originate from a benign melanoma. Malignant melanomas are progressive, and they will extend into the filtration angle. They typically have blood vessels, and the pupil may be distorted.

ANATOMICAL STRUCTURE/PHYSIOLOGICAL STATUS

Normal Clinical Picture (2,6)
The irides should be structurally intact, symmetrical, and free of extra tissue. The circumcornal zone should appear whitish, nonedematous, and free of hypervascularization. The anterior chamber should be clear and transparent. The pupils should display normal size, location, and reflexes.

The neonate's pupils are small, about 2 mm in diameter under "average" room illumination. They do not ordinarily achieve adult size (about 3.5 to 4 mm) until the child is about 6 months old, this occurring when the dilator muscles of the iris begin to equal the sphincter muscles in strength and efficiency. It is not unusual for the neonate's pupils to be unequal in size. In some children, this condition may persist up to about the age of 3 years.

Examination Procedures

Direct visual inspection with naked eye and slit lamp is recommended. Furthermore, light reflexes should be tested. The two light reflexes, the direct and the consensual, test the anterior arc. A light shone in one eye should produce equal constriction of both pupils. This is evidence that the optic tract is functioning on the side being tested, and that the pupillomotor fibers of both eyes are functioning. If neither eye responds, it is likely that the eye being stimulated does not see. This is confirmed if stimulating the opposite eye causes binocular pupil constriction (6) (see amaurotic pupil, below).

Near reflex is not a true reflex. Rather, it is an associated movement, a synkenesis. The III nerve innervates the medial rectus muscle, the ciliary muscle, and the sphincter pupillae. It is not surprising, therefore, that shifting fixation from distance to near stimulates not only accommodation and convergence, but also pupil constriction.

The swinging light routine (17,29) is achieved by following the procedure described above for testing the light reflexes, but by doing it more rapidly. That is, move the light stimulus back and forth, from one eye to the other, fairly quickly and rhythmically. Observe reactions of both pupils. A normal response is constriction of both pupils. An unexpected response—but one that the test is designed to identify—is a paradoxical reaction in one pupil: it appears to constrict when the opposite eye is stimulated, but it dilates when the light is centered on it. (In fact, it does not dilate; it simply does not constrict; hence it appears to be dilating as it returns to habitual size.) (See Marcus Gunn pupil, below.)

Abnormalities and Their Possible Causes (6,12,28)

Aniridia.   This abnormality is often associated with vascularized corneal pannus, lens opacities, and lens coloboma. Aniridia may be inherited, congenital, or traumatic.

Coloboma.   Coloboma may be acquired (e.g., trauma, surgical), genetic, congenital, or idiopathic.

Persistent Pupillary Membrane.   This condition may be idiopathic or caused by fetal iritis, heredity, or oxygen in a premature nursery.

Polycoria.   Polycoria, or multiple pupils, each with its own sphincter, is very rare. The condition is congenital.

Corectopia.   This eccentric displacement of the pupil is genetic, and is usually related to other anomalies.

Microcoria.   This condition, characterized by unequal-size pupils, is caused by congenital miosis. The condition is usually related to ophthalmoplegia.

Anisocoria.   Unequal-size pupils is frequently indicative of central nervous system involvement; it may be idiopathic.

Miosis.   Characterized by pupils less than 2 mm in diameter, miosis has two primary causes:

   1. Drugs (e.g., parasympathomimetics that activate the sphincter muscle, such as pilocarpine and neostigmine; sympatholytics that relax the dilator muscle, such as reserpine, alpha methyldopa, histamines, and morphine)
   2. Neurogenic disorders (e.g., meningitis, encephalitis, Horner's syndrome, Argyll-Robertson pupil)

Mydriasis.   Pupils larger than 5 mm in diameter may be due to any of the following:

   1. Drugs and toxins (e.g., sympathomimetics that activate the dilators; parasymphatholytics that immobilize the sphincters, such as cyclopentolate and tropicamide)
   2. Bovine milk protein (in infants with allergic malabsorption)
   3. Ocular trauma or foreign body
   4. Neural lesion
   5. Idiopathic causes

Hippus.   These irregularly rhythmic, visible pupillary oscillations, 2 mm or more in amplititude, may be a normal variation or neurogenic (e.g., III nerve palsy; myasthenia gravis; cerebral tumor)

Amaurotic Pupil.   This condition results in a blind eye that does not respond to direct light stimulation but does demonstrate an intact consensual response. It indicates monocular blindness.

Light-near Dissociation.   Characterized by relatively large pupils that respond appropriately to a near stimulus but not to light; light-near dissociation indicates a lesion in the pretectal area of the upper midbrain. The condition may be caused by encephalitis, gliomas of the quadrigeminal plate, and vascular disease. It may be part of Parinaud's syndrome if accompanied by an inability to shift the gaze upward and a retraction nystagmus.

Argyll-Robertson Pupil.   This condition involves dissociation of light and near reflexes, but it is different in that the habitual pupil size is relatively small. There may be a lesion in the pretectal neurons above the Edinger-Westphal nucleus, due to lues, encephalitis, etc.

Marcus Gunn Pupil.   This condition indicates an afferent defect in which the "swinging light" routine (see above) causes both pupils to constrict in response to a light stimulus in one eye, and to dilate (or, in fact, simply to not constrict) when the light is moved to the other eye. This is an extremely sensitive indicator of optic nerve dysfunction. It is often associated with optic nerve tumor and retro-bulbar neuritis.

Tonic Pupil. Not ordinarily found in prepuberty-aged children, this is typically a unilateral condition. The affected pupil fails to react to light and does react very slowly to a near stimulus. Redilation then also takes an unusually long time—up to 1 minute. Dysfunction of the autonomic nervous system is due to a lesion of the ciliary ganglion. It may be viral in origin. It also may be an indication of Adie's syndrome, which includes loss of patellar and Achilles reflexes.

STATUS OF ADJACENT COMPONENTS

Normal Clinical Picture
The circumcorneal zone should appear relatively white, nonedematous, and free of hypervascularization. The peripheral retina, including the vitreous base near the ora serrata, should be free of exudates (24). The anterior chamber should be clear and transparent.

Examination Procedures
Conduct direct visual inspection of the perilimbal zone and the pupil. Use a slit lamp, which is essential for assessment of the anterior chamber. Additionally, binocular indirect ophthalmoscopy should be used for inspection of the peripheral retina.

Abnormalities and Their Possible Causes (11,12,26)
Iritis. Inflammation of the iris, is characterized by marked injection of the peri-limbal vessels (ciliary flush), flare and cells in the aqueous, miosis, pain, and photophobia. Its cause is often obscure but has been related to trauma, rheumatoid arthritis, sarcoid, syphilis, and ulcerative colitis.

Cyclitis. Most involvements of the anterior uveal tract encompass both the iris and the ciliary body and manifest as an iridocyclitis. However, there are certain instances where only the ciliary body is involved. Cyclitis free of iritis presents as a very mild phenomenon: no significant injection, normal pupillary signs, very mild reaction in the anterior chamber but many cells in the anterior portion of the vitreous body, mild edema of the disc, sheathing of the retinal vessels, en-gorgement of the veins, and exudation at the vitreous base near the ora serrata. The cause of cyclitis is usually unknown.

Cysts of the Pigment Epithelium. These cysts may occur anteriorly through the stroma or fall free in the anterior chamber. They are often associated with miotic strabismus therapy (see Chapter 10).

Cysts of the Ciliary Epithelium.   These tend to present in the pupil, or they may exert pressure on the iris and be identified in that fashion.

□ The Crystalline Lens

SIZE

Normal Clinical Picture (6)
The lens grows throughout life. The adult, unaccommodated lens measures about 9 mm in horizontal diameter, 8 mm in the vertical, and is about 4 mm thick. This is about twice the mass of the newborn's lens.

Examination Procedures
Ophthalmoscope and slit lamp examinations should be performed.

Abnormalities and Their Possible Causes
Congenital Aphakia.   This is an extremely rare developmental anomaly.

Apparent (or secondary) Aphakia.   The lens appears as a whitish, membranous mass supported by poorly formed zonular fibers. The capsule is wrinkled; the vitreous may be clear. This, too, is a developmental anomaly.

Microphakia.   This condition is characterized by a small, round lens, reminiscent of a fetal lens. It is very rare and is familial or due to arrested fetal development.

SHAPE

Normal Clinical Picture (27)
The newborn's lens is approximately spherical. It assumes a disc shape as it grows, due to the significant increase of the equatorial circumference in contrast to virtually no sagittal growth.
   The lens surface of the adult unaccommodated lens is convex, the anterior surface radius measuring 11 mm and the posterior, 6 mm. Only the central region of these surfaces displays spherical curves, a region approximately 4 mm in diameter. Peripherally, the surfaces flatten until they reach the steep equatorial curve.

Examination Procedures
Conduct slit lamp examination.

Abnormalities and Their Possible Causes (1,2,11)
Lenticonus Posterior.   This condition is characterized by a conical projection of the lens from the region of the posterior pole. It is sometimes accompanied by an opacity in the region of the conus and adherent hyaloid remnants. It is due to a developmental anomaly.

Lenticonus Internus. A bulge in the posterior part of the lens that does not cause a change in the curve of the lenticular posterior surface is indicative of lenticonus internus. It is due to a developmental anomaly.

Coloboma of the Lens. This condition typically presents as a concavity (a notch) in some portion of the lens circumference. Most colobomas occur in the lower part of the lens, but they have been observed in other locations and also have been known to present merely as flattenings rather than concavities. They are due to developmental anomalies.

POSITION

Normal Clinical Picture
The lens should be positioned immediately behind and adjacent to the iris, centered so that mydriasis does not expose any portion of the lens.

Examination Procedures
Conduct direct inspection, including a slit lamp examination.

Abnormalities and Their Possible Causes
Ectopia Lentis. These congenital dislocations of the lens are usually bilateral, symmetrical, upward, and nasal. They may cause monocular diplopia, depending upon the relationship of the lens edge to pupil size. The condition is inherited and also has been associated with Marchesani's and Marfan's syndromes.

Spontaneous Dislocation of the Lens. This condition appears to be part of a congenital involvement or some postnatal event. It has been linked with buphthalmos, staphylomas, and highly myopic eyes, where enlargement of the globe stretches the zonule to the breaking point. It may also be caused by the growth of an intraocular tumor.

Traumatic Dislocation of the Lens. This condition is relatively common following a contusion. The lens is apt to retun to its normal position and status as the eye recovers.

TRANSPARENCY

Normal Clinical Picture (6)
The crystalline lens earns its name from its clarity and transparency. Its primary chemical ingredient is water (about 65%), with most of the remainder being protein. Its main substance comprises fibers contained in a homogeneous, interfibrillar material. The lens is contained within a hyaloid envelope.

Examination Procedures
Slit lamp and ophthalmoscopic examinations are essential.

Abnormalities and Their Possible Causes
Cataracts (11,12).   Cataracts may be congenital, or they may develop postnatally. In either event, because the lens continues to develop throughout life, cataracts are usually identified as developmental unless they are sequelae of trauma, metabolic dysfunction, ocular inflammation, or a degenerative lesion. Within the developmental category, cataracts may be classified as inherited (i.e., genetically influenced) or simply congenital. They may also be classified according to their appearance and location within the lens. Developmental cataracts appearing in the axial position of the lens tend to be congenital; those in the equatorial region are more apt to be inherited.

Mittendorf's Dot.   This relatively large (1-mm) opacity on the posterior pole of the lens capsule is fairly common (it occurs in about 2 percent of the population). It has no effect on sight. This condition is congenital; the Mittendorf's dot is an embryological remnant.

□ The Vitreous Body

CLARITY

Normal Clinical Picture (2,6)
The vitreous (or hyaloid) body is a transparent and colorless gel that fully occupies the posterior cavity of the globe. In the fetal stage, the glove contains a vascular system (hyaloid vessels) that runs through the canal from the optic nerve to the back of the lens, there forming the tunica vasculosa lentis, the vascular network of the embryonic lens. This vascular system usually atrophies by the time of delivery. The atrophy may be incomplete, however, with portions of the artery remaining. In very rare cases, the entire hyaloid artery may persist.

Examination Procedures
Slit lamp and ophthalmoscopic examinations should be conducted.

Abnormalities and Their Possible Causes
Muscae Volitantes.   These floating "specks" are often noted when looking at a brightly illuminated field, such as a blue sky. They are attributed to small fixed flecks of protein, and are benign.

Hemorrhages.   Hemorrhages initially appear as red threads or veils. Over time (a few weeks), these are replaced by a gray-white residue, which, in transmitted light, appears as dark points, lines, or floccules. Hemorrhages may be caused by trauma, inflammation (e.g., chorioretinitis, syphilis), hematologic disorders (e.g., leukemia), and subarachnoid hemorrhages.

Cellular Opacities.   These gray-white punctate or linear opacities often form a gray veil. They are frequently seen in association with ocular inflammation; e.g., iritis, vitreous abscesses, endophthalmitis, perphlebitis.

Tumor Cells.   Tumor cells may present as small, multiple tumor seeds.

Pigment.   Pigment appears as small yellow or brown punctate deposits. Its presence signals retinal detachment, cyclitis, retinitis, or trauma.

Synchisis Scintillans.   These are glistening yellow-white cholesterol crystals that tend to appear following hemorrhages.

Siderosis.   These usually appear as brown-yellow or blue-green–gray pigment deposits. Color depends upon the metal that precipitated the condition. Siderosis is the outcome of an intraocular metallic foreign body.

Pseudogliomas.   These opacities cause a gray-white pupillary reflex (amaurotic cat's eye pupil) and blindness. These arise from a number of sources, including persistent hyaloid artery, persistent hyperplastic primary vitreous, retinal dysplasia, congenital progressive oculoacousticocerebral degeneration (Norrie's disease), and retinopathy of prematurity.

□ The Fundus

OPTIC DISC

Normal Clinical Picture (2,6,27)
The optic disc measures approximately 1.5 mm across and a trifle more than that in the vertical dimension. It is located about 3 mm from the fovea, measured center to center. Thus, the distance from disc edge to fovea is about 2 to 2.5 disc diameters, a condition that remains constant from birth onward.

During the first year of life, the disc's color changes from grayish-white to pink; disc margins, initially ill-defined, become distinct. The physiological cup deepens and widens, and becomes more apparent; the lamina cribrosa becomes better established as medullation of the optic nerve is completed; and the retinal vessels, instead of emerging from the center of the cup, assume a nasally oriented position.

Examination Procedures
Examination should include ophthalmoscopy, visual fields (see Practical Suggestion 4-3), and slit lamp with Hruby or 90 diopter lens.

Abnormalities and Their Possible Causes (28,29)
Hypoplasia and Aplasia.   These abnormalities are congenital and are often associated with endocrine disorders and other anomalies (e.g., anencephaly, hydrophthalmos, colobomata, aniridia).

Papilledema. Papilledema is a sign of increased intracranial pressure caused by cerebral tumor, sinus thrombosis, limited intracranial capacity (e.g., Crouzon's disease), subdural or extradural hematoma (trauma), and infection (meningitis).

Edema of Optic Disc. Edema presents the same clinical picture as papilledema but stems from causes other than increased intracranial pressure. Ocular causes include a sudden increase in intraocular pressure, neuroretinitis, uveitis, orbital tumor, abscess, aneurysm, and nerve sheath hemorrhage. Systemic causes include vascular hypertension and endocrine disorders.

Pseudopapilledema. This condition resembles papilledema superficially; however, it is not a true edema. Pseudopapilledema can be a normal variation or due to heredity, medullated nerve fibers, tumor of the disc, or hyaline bodies.

Optic Neuritis. This abnormality is also termed, under certain conditions, papillitis, intraocular optic neuritis, neuroretinitis, perineuritis, axial neuritis, retrobulbar optic neuritis, and purulent neuritis. These labels refer to the site, the cause, or the scope of the involvement. Only two designations are used here: papillitis and retrobulbar optic neuritis.
   Papillitis is evidenced by a lesion of the disc characterized by exudate in the vitreous, swelling of the disc, obliteration of the physiological cup, and vessel congestion.
   Retrobulbar optic neuritis, a lesion of the optic nerve that causes none of the above-mentioned signs and symptoms, manifests a Marcus Gunn pupil phenomenon.
   In both types, there usually is an abrupt loss of visual acuity, an accompanying field defect, and some pain on eye movement. Visual acuity may start to improve within a month, at which time the nerve head may develop a pallor. Causes include hereditary factors, toxic agents, inflammation, demyelinization, or degeneration of optic nerve fibers stemming from intraocular or orbital involvements.

Optic Atrophy. This abnormality is characterized by pale disc (ranging from chalk white to subtle, less-than-usual pink), reduced visual acuity, and visual field changes resulting from decreased vascularization and glial proliferation of the optic disc following ganglion cell atrophy.
   Optic atrophy is caused by lesions that interrupt the optic nerve, chiasm, or optic tract. These may be congenital or may be due to postnatal trauma; inflammation (e.g., meningitis, scarlet fever); demyelinating disease (e.g., postinfectious encephalitis); blood dyscrasias (e.g., leukemia, polycythemia); allergy (e.g., food, insect bites); metabolic disorder (e.g., endocrine exophthalmos); toxic agents (e.g., dilantin, streptomycin); and syndrome-related conditions (e.g., Crouzon's syndrome, Albright's syndrome).
   Tumors. Usually, these are optic nerve gliomas that cause slowly developing axial exophthalmos, or—on the disc—melanocytoma.

Pigment Changes in the Disc Region. The following pigment changes may be observed:

1. *Choroidal nevi* tend to be round, elevated, and slate gray.
2. *Retinal pigment epithelium proliferation* is characterized by dustlike pigment that covers the disc, either partially or completely. It may be surrounded by an annulus of thickened gray-white retina.
3. *Melanocytoma* is benign, but it may become malignant. It resembles melanoma. This abnormality occurs most often in dark-pigment racial groups. It appears as dark black tumors with feathery borders on or adjacent to the disc.
4. *Hemosiderin deposits.* These crystals accumulate on the disc following a vitreous hemorrhage.
5. *Malignant melanoma.* These brown to slate-gray lesions are shiny with bumpy surfaces. They have a tendency to grow and are frequently accompanied by an overlying serous retinal detachment.

Deep and/or Wide Physiological Cup. This refers to a C/D ratio greater than 1:3 and a depth greater than 1 mm (3 diopters with the ophthalmoscope). Causes include congenital glaucoma, hereditary disorders (e.g., Marfan's syndrome, various chromosomal disorders, syphilis, infantile phyoglycemia, toxoplasmosis), trauma, inflammation, and idiopathic factors.

BLOOD VESSELS OF THE FUNDUS

Normal Clinical Picture (2,6,26)
The walls of the retinal vessels are normally transparent; they are visible only because they contain blood. This is especially so in young, healthy eyes where the effects of age—e.g., thickening of the vessel walls—have not yet occurred.

The blood vessels of the neonate are so narrow that distinguishing between artery and vein is difficult. This changes fairly quickly, however, so that by the age of 6 months the arteries and veins have achieved a normal size relationship (2:3) and are gracefully and symmetrically distributed throughout the inner globe.

Choroidal vessels are usually visible by ophthalmoscopy during the first 6 months of life and thereafter in children with light pigmentation.

Examination Procedures
The following procedures are recommended:

1. ophthalmoscopy
2. slit lamp with Hruby or 90 diopter lens
3. fluorescein angiography (17,30,31)

Abnormalities and Their Possible Causes
Tortuous Blood Vessels. These may be a normal variation or due to a congenital or hereditary disorder (e.g., Osler's disease, sickle-cell disease, chronic glaucoma, Eales's disease, cri du chat syndrome, Coat's disease).

Retinal Artery Occlusion. This abnormality is characterized by sudden blindness, diffuse retinal pallor, and a cherry-red spot in the macula. It may be caused by embolism due to postrheumatic vegetation, cardiac caterization, valvotomy; ocular trauma combined with secondary glaucoma; sickle-train hemoglobinopathy; syphilis.

Arterial Narrowing. *Localized* narrowing may result from trauma, inflammation, and dystrophy. *General* arterial narrowing results from congenital microphthalmos, trauma, infection, edema (as with orbital cellulitis), and central nervous system disorders (e.g., Tay-Sachs).

Sheathing of Retinal Veins. White or gray envelopes around vessels, hemorrhage, and exudate may be present in this condition. Sheathing may be caused by developmental disorders. In those instances, sheathing occurs in the vicinity of the disc only. Eales's disease, brucellosis, and viral infection (e.g., herpes, influenza) also have been implicated.

Dilated Veins. These veins exceed the normal A/V 2:3 ratio and are caused by trauma and congenital disease.

Macroaneurysms of Retinal Artery. These often present in conjunction with localized hemorrhage and exudation. The causes may be congenital or idiopathic.

Retinitis Proliferans. This abnormal growth of new vessels into the vitreous tends to be stimulated by hemorrhage and irritation in association with diabetes mellitus, sickle-cell disease, syphilis, and trauma.

Temporal Displacement of Retinal Vessels. This condition may be caused by retinopathy of prematurity, sickle-cell disease, vitreous retinopathy, inflammation, trauma, and familial factors.

Choroidal Neovascular Ingrowth Through Breaks in Bruch's Membrane into the Macular Area. These ingrowths are caused by trauma, macular drusen, choroidal neovasculature, and idiopathic factors.

Choroidal Nevus Ingrowth at Optic Nerve Head Margin. These growths may be idiopathic, due to macular drusen, or due to hyaline bodies of the disc.

PERIPHERAL FUNDUS

Normal Clinical Picture (2,6,27)
Like the disc, the rest of the fundus changes significantly during the first 6 months of postnatal life. It is relatively free of pigment, causing the choroidal vessels to stand out prominently against the light background. Then, gradually, pigment deposits within the choroidal intervascular spaces, eliminating this condition, and the vasculature contrast commences to resemble the adult's.

The retinal periphery is not completely developed at the time of birth. The retina is thicker at the ora serrata, forming a redundant fold: Lange's fold. In addition, the peripheral retina vasculature does not develop fully until the infant achieves a weight of about 1900 grams. Once that level of development is achieved, there is consolidation. Until that point, the retina is highly vulnerable to the development of retinopathy of prematurity.

Examination Procedures
Use the following procedures to examine the fundus:

1. ophthalmoscopy
2. slit lamp with Hruby or 90-diopter lens
3. ERG (17,30,31)
4. EOG (17,30,31)
5. fluorescein angiography

Abnormalities and Their Possible Causes (30, 31)
Hemorrhages.   Intraretinal or preretinal bleeding, can be stimulated by congestion of head and neck, trauma, inflammation (e.g., perivasculitis), toxic states, vascularized neoplasms (e.g., hereditary hemorragic telangiectasia as in Rendu-Osler-Weber disease), sickle-cell anemia, and diabetes mellitus.

Large Hemorrhage in Infants.   This condition may be caused by subdural hematoma, hygroma, or subarachnoid hemorrhage.

Retinal Hemorrhage with Central White Spot.   Hemopoietic disease (anemia, leukemia), diabetes mellitus, and intracranial hemorrhage are possible causes of this abnormal condition.

Microaneurysms of Retina.   These are characterized by punctate red spots scattered about the posterior pole of the globe; possible causes include diabetes mellitus, sickle-cell anemia, leukemia, Eales's disease, and Osler's hemorrhagic telangiectasia.

Retinal Falciform Folds.   These may be several millimeters high; they emanate from the disc and course inferiorally and temporally toward the ciliary process. The folds may be unilateral or bilateral. The effect of acuity depends on the extent of macular involvement. This defect has been associated with retinal detachment and macular degeneration.

Cotton-wool Spots.   Characterized by soft exudate and fluffy, white, superficial deposits on retina, cotton-wool spots are caused by hypertensive retinopathy and lupus erythematosus.

Hard Exudates.   These are yellowish-white discrete masses located deep in retina, caused by diabetes mellitus, Coats' disease, circinate retinopathy, and xanthomatosis.

Single White Lesion.   Causes of single white lesions include retinoblastoma, glioma of the optic nerve, and toxocara canis.

Pale Fundus Lesion.   General pallor is associated with albinism, retinal ischemia, vascular retinopathy, and leukemia. Localized pallor is seen in connection with opaque nerve fibers, retinopathy of prematurity (ROP), retinal detachment and schisis, and retinoblastoma; and also as a normal variation.

Pigmented Lesion.   A single, dark lesion on the retina may indicate detachment or Coats' disease. Such a lesion in the vitreous indicates vitreous hemorrhage or abscess.

Multiple Pigmented Lesions.   These may be racial characteristics or indicative of nevus of Ota.

Flat Lesion.   If the lesion is bluish-gray or black it is probably a benign melanoma. If there is patch of dense pigment, atrophic in center it suggests a pigmented scar. If the lesion is in the macular region with other atrophic changes, suspect Fuchs' dark spot.

Raised Lesion.   These suggest detachment, malignant melanoma, and choroidal hemorrhage.

Widely Disseminated Pigment Changes.   These changes may be due to genetic factors or to retinitis pigmentosa.

Peripheral Fundus Lesion.   If the lesion is pale and raised, suspect vitreous opacities, ROP, toxocariasis, or retinoblastoma. If flat, consider coloboma, chorioretinitis, or peripheral degeneration. Dark and raised lesions suggest choroidal detachment, simple detachment, cysts, scleral indentation, ciliary body neoplasm, and choroid neoplasm.

Angioid Streaks.   Rupture of Bruch's membrane, evidenced by brownish lines surrounding the disc and radiating toward the periphery, are characteristic of this abnormality, which is caused by sickle-cell disease and acromegaly.

Choroidal Folds.   These folds of the posterior pole at the choroid level can be seen with a Hruby (or 90D) lens and/or as a pattern of alternating light lines on fluorescein angiography. Possible causes include high hyperopia, orbital mass, uveitis, papilledema, exophthalmos, and idiopathic factors.

Choroiditis. Toxoplasmic retinochoroiditis, herpes simplex retinochoroiditis, toxocara retinochoroiditis, and syphilitic retinochoroiditis are possible causes of choroiditis.

MACULA

Normal Clinical Picture (2,6,27)
The macula is approximately the same size as the disc; i.e., 1.5 mm in diameter. At the center of macula is a small depression, the fovea. It lies about 3.5 to 4.0 mm lateral to the edge of the disc and just below its middle.

Examination Procedures
Examination of the macula should include the following:

1. ophthalmoscopy
2. slit lamp with Hruby or 90-diopter lens
3. visual acuity
4. amsler grid
5. color vision (unilateral)

Abnormalities and Possible Causes (30,31)
Pseudomacular Edema. This abnormality is caused by serous detachment of the retinal pigment epithelium and central serous retinopathy.

Macular Edema. Trauma associated with uveitis, hemangioma of the choroid, telangiectasis of the retina, peripheral uveitis (pars planitis), and Fabry's disease are known causes of macular edema.

Retinoschisis. This split of the retina in the nerve fiber layer may extend from the disc to the ora serrata. The macula takes on the appearance of a spokelike configuration, and vitreous membrane is often visible. Possible causes include primary and secondary detachment.

Macular Pucker. This condition is characterized by tiny folds arranged in a stellate pattern around the macula; it is usually associated with a preretinal membrane. Macular pucker is associated with vitreous blood, retinal detachment, detachment of the macula, and multiple perforations.

Cherry-red Spot in the Macula. Spingolipidosis (e.g., Tay-Sachs disease, Gaucher's disease) is linked with this abnormality.

Macular Hole. These are caused by cystic degeneration and histoplasmosis.

Elevated Macular Lesion. Malignant melanoma, central serous detachment of the retina, angioplastic retinopathy, and chorioretinitis should be suspected when elevated macula lesions are observed.

White or Yellow Flat Macular Lesions and Pigmentary Changes. These lesions are associated with post trauma or inflammation, coloboma of the macula, radiation injury, Fuchs' spot (degenerative myopia), Best's disease (occurs in children up to about age 7 years: egg yolk lesions at macula, later absorbed to leave an atrophic scar), and Stargardts' disease (occurs in children between the ages of 8 to 14; variable appearance depending upon inherited characteristics; same general picture as Best's disease).

□ The Oculomotor System

The oculomotor system comprises the extraocular muscles and the nerves that innervate them. Obviously, these do not function independent of the sensory components of vision. The opposite is closer to the truth; the oculomotor system is driven, stimulated to act, by the sensations detected by the ocular sensory components. Therefore, a deficit in one system, either one, is likely to affect the other.

The integrity of the oculomotor system is revealed through its function: the ability of the eyes to perform certain actions both separately and in concert. Discussion in this section is limited to the detection of abnormalities and, where appropriate, a listing of possible causes. Diagnosis of oculomotor disorders is presented in Chapter 6.

FIXATION ACCURACY

Normal Clinical Picture
The tendency to direct the eyes toward a specific sensory stimulus, and to make the postural adjustments needed to do this, appears to be innate. Infants demonstrate it very early in their postnatal life, usually during the first week or so after birth, as they direct their eyes toward the various light sources in their environment (19,27). It is this characteristic that makes possible the OKN and PL methods of measuring visual acuity (see Chapter 3).

By age 3 months, the average child is able to maintain accurate fixation in a field of gaze with either or both eyes, and, if fixation is disrupted, he is able to reestablish it easily.

At some point in early life this ability becomes established at the reflex level. But until that stage is reached, the function is vulnerable to erosion through deprivation; without central vision stimulation, it will deteriorate (32). This is corroborated by the fact that children whose visual acuity is reduced markedly during the first 2 years of life will develop nystagmus (see Chapter 6).

Examination Procedures
Visual Acuity. This is one of the most valid indices of monocular fixation accuracy, for very obvious reasons. The child who displays 20/20 acuity or better (corrected or uncorrected), in each eye, is also displaying precise fixation with each eye. No additional documentation is required.

Stereoacuity.   Detection of small amounts of retinal image disparity within Panum's area requires precise, simultaneous bifoveal alignment (see Chapter 6 for a more detailed discussion of stereopsis and stereoacuity testing). It follows, therefore, that a stereoacuity test may be used as a valid assessment of binocular fixation accuracy, which, if present, assures fixation accuracy of each eye.

There are a number of commercially produced tests available, many of which would serve here. For discussion purposes, consider the Random-dot E stereotest (RDE) (33). It is effective with children as young as 3 years and has been shown to be highly sensitive to minimal binocular deviations when used at a 1.5-meter testing distance (34); this despite the fact that the disparity represented at that distance is in excess of 150 seconds of arc.

Passing performance with the RDE at 1.5 meters implies precise bifoveal alignment; no additional testing is necessary. Failure, however, is not certain evidence of bifoveal misalignment. It may very well be due to substandard visual acuity or simply a lack of understanding (see Chapter 6).

Ancillary Tests.   These tests are to be used when visual acuity and stereoacuity test outcomes are unobtainable or unreliable. They include visuscopy, unilateral cover test, Hirschberg method, and entoptic phenomena.

Visuscopy is an appropriate follow-up in the event that the patient does not display 20/20 visual acuity in each eye. It requires an ophthalmoscope that is capable of projecting a fixation target onto the patient's fundus. Virtually all ophthalmoscopes now come equipped with this feature, varying mainly in the design of the target. Most project a set of concentric rings with a central "bull's eye."

Direct the patient to cover one eye with his palm and "look at the center of the target with the other." Locate the position of the patient's macula in relation to the projected pattern's center. If the two coincide, you may assume that the patient is capable of precise monocular fixation. If the two do not coincide, it is evidence of eccentric fixation (see Chapter 6). Repeat the process with the other eye (see Practical Suggestion 4-13).

The unilateral cover (cover/uncover) test is especially useful when the patient's response to the stereoacuity test is inconclusive and/or unreliable, not an unlikely situation with very young children (see Eskridge [35]).

Present a detailed farpoint fixation target; e.g., 20/30 letters (if legible) or, with the preschooler, a line drawing that contains discussible details.

Direct the patient to look at the target, urging him to keep it clear.

Cover one of the patient's eyes with an occluder while you watch his other eye for signs of a shift, a realignment to obtain more central fixation. (Note: An infant may object to an occluder held against his face; some examiners prefer to postion their thumb so that it obstructs the vision of one eye.)

Keep the cover in place for a few seconds (or longer if you have reason to suspect a deviation), then remove it, all the while watching the other eye for any signs of a fixation shift.

Repeat the procedure with the occluder before the opposite eye.

Repeat the procedure at nearpoint.

Repeat the procedure at farpoint, but this time use a nondetailed fixation target, such as a fairly large spot of light.

The reason for using two types of fixation targets is probably obvious. The detailed targets will stimulate accommodation. This could trigger strabismus in a patient with a high AC/A ratio and a tendency toward esotropia. The nondetailed target, on the other hand, may sponsor strabismus in the patient with (intermittent) exotropia, for a related reason; eliminating the accommodation demand reduces the stimulus to convergence to the point where some patients no longer retain bifoveal alignment (see Chapter 6).

Repeat the procedure at nearpoint.

If you see no movement of the uncovered eye as you cover and uncover the partner eye in these four conditions, assume that there is simultaneous bilateral fixation accuracy; that both eyes align simultaneously and accurately; or, that misalignment is too small to be detected with this method. It is not fail-safe (see Chapter 6 in regard to small-angle strabismus).

The Hirschberg method (36) is not a precisely accurate method for determining binocular fixation accuracy. However, if the patient is too young to respond reliably to the visual acuity test, the Random-dot E stereotest, visuscopy, and the unilateral cover test, then Hirschberg method for measuring binocular alignment is probably the best remaining option.

The principle of the test is simple. A light source (penlight) positioned in front of the patient will be reflected from both corneas. If the eyes are in alignment, these reflections ("reflexes") will be situated symmetrically; if the light source is held centrally, the reflexes will appear fairly close to the center of the respective corneas. (The pupil is used as a reference point.) If something different is observed—if, for example, the reflex is centered on one cornea and displaced laterally on the other—then a misalignment of the two eyes may be inferred, with the one presenting the displaced reflex as the one that is misaligned. (Technical accuracy requires that attention also be given here to the measurement of angle kappa. For practical purposes, this is discussed in the section devoted to diagnosis of strabismus, along with the method to be used for quantifying the misalignment of the corneal reflexes [see Chapter 6]. At this stage of the examination, it is sufficient simply to identify whether or not there is apparent misalignment.)

Entoptic phenomena, Maxwell's spot and Haidinger's brushes, aid in documenting fixation accuracy. By definition, however, both of these involve the perception of illusions. It is highly improbable that a child too young to respond reliably to a visual acuity test and a stereoacuity test would be able to communicate appropriately about an entoptic phenomenon. In fact, it is inconceivable. Hence, there is no practical reason for discussing these here.

Abnormalities and Their Possible Causes

Eccentric Fixation. Possible causes include central scotoma, macular edema, ectopic macula, and abnormal fixation reflex—the outcome of a sensory-motor maladaptation.

Strabismus.   Possible causes of strabismus include neurological deficit (e.g., extraocular muscle palsy, central nervous system lesion), structural anomaly, and neuromotor functional disorder.

Head Turn or Tilt.   Possible causes of this abnormality include strabismus, nystagmus, nystagmus blockage syndrome, ptosis, and extraocular muscle palsy (see below).

FIXATION STABILITY

Normal Clinical Picture
When the eyes fixate, they should appear to be stationary. This is true at all ages, whether one eye or both are open, and regardless of the relative position of the stimulus within the field of vision. Anything to the contrary is not normal and requires careful investigation.

Examination Procedures
Examination should include the following:

1.   Direct visual inspection. Naked-eye observations, a few seconds at each of the diagnostic positions of gaze, are usually sufficient. If magnification is desired, position a magnifying lens peripheral to the visual axis and watch the limbus, or some other landmark, for signs of movement.
2.   Assess the patient under monocular and binocular viewing conditions. Not as many observations are needed under monocular conditions; the primary concern is whether there is any deterioration of fixation stability in comparison with when both eyes are open (see discussion regarding latent nystagmus, Chapter 6). Assess with fixation at nearpoint and again at farpoint. Once more, the latter need not be explored in great depth. The essential concern is whether there is a deterioration in fixation stability when the visual axes are parallel as compared with when they are converging (see Chapter 6).

Abnormalities and Their Possible Causes
Pendular Nystagmus.   Possible causes of this condition include defective vision and heredity (see Chapter 6).

Jerky Nystagmus.   Possible causes include central nervous system disorders and drugs (see Chapter 6).

MOTILITIES

Normal Clinical Picture (37)
The movement of a single eye referred to as a duction. The conjugate movement of both eyes (in the same direction) is referred to as a version. The disjugate movement of both eyes (in opposite directions) is referred to as vergence. A normal eye can move freely and voluntarily within a fairly wide area, ranging from 10

mm horizontally (laterally and nasally, from center), 7 mm upward, and 14.5 mm downward. When both eyes are open (and aligned), version movements should appear to be yoked, both eyes maintaining their relative positions in all directions of gaze. Nearpoint of convergence should be within 8 cm of the bridge of the nose, and a shift in fixation from near to far, in the primary position of gaze, should be accomplished by synchronous divergence.

Examination Procedures
The following assessments should be made during examination:

1. Ductions. Observe one eye (the other is occluded) as it follows a fixation target to all diagnostic positions of gaze. Repeat with the other eye. (Note: With young children, it is often simpler to use a stable fixation target and move the child's head, gently but with authority, vertically and horizontally.) Table 4.1 shows the extraocular muscles and their respective roles in various duction movements.

2. Versions. Repeat duction assessment procedure under binocular viewing conditions. (Note: The RDE may be used for this purpose, but it is not ordinarily worth the extra time. To accomplish this, test the child's stereoacuity with the RDE stereograms held in all diagnostic positions of gaze. If versions are adequate, stereoacuity should be unaffected by altered gaze positions. If versions are faulty, it should become evident through a breakdown in stereoacuity in those positions of gaze.)

3. Nearpoint of convergence. Observe patient's ability to maintain binocular fixation on a target as it is brought closer to him (see Chapter 7 for complete description and variations in testing procedures).

Abnormalities and Their Possible Causes
Restricted Motilities in One or More Action Fields. Possible causes include extraocular muscle damage or dysfunction, oculomotor nerve involvement, and syndrome-linked anomalies such as the following:

Cardinal Direction of Gaze	Muscle Predominantly Active		Cranial Nerves Involved	
	O.D.	O.S.	O.D.	O.S.
Right	LR	MR	VI	III
Left	MR	LR	III	VI
Up and right	SR	IO	III	III
Up and left	IO	SR	III	III
Down and right	IR	SO	III	IV
Down and left	SO	IR	IV	III

Table 4.1 Action of Extraocular Muscles in Six Cardinal Positions

Duane's retraction syndrome: usually characterized by an absence of abduction ability and globe retraction on adduction. May be bilateral, but most often involves one eye only.

Brown's syndrome: characterized by inability to elevate an adducted eye, resembling paresis of inferior oblique muscle. No difficulty in elevating abducted eye. Attributed to superior oblique tendon anomaly (or the tendon sheath) that limits action of inferior oblique.

Mobius syndrome: characterized by an inability to abduct either eye. Vertical versions and convergence remain intact. Esotropia is common. Frequently accompanied by bilateral seventh cranial nerve palsy affecting the obicularis muscles of the lower lid, and causing an expressionless face, a round mouth, and an inability to grin normally or wrinkle his forehead.

Head Turn or Tilt. This reaction is considered abnormal when the patient is presented with a centrally situated stimulus; i.e., when there should be no head turn/tilt. Possible causes include extraocular muscle or nerve paresis, with the head turned in the direction of the action of the involved muscle (e.g., a head turn to the right, so that the left eye is forward of the right, implicates the right lateral rectus or the left medial rectus). The rationale for this: when an extraocular muscle is paretic—unable to contract fully—its direct antagonist will overact, thereby causing the eye to deviate from alignment when both eyes are open. The magnitude of deviation will increase as binocular gaze is shifted in the direction of the action of the involved muscle. One outcome of binocular misalignment is diplopia, with the image belonging to the deviated eye displaced in the direction of the action of the involved muscle. In order to reduce the diplopia, the patient turns his head, thereby enabling him to look "straight ahead" while actually looking in the direction opposite to the action of the involved muscle.

A head tilt to one side, with or without accompanying head turn, can be explained by the same rationale and typically signals an involvement of one of the muscles responsible for vertical eye movements: superior and inferior recti, superior and inferior obliques. The so-called three-step method is effective in identifying which of these is involved through a deductive process (see 36,37,38).

A head tilt upward or downward usually indicates an "A" or a "V" pattern, wherein the binocular deviation is greater on upward or downward gaze. In these instances, it is most often attributable to impaired function of one of the obliques (37).

Receded Nearpoint of Convergence. Possible causes of this abnormality include a functional deficit often accompanied by low AC/A. Covergence paralysis stemming from local or central nervous system involvement should also be suspected (see Chapter 6).

Esotropia Provoked by Convergence. This condition is probably due to a high AC/A (see Chapter 6).

■

B. ABNORMALITY NOTED?

The assessment of ocular health and structural integrity is usually a straightforward process. There are times, however, when an abnormality is observed that necessitates more in-depth investigation. Before doing this, the optometrist engages in a subset of actions indicated on the Figure 4.1 flow diagram as steps C through H. In brief, these represent the steps leading to the decision regarding whether to focus attention on the abnormality and to depart from the standard examination sequence, or whether, instead, to set the information aside (but not out of mind) for the moment, to continue with the standard procedures, and to address it after a more thoroughly developed clinical picture has been assembled.

■

PRACTICAL SUGGESTIONS

4-1. If you have difficulty getting the child to fixate adequately while testing near point of convergence (NPC) or ocular motilities, try a penlight: identify it as a "candle," and urge the child to try to "blow it out." Obviously, you must control the off/on switch appropriately if you wish to have the child sustain this behavior very long.

4-2. A small toy mounted on a tongue depressor serves well as a fixation target when conducting nearpoint cover tests. Hold the tongue depressor between your teeth, thus freeing your hands for the occluder and prisms.

4-3. "Confrontation" visual fields may be more reliably tested with young children by presenting two stimuli (in opposing fields) and having the child identify which of the two ("the one on *this* side or *that* side") moved.

4-4. When doing ophthalmoscopy on a babe-in-arms, have the mother hold the child in a supine, breast-feeding position so that one of his eyes is adjacent to his mother's chest and the other is available to your ophthalmoscope. Then, when ready to examine the other eye, have the mother hold the child in the opposite orientation. Offering the child a bottle at this time is also often very helpful.

4-5. A very young child may fall asleep during the course of the examination. Take advantage of the situation by conducting (direct/indirect) ophthalmoscopy as she sleeps.

4-6. It is often easier on the examiner's lower back to have the child stand (on the floor, or on the foot rest of the examination chair) as direct ophthalmoscopy is done.

4-7. Direct ophthalmoscopy of children with significant myopia is typically non-productive because of the magnified image available to the clinician. To overcome this, place a neutralizing (minus) lens in front of the eye (or, if the patient already wears glasses, have him wear them) as you conduct ophthalmoscopy.

4-8. If you observe an unusual (and potentially clinically significant) anatomical feature in a child's eyes, take a moment to look for a similar feature in the accompanying parent's/sibling's eyes. For example, if the patient's C/D ratio is unusually large, but is similar to what you observe in her mother/father/brother/sister, then you have reason to be less anxious. (Obviously, the presence of similar characteristics in other family members does not absolve you from the obligation of appropriate actions, but it does provide one "reasonable explanation" for the phenomenon.)

4-9. When instilling drops in a child's eyes, have him use his own hand as a fixation target. In other words, if you want him to "look up," then have him fixate his hand as he elevates it to the appropriate location.

4-10. Many children become very apprehensive when eye drops are to be instilled. It may help to present them with a distracting task; e.g., "I want you to start breathing in through your nose and out through your mouth, slowly and loud enough so that I can hear it. Like this: breathe in . . . breathe out . . . breathe in . . . breathe out . . . etc."
  Another tactic: "I want you to listen to me say numbers and tell me every time I say the number *three*. Ready; listen: 1 . . . 2 . . . 4 . . . 6 . . . 3 . . . etc." The goal, of course, is to center the child's attention on something other than the eye drops. (These same tactics may be applied when attempting to carry out ophthalmoscopy with an anxious, photophobic child.)

4-11. Some children have to be physically restrained when certain procedures are to be conducted; e.g., when instilling drops, everting an eyelid. To do this:

  1. Have the child sit on her parent's lap, facing forward (back to parent).
  2. Instruct the parent to cross one of his legs over the child's two legs and wrap his arms around the child's arms, thus effectively restraining the child.
  3. The examiner now needs only to control the child's head/eyelid as the procedure continues.
  4. When instilling drops, make certain to prevent the child from blinking (and thereby expelling the drug) until a second or two *after* the drop makes contact with the globe. Do this by stabilizing both the upper and lower eyelids with the fingers of your one hand.

4-12. Consider omitting the topical anesthetic as preliminary to instilling a cycloplegic or mydriatic if the patient is young and/or very apprehensive about having drops administered in his eyes. Too often, it is very difficult to instill a second drop. In those cases, it is preferable that the first drop be the cycloplegic or mydriatic.

4-13. When conducting visuscopy, first project the target onto the child's palm and ask her to place her index finger (of the other hand, of course) on the center of the "bull's eye." This serves two purposes. One, it tends to reduce her anxiety about the procedure, and, second, it illustrates that the child understands what she will be asked to do when the procedure is carried out.

REFERENCES

1. Ellerbrock VJ. Developmental, congenital, and hereditary anomalies of the eye. In: Hirsch M, Wick R, eds. Vision of children. Philadelphia: Chilton Books, 1963.
2. Duke-Elder S. Systems of ophthalmology. Vol. III. St. Louis: Mosby, 1970.
3. Smith C. The development of the eye. In: The Ophthalmology Staff of the Hospital for Sick Children, Toronto. The eye in childhood. Chicago: Year Book Medical Publishing, 1967.
4. Woodruff ME. A systems examination of the infant's visual function. JAOA 1973; 45(3):410–15.
5. Harvey AM, Barondess JA, Bordley J III. Differential diagnosis. 3rd ed. Philadelphia: Saunders, 1969.
6. Spooner JD. Ocular anatomy. London: Butterworth, 1957.
7. Spaeth EB, Harley RD. Diseases of the orbit. In: Harley RD, ed. Pediatric ophthalmology. Philadelphia: Saunders, 1975.
8. Kroll AJ, Casten VG. Diseases of the orbit. In: Leibman SD, Gellis SS, eds. The pediatrician's ophthalmology. St. Louis: Mosby, 1966.
9. Crawford JJ. Diseases of the orbit. In: The Ophthalmology Staff of the Hospital for Sick Children, Toronto. The eye in childhood. Chicago: Year Book Medical Publishing, 1967.
10. Nover A. Orbital tumors in infants. Z. Kinderheilk 1967; 100(4):343.
11. Pau H. Differential diagnosis of eye diseases. Philadelphia: Saunders, 1978.
12. Helveston EM, Ellis FD. Pediatric ophthalmology practice. St. Louis: Mosby, 1980.
13. Roy FG. Ocular differential diagnosis. 2nd ed. Philadelphia: Lea and Febiger, 1975.
14. Catania LJ. Lumps and bumps of the eyelids or "What is that thing?" So J Optom May 1979:16–19.
15. Flanagan J. Diseases of the lacrimal apparatus. In: Harley RD, ed. Pediatric ophthalmology. Philadelphia: Saunders, 1975.
16. Crawford JC. The lacrimal apparatus. In: The Ophthalmology Staff of the Hospital for Sick Children, Toronto. The eye in childhood. Chicago: Year Book Medical Publishing, 1967.
17. Keeney AH. Ocular examination: basis and technique. St. Louis: Mosby, 1976.
18. Shusterman M. Inflammation of the conjunctiva. In: the Ophthalmology Staff of the Hospital for Sick Children, Toronto. The eye in childhood. Chicago: Year Book Medical Publishing, 1967.
19. Catania L, Fingeret M, Beatty RL, White KG. Primary eye care for the pediatric patient. JAOA 1979; 50(11):1201–06.

20. Furgiuele FP. Disorders of the conjunctiva. In: Harley RD, ed. Pediatric ophthalmology. Philadelphia: Saunders, 1975.
21. Borish IM. Clinical refraction. 3rd ed. Chicago: Professional Press, 1970.
22. Allen JH. External diseases of the eye. In: Leibman SD, Gellis SS, eds. The pediatrician's ophthalmology. St. Louis: Mosby, 1966.
23. Callahan WP. The cornea. In: The Ophthalmology Staff of the Hospital for Sick Children, Toronto. The eye in childhood. Chicago: Year Book Medical Publishing, 1967.
24. Amos MA, Amos DM. Anterior segment and external ocular manifestations of infectious diseases in children. JAOA 1979; 50(11):1291–99.
25. Van Herrick W, Shaffer CA, Schwartz A. Estimation of width of angle of anterior chamber. Am J Ophthal 1969; 68:626.
26. Giles CL. Inflammatory diseases. In: Leibman SD, Gellis, SS, eds. The pediatrician's ophthalmology. St. Louis: Mosby, 1966.
27. Parks MM. Growth of the eye and developmental of vision. In: Leibman SD, Gellis SS, eds. The pediatrician's ophthalmology. St. Louis: Mosby, 1966.
28. Griffin JF. Pediatric neuro-ophthalmology. In: Fenman SS, Reinecke RD, eds. Handbook of pediatric ophthalmology. New York: Grune & Stratton, 1978.
29. Levatin P, Prasloski PF, Collen MF. The swinging flashlight test in multiphasis screening for eye disease. Can J Ophthal 1979; 8:356.
30. Shusterman M. The retina, including the vitreous. In: The Ophthalmology Staff of the Hospital for Sick Children, Toronto. The eye in childhood. Chicago: Year Book Medical Publishing, 1967.
31. McMeel JW. Degenerative diseases of the retina. In: Leibman S, Gellis S, eds. The pediatrician's ophthalmology. St. Louis: Mosby, 1966.
32. Parks MM. Ocular motility and strabismus. New York: Harper & Row, 1975.
33. Reinecke RD, Simons K. A new stereoscopic test for amblyopia. Am J Ophthal 1974; 78(4):714.
34. Rosner J. The effectiveness of the random-dot E stereotest as a preschool vision screening instrument. JAOA 1978; 49(10):1121.
35. Eskridge JB. The complete cover test. JAOA 1973; 44(6):602.
36. Krimsky E. The corneal light reflex. Springfield, Ill.: Thomas, 1972.
37. Parks MM. Ocular motility diagnosis. In: Apt L, ed. Diagnostic procedures in pediatric ophthalmology. Boston: Little, Brown, 1963.
38. Koch PS. An aid for the diagnosis of a vertical muscle paresis. J Pediatr Ophthal Strab 1980; 17(40):272.

5

Question 5
What Is the Patient's
Refractive Status?

□

In addressing this question (see Figure 5.1) the clinician seeks information that will enable him to:

1. Explain at least some, if not all, of the observed and reported signs and symptoms that have been noted up to this point in the examination, such as:
   a. reduced visual acuity
   b. binocular anomaly
   c. visual discomfort
   d. inefficient performance in certain visual tasks
2. Predict the continuation of clear, comfortable, efficient binocular vision in those cases where it is the current condition.

As such, the balance of this chapter deals with the following topics:

1. The expected refractive status of the young child; the extent to which age has been shown to influence a child's refractive status.
2. The currently prevailing notions regarding the etiology and pathogenesis of ametropia.
3. Methods for measuring refractive status when standard, adult-appropriate procedures are not suitable or sufficient.
4. Conditions that should be ruled out when marked changes in refractive status are noted and/or when 20/20 visual acuity cannot be achieved in both eyes.

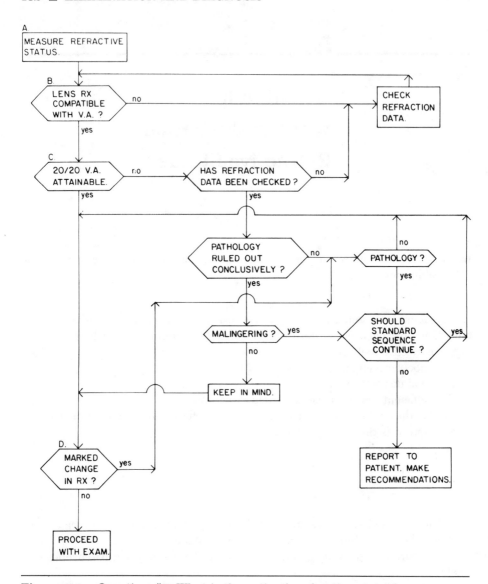

Figure 5.1   Question #5: What is the patient's refractive status?

■

THE REFRACTIVE STATUS
OF CHILDREN

□ First Year of Life

SPHERICAL REFRACTION

Healthy, normal, full-term neonates are likely to be hyperopic. Virtually all reports indicate that. What is not so well agreed upon is the amount of hyperopia they will normally display.

One investigator, Goldschmidt (1), for example, analyzing data from a sample of 356 newborns, cites a mean refraction of +0.60D (S.D. = 2.2), while another study by Gonzales (2), involving 83 neonates, reports a mean of +2.60D (S.D. = 1.9). More recently, Zonis and Miller (3), reporting on 300 Israeli newborns—the offsprings of mothers from different ethnic backgrounds (Sephardic, Ashkenazic, Arab)—found a mean refractive state of +1.10D (S.D = 1.6). Banks (4) combined the data from 11 different reports dating from 1892 to 1974, including the three cited above, comprising a total of 3057 children ranging in age from 1 day to 10 days, and calculated a mean refractive state of +2.00D (S.D. = 2.0; range of means = from + .0.60D to +2.60D). Banks noted also that the distribution of these data conformed to a binomial, or "normal," curve.

In sum, then, it appears that most full-term, normal children are moderately hyperopic at birth—somewhere between emmetropia and 3 diopters—with the main sources of variance being their parentage and the measurement method used to determine the refraction.

PREMATURE NEWBORNS

Infants whose birth-weights are less than 2500 g do not present a similar picture. They usually are neither quite so hyperopic nor so normally distributed. Banks (4), combining the data from four reports (N = 487) (5, 6, 7, 8), calculated a mean refraction of approximately +0.87D, accompanied by a broad variance (S.D. of means = 2.7; range of mean = −1.30D to +1.10D). Representative among these is a study by Scharf and associates (8), based on 353 eyes (177 newborns; one congenital cataract) of children whose respective birth-weights ranged between 1000 and 2500 g. They found approximately 45 percent to be myopic (ranging from −1.00D to −10.00D; mode = −4.00D) and the others to be either emmetropic or moderately hyperopic (ranging up to +5.00D; mode = −1.00D), with no apparent relationship between birth-weight and refraction. (It is also worth noting that, as the premature, myopic children in this study grew, they tended to become less myopic. Eighty of the babies were reexamined at the age of six months; 25 of the 65 originally myopic eyes had become emmetropic, while most of the remaining myopes showed at least some shift toward emmetropia.) Similar data have been reported by other investigators (9,10), and one has also noted that many prematurely born children continue to show evidence of visual deficits when they reach adolescence (11).

ASTIGMATISM

The prevalence of astigmatism in newborns appears to be a less firmly established statistic. On the one hand, there are reports that claim astigmatism to be "exceedingly rare in children under the age of six years," (Payne [12], as cited in [13], p. 158; [14]), while others report a very high prevalence of astigmatism in the first year of life (as much as 45 percent [15]) and point out that in the vast majority of those manifesting astigmatism at this age, it is against the rule (16,17,18). (Most of these reports are based on randomly drawn samples comprising mainly white children. There is clear evidence of astigmatism being even more prevalent—and permanent—among certain other racial groups; e.g., American Indians [19].)

Two relatively recent studies bear special mention, both because of their findings and the novel methods they employed to measure astigmatism in babies. Howland and his group (20) observed that 50 percent of the newborns they examined (N = 15) by means of a photorefraction procedure showed more than 0.75D astigmatism, whereas, in contrast, they found only 8 percent prevalence among the adults (N = 26) they tested with the same procedure.

Mohindra and her collaborators (21) cite about a 20-percent prevalence of 1.00D or more astigmatism among their newborns (N = 17) and a surprising 40 percent in their 1-to 10-week-old group (N = 86). Their method (near retinoscopy) was less unique than Howland's. It is a variation of the standard retinoscopy procedure that, according to Mohindra, yields findings very similar to what one measures with standard cycloplegic refraction methods. (Near retinoscopy procedure is described later in this chapter.)

By the age of 1 year, the prevalence of astigmatism appears to diminish. For example, both Howland and Mohindra, in their aforementioned studies, observed a reduction in mean astigmatic error at age 1, even though the prevalence figures from both groups tended to remain about the same as they were with the newborn group. Ingram and Barr (22) reported a 29 percent prevalence of astigmatism (1.00D or more) among this age group. Finally, Atkinson and colleagues (23) reported a marked falling off in the prevalence of astigmatism among children between the ages of 12 and 18 months. Thus, whatever the cause, it appears that astigmatism is not uncommon among children during their first year of life but tends to be much less common as they grow older (24).

ANISOMETROPIA

Anisometropia appears to be relatively common among very young children, although this statement is based on skimpy data drawn from just a few sources. Zonis and Miller (3), for example, report that 17.3 percent of the 300 Israeli newborns they examined manifested significant anisometropia (more than 1.00D), while Ingram and Barr (22), reporting on 1-year-olds, found anisometropia in about 8 percent of the group they studied.

□ Three- to Five-Year-Olds

SPHERICAL REFRACTION

Relatively little normative data have been published about this age group, but what is available suggests a continuation of the trend that was noted among the younger children. For example, Ingram and Barr (22) report a mode refraction among their 3 1/2-year-olds of approximately $+0.50D$, with significantly reduced variance as compared with the distribution obtained from the same children when they were 1-year-olds. Thus we note that the distribution that, at birth, conformed to a normal curve commences to be leptokurtotic—peaked—and slightly skewed in the direction of hyperopia.

ASTIGMATISM

Here, again, Ingram and Barr's data (22) are helpful. They report approximately 8 percent prevalence of astigmatism among a group of 3 1/2-year-olds. This is far less than the 29 percent they found among the same children when they were 1-year-olds. The report states: "There is quite clearly a highly significant decrease in the incidence of astigmatism both in individual eyes and in the number of children who have astigmatism of $+1.50D$ or more in either or both eyes" (p. 341). This is consistent with Howland's observation (23) that "many individuals must lose their astigmatism between the age of one year and later childhood" (p. 332). It also appears to be supported by Woodruff (24), who reported a relatively low prevalence of astigmatism in 3-year-old children.

ANISOMETROPIA

Ingram and Barr (22), reporting on 186 English children who were examined at age 1 year and again when they were 3 1/2 years old, found about 7 percent to be anisometropic at both ages. It is noteworthy, however, that although the prevalence statistics remained quite stable over those 2 1/2 years, the makeup of the group did not. Among the twelve 1-year-olds with anisometropia, only five continued to display it at age 3 1/2, and eight children who were anisometropic at 3 1/2 had not been when they were 1 year old.

□ Six- to Ten-Year-Olds

Hirsch (13, p. 149), in comparing the refractive status of newborns (25) with children between the ages of 6 to 8 (26), identified two "clear trends" that characterize the changes that occur in refraction of 6-year-olds when compared with newborns:

1. A one diopter reduction in hyperopia; he cites a newborn mean of $+2.07D$ as contrasted with a mean of $+1.00D$ for the young schoolchild.

2. A marked decrease in variability. Standard deviation for the newborn is 2.73; for the young schoolchild, it is 1.62.

Others also have reported pertinent data on this age group. In essence, they corroborate Hirsch's observations, not only in regard to spherical refraction but to astigmatism and anisometropia as well (27,28).

□ Adolescence

At this stage, the distribution of spherical refraction continues to show a marked leptokurtosis, but it is now skewed negatively. In other words, most adolescents are relatively emmetropic, but those who are not are more likely to be myopic than hyperopic (27). Once again, Hirsch (29) offers some pertinent information, reporting that among a sample of about 200 children examined at ages 5 to 6 years and again 8 years later, at ages 13 to 14: (a) all who were myopic at ages 5 to 6 continued to be myopic 8 years later; (b) about half of the 185 who were emmetropic at ages 5 to 6 had become myopic by ages 13 to 14, a few manifested hyperopia, and the remainder continued to be emmetropic; (c) about 20 percent of those who were hyperopic at ages 5 to 6 were myopic 8 years later, another 20 percent were emmetropic, and the remainder continued to manifest hyperopia.

In summing up these data, Grosvenor (30) cites Hirsch's conclusions as follows:

1. If a child is myopic at ages 5 to 6, the myopia is sure to remain and will probably increase.

2. If a child is more than 1.50D hyperopic at ages 5 to 6, she is very likely to remain hyperopic at ages 13 to 14, but perhaps of a lesser magnitude.

3. If a child has a spherical refraction between $+0.50$ and $+1.25D$ at ages 5 to 6, she has the greatest chance of being emmetropic at ages 13 to 14.

4. A child having a spherical refraction between 0.00 and $+0.50D$ at ages 5 to 6 has a high probability of becoming myopic by ages 13 to 14; the probability is even greater if against-the-rule astigmatism is present.

□ Summary

A retrospective inspection of the patterns of change in the refractive states of children from birth to adolescence reveals a clear trend. Stated simply, the distribution of spherical refraction for newborns tends to assume a Gaussian curve, a normal distribution, although some investigators would argue that even at that age the curve is slightly leptokurtotic and skewed positively. The distribution for 6-year-olds shows a distinct leptokurtosis and a slight decrease in the positive skewedness. In other words, as children mature, between birth and age 6, variance in refractive states reduces markedly, with far fewer moderate hyperopes and myopes being evident than there are among the newborns. The trend continues so that, by adolescence, although emmetropia continues to be prevalent, myopia is more common than hyperopia, and the number of high myopes exceeds the number of high hyperopes (13).

This phenomenon—a marked increase in the prevalence of emmetropia and a reduction in variance—has been termed "emmetropization" (31; as cited in Hirsch, 13). It will be discussed more fully in the next section. At this point, however, it is useful to introduce an interesting, tentative explanation for emmetropization that has been offered by Glickstein and Millodot (32). They point out that since retinoscopy is based on light reflected from the retina, the accuracy of a retinoscopic measurement depends upon the proximity of the retina's reflecting and receptive layers. The greater the distance between the two, the larger the measurement error. They then go on to explain that because the reflective layer of the retina lies anterior to the receptor layer, an overestimation of hyperopia results. This is especially so in the short eyeball of the newborn, where the separation between the two layers is relatively greater than it would be in a larger eye. Millodot and O'Leary (33,34), on the basis of this, suggest that the average newborn may, in fact, be emmetropic despite what the retinoscope reveals.

Their explanation, however, does not appear to apply to the premature infant data cited earlier (8). Thus, although it warrants mention, the hypothesis falls short of providing a satisfactory explanation for the phenomenon of emmetropization wherein a reduction in myopia is noted during the first year of postnatal life.

■
FACTORS THAT INFLUENCE REFRACTIVE STATUS

Traditionally, ametropia was attributed to axial length. Short eyes were linked with hyperopia; long eyes with myopia; eyes of the "correct" length were destined to be emmetropic. To this was added the notion that some ametropia was caused by one of the refractive elements of the eye, other than axial length, being too "strong" or too "weak." Hence the emergence of the classifications: axial and refractive ametropias, and the concept that there was a "normal" or ideal axial length, a normal corneal power, and so on:

Early in this century, Steiger (35) proposed that the refractive states of a randomly drawn normal sample of humans would distribute as a normal curve. He based his proposition on the observation that healthy, normal-appearing corneas varied from 39D to 48D, distributing in conformance with a Gaussian curve. No single power within this range necessarily signaled either emmetropia or ametropia. He reasoned that all of the refractive elements of the eye would follow this familiar biological pattern, and, thus, if they were combined at random, the total refraction of a randomly drawn sample of eyes would also display similar normal variability.

As already noted, the data do not support Steiger's hypothesis. The distribution of refractive states among children beyond the infancy stage does not conform to a normal curve; it is leptokurtotic. That is, there are far too many emmetropes in comparison with ametropes, and there are far more high myopes than there are high hyperopes among persons beyond the age of 8 or 10 years.

Later, Tron (36) measured the anterior chamber depths of a number of eyes, along with corneal powers and lens surfaces and thicknesses, and, from these, computed axial length, using Gullstrand's index of refraction for the lens. His data showed a normal distribution for all elements except axial length; and even that element distributed along a Gaussian curve when all very myopic eyes (greater than $-6.00D$) were excluded from the sample.

By 1946, a procedure had been developed to measure axial length with x-ray. Stenstrom (37) measured 1000 adult right eyes with this procedure and, like Tron, showed that axial length was not normally distributed but did assume such a curve when all eyes showing fundus changes characteristic of high myopia (myopic crescents, for example) were excluded from the sample.

In essence, these studies support the following statements:

1. Corneal powers vary normally, with the vast majority ranging from 39D to 47.6D.

2. Anterior chamber depths vary normally, with the vast majority ranging from 2.5mm to 4.2mm.

3. Lens powers vary normally, with the vast majority ranging from 15.5D to 23.9D.

4. Axial lengths vary normally *in eyes with total refractive states between $-6.00D$ and $+4.00D$*, with the vast majority ranging from 22mm to 26mm. If ametropic eyes beyond $+4.00D$ and $-6.00D$ are included in the sample, however, then the distribution departs from the Gaussian curve.

In effect, then, most eyes are emmetropic by virtue of being "fully coordinated" (38,39). That is, emmetropia derives from a combining of compatible corneal power, lens power, anterior chamber depth, and axial length. When ametropia occurs, it may be due to a correlation error (a breakdown in the aforementioned emmetropization phenomenon) or to one or more deviant components. The former, known as *correlation ametropia*, results from a condition where all the components fall within normal ranges yet the combination yields ametropia, typically ranging between $+4.00D$ and $-6.00D$. The latter, known as *component ametropia*, derives from a condition where one or more of the optical elements falls outside the normal range. Most often, this is due to axial length and, again most often, the amount of ametropia is marked: greater than $+4.00D$ or $-6.00D$. Thus, the alternative ametropia classifications: physiological and pathological (40).

A new classification system for myopia recently has been proposed by Grosvenor (41), who argues that systems based on etiological assumptions (e.g., component vs correlation, functional vs structural) interfere with our ability to understand myopia. He proposes, instead, that myopia be classified according to age of onset: (a) congenital; (b) youth onset; (c) early-adult onset; (d) late-adult onset. This appears to be compatible with some of the research that has been published lately in respect to certain differences among refractive groups (42,43,44).

□ Etiology and Pathogenesis of Ametropia

Many etiologies have been proposed. Some investigators argue that refractive status is genetically determined. Others contradict, and seek to show the prevailing influences of environment. The evidence to support either argument to the exclusion of the other is not substantial (45). It seems probable that there are many etiologies. Indeed, heredity does seem to influence an individual's refractive status, but is not independent of the influence of prenatal, perinatal, and postnatal environmental factors.

Listed below are some of the currently held rationales for ametropia.

HEREDITY

There are a number of studies that seem to indicate a strong link between heredity and refractive status (46,47,48). The most compelling arguments for the influence of heredity on refractive state are based on twin studies. Starting with Jablonski (49), there is an accumulation of data showing a significantly higher degree of concordance in uniovular twins than in binovular twins. In other words, the refractive states of a pair of monozygotic twins is much more likely to be the same, or at the least similar, than is the case with fraternal twins. Hoste (50) corroborated Jablonski, drawing his data from 60 pairs of uniovular and 60 pairs of binovular twins. Wixson (51) found +0.99 correlations in the spherical refractive status of a cohort of identical twins, +0.67 with fraternal twins, and +0.54 between siblings. Sorsby and associates (52) followed up with a study comprising 78 uniovular and 40 binovular twins of the same sex. Not only did their data support Jablonski's earlier observations regarding the greater likelihood of uniovular twins manifesting similar refractive states, but Sorsby's group also showed that the separate optical elements of uniovular twins were more alike than those of binovular twins. More recent twin studies (53) continue to echo what is cited above. One of these is particularly interesting in that it reports the refractive data derived from a set of triplets, age 6, two of whom are monozygotic twins while the third is fraternal (54). The monozygotic pair are remarkably similar in their physical characteristics—height, weight, refractive error (both manifest significant myopic astigmatism and anisometropia of very similar magnitudes), axial length, and so on. Their sister, the third child, displays hyperopic astigmatism. Data such as these are difficult to explain except on the basis of heredity.

Many of these aforementioned studies, however, also showed that discordance among uniovular twins is hardly rare. True, monozygotic twins often do reveal very similar refractive states but this is by no means invariant. Many uniovular twins differ markedly in their refractions. In fact, this occurs often enough to temper the enthusiasm of those who try to explain refractive status solely on the basis of genetic factor.

ENVIRONMENTAL FACTORS

Prenatal
Gardiner and James (55) linked myopia with maternal illness during pregnancy. Their argument is weakened, however, by the fact that approximately 40 percent of the myopic infants in their study were born premature and/or had a familial history of myopia.

Perinatal
Myopia and premature birth have been shown to be closely interrelated. In addition to the already cited studies, there are reports by Birge (56), Fletcher and Brandon (57), and others. Indeed, Curtin (58), citing Weekers and colleagues (59), points out that prematurity has been acknowledged as a primary factor in the discordance of refraction in uniovular twins.

Postnatal
Acquired Systemic Disease. Myopia has been associated with syphilis, tuberculosis, and hypothyroidism (58), as well as such childhood febrile diseases as measles and scarlet fever. Collagen disorders stemming from disturbances in enzyme control also have been implicated by some investigators (28, pp. 72–75).

Glaucoma. Infantile glaucoma often results in axial elongation and a resultant myopia. Such changes in refraction are well documented among older children (60,61,62).

Nutrition. Gardiner (63) cites evidence that, he proposes, links the development of myopia to diets lacking in sufficient protein.

Functional: Use-Abuse
Many investigators have pointed out a close relationship between myopia and prolonged close work (46,47,64,65,66). Even within this group, however there is disagreement over the source of myopia due to excessive close work.

Sato (67), for example, proposed that the myopia that stems from prolonged close work is attributable to an increase in the refractive power of the crystalline lens.

Otsuka and Kondo (68) focused on the hypertonicity of the ciliary muscle and reasoned that the increased ciliary tonus imposes excessive stress on the choroid. This, in turn, produces such myopia-related pathologies as chorioretinal degeneration and scleral atrophy.

Young (69,70,71,72) and others (73) offer a variation of this explanation, suggesting that myopia caused by excessive close work is due to the fact that the intraocular pressure increases as the eye accommodates. Hence, excessive close work means extended periods of elevated intraocular pressure, which, in the young, relatively plastic eye can lead to increased axial length. Young (74) produced myopia in a group of monkeys by placing them in hoods that limited their gaze to nearpoint and cites this as evidence in support of his proposition. Young also has published data showing that myopia is much more prevalent among Barrow (Alaska) Eskimo children than it is among their parents (75). He attributes this to the relatively recent advent of compulsory education in that community. His argument is that with the arrival of this new phenomenon, regularly scheduled school for all children—something their parents were spared—comes the inevitable: myopia due to excessive close work.

Van Alphen (76) poses an intriguing theory that combines genetic and environmental influences. He reanalyzed Strenstrom's data (37), using single order and multivariate procedures and ultimately identified three basic (statistical) factors that relate to refractive status.

One, Factor S, pertains to the inherent differences in the size of the eye. It operates in corneal power and axial length and does not contribute to the variance of anterior chamber depth, lens power, or, indeed, total refractive power of the eye. In short, Factor S simply attests that there is naturally derived difference in eyesize; that large eyes tend naturally to have flat corneas. Van Alphen suggests that Factor S is a "growth" factor, largely determined by genetic influences, and includes in his arguments evidence regarding the inheritability of corneal curvature and corneal diameter.

A second factor, Factor P, represents an underlying interrelationship among axial length, anterior chamber depth, and lens thickness. Van Alphen terms this a "stretch" factor and reasons that it supports the notion of a mechanism, independent of inherent (and inherited) differences in globe size, which causes the eye to stretch, to adjust axial length to total refractive power.

The third factor, Factor R, loads on all of the ocular component variables and represents the extent to which stretch is compatible with total refractive power: the degree of emmetropization.

Van Alphen uses these three factors to propose a theory of emmetropia/ametropia. In doing so, he makes two assumptions, offering some experimental evidence to suport the first and some correlation-based speculations for the second.

The first assumption: ciliary muscle tone is reflected in the tension of the choroid: contraction of the ciliary muscle pulls the choroid forward. (This is no longer so speculative. See [77,78,79].) Intraocular pressure on sclera elevates as the tension of the ciliary muscle-choroid layer is relaxed. Therefore, a reduced ciliary muscle tone results in elevated intraocular pressure, which, in turn, causes a nonrigid (young) sclera to stretch. (Simultaneously, a relaxed ciliary muscle-choroid layer results in a posterior displacement of the iris diaphragm, thereby causing a deepening of the anterior chamber and, at the same time, a flattening of the lens; i.e., Factor P.)

The second assumption: ciliary muscle tone plays a central role in the self-focusing (emmetropization) process wherein the hyperopic newborn's eye expands until the axial length corresponds properly with total refractive power. Ciliary muscle tone is controlled by both parasympathetic and sympathetic nervous systems. Hence, the emmetropization process might well be affected by psychological factors; emotional stress might impact on refractive state on the basis of its intimate linkage with the sympathetic nervous system. He cites certain correlational evidence to support this thesis.

In other words, the assumptions propose that the growing hyperopic eye of the young child will continue to grow in length so as to maintain appropriate correlation with the other optical elements of the eye. The key determinant in stopping the growth process is not genetically determined; rather it is the clarity of the retinal image, as registered in the visual cortex. As evidence of this, Van Alphen points out that eyes with inborn structural faults that prohibit clear acuity, such as congenital corneal astigmatism, rarely end up emmetropic. (Since then, others have contributed evidence supportive of this position [80,81,82].) Hence, reduced ciliary muscle tone has two effects. One, the emmetropic eye will behave as hyperopic when the ciliary muscle is not being stimulated. Second, when ciliary muscle tone is reduced, the eye is more vulnerable to the stretching influence of elevated intraocular pressure. These two effects, in combination, predict an eye that stretches to the point where it is myopic and/or the sclera becomes less plastic through maturation.

Since the publication of the Van Alphen monograph, a number of investigators have focused their efforts on studying the potential links between accommodation and myopia, paying special attention to: (a) the connection between accommodation and elevated intraocular pressure in the vitreous chamber and the impact of this phenomenon on the eventual size and shape of the globe; (b) the potential contribution of tonic (dark focus) accommodation to the development of myopia; (c) the interacting roles of the sympathetic and parasympathetic nervous systems in ocular accommodation. These studies have demonstrated that (a) intraocular pressure does increase in the vitreous chamber when the eye accommodates (73, 83); this, in turn, causes the eye to stretch, but only along the anterior-posterior axis (84); (b) there appears to be a relationship between an individual's refractive status and tonic accommodation (TA): late-onset myopes typically demonstrate lower TA than do hyperopes, emmetropes, and early-onset myopes (44,85); (c) the ciliary muscle is innervated by both the sympathetic and parasympathetic nervous systems, with the sympathetic input being mediated by inhibitory beta receptors (86).

One proposed role of the sympathetic system is to attenuate excessive shifts in the TR accommodative state produced by sustained near-vision tasks (86). As such, sympathetic innervation—in conjunction with parasympathetic—is presumed to play a significant role in determining an individual's TA status (87). Bullimore and Gilmartin investigated the influence of a cognitive demand on the TA of emmetropes and "late-onset" myopes and observed that a cognitive task (backward counting) induced a positive shift in TA that was significantly greater in the myopic group than it was in the emmetropic group (88). They interpreted this as an indication that individuals with relatively high values of TA have a sympathetic facility that is augmented by substantial levels of concurrent parasympathetic activity.

McBrien and Millodot (85) also showed a strong correlation between the accommodative response gradient and refractive error, thereby again suggesting that hyperopes accommodate more to a particular near target than do emmetropes or myopes. They, too, interpret their observations in the context of dual-innervation of the ciliary body.

Green (89) also focused on the relationship between intraocular pressure and myopia, but from a different viewpoint. He suggests that it is transmural pressure that weakens scleral fibers, thereby allowing a detrimental increase in "creep rate," which Green, a bioengineer, relates to a stretching of the globe. (Green defines transmural pressure as the difference between intraocular and intraorbital pressures.) According to Green, when an individual accommodates, tension on the choroid increases, intraocular pressure elevates, pressure in the suprachoroid space decreases, and intraorbital pressure rises, thus placing the sclera under *compressive stress*. Then, as the situation reverses, the sclera experience *tensile stress*. This fluctuation between tensile and compressive stress eventually weakens the scleral tissue, just as bending a piece of sheet metal back and forth weakens the metal. The result? When the scleral tissue has been sufficiently weakened, the globe is more susceptible to stretching.

Thus far, no major "breakthroughs" have been achieved in revealing the key causal links between refractive status and underlying visual processes, but it is plain that the speculations of van Alphen were closer to the mark than they were thought to be when he originally expressed them.

_____ ■ _____

A. MEASURE THE REFRACTIVE STATUS

□ Child-Appropriate Methods for Measuring Refractive Status

As pointed out in the introduction to this book, we make the assumption that the reader comes to these pages already familiar with standard procedures for the clinical management of adult patients. This volume is intended to provide whatever additional information is needed for the effective clinical care of children too young to be treated as adults. As such, the material that follows does not deal with standard, adult appropriate methods. Rather, these will be either modifications of standard procedures or techniques that are not customarily used with adults, but that may be useful with children because of the malleable quality of the young eye.

OPHTHALMOMETRY

The standard ophthalmometer is appropriate for most school-aged children. This is not the case, however, with the very young child or with the older child who is unable to maintain the posture required by the instrument. In those cases, a hand-held, albeit less precise, instrument is needed: one that exploits the principles of the ophthalmometer without imposing so many demands.

Placido Disc

The initial version of the keratoscope is attributed to Goode ([90], reported by Borish [45]). It used a small, luminous square as the stimulus. The examiner simply investigated the reflection of this stimulus from the cornea. Placido (91) subsequently developed a similar instrument that took the form of a flat disc on which appeared black and white concentric rings. This design was universally accepted and continues to be identified with its designer, as the *placido disc*. In its current form, the placido disc usually is 16 cm in diameter and comprises 10 black and white alternating concentric rings. There is a small aperture in the center of the disc. Ordinarily, the device contains no illumination source. It depends, instead, on external illumination, such as a lamp placed behind the patient so that it will illuminate the face of the disc.

Illuminated Keratoscope

A keratoscope is nothing more than a placido disc with a built-in source of illumination. It tends to be somewhat smaller (about 7.5 cm in diameter) than the standard placido disc, with the power supply located in a handle designed to house flashlight batteries. This instrument provides flexibility not available in the basic instrument and therefore warrants inclusion in the examiner's inventory of instruments (see Figure 5.2).

Also worth considering is a relatively uncomplicated and inexpensive photokeratoscope that has been described by Sivak (92). It is an adaptation of the keratoscope that makes use of a standard 35mm camera to record keratoscopic reflections from the patient's cornea.

RETINOSCOPY

The retinoscope can be used in various ways with young patients. In this section the following procedures are considered:

1. Static retinoscopy
   a. Manifest
   b. Cycloplegic
2. Dynamic retinoscopy
   a. Book retinoscopy
   b. Bell retinoscopy
   c. Monocular Estimate Method (MEM)
   d. Chromoretinoscopy
   e. Near retinoscopy

Figure 5.2
The keratoscope.

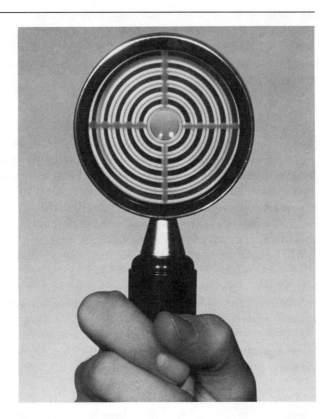

Static Retinoscopy

Manifest (or physiological) and cycloplegic (or pharmocological) retinoscopy methods differ in how the examiner attempts to control the influence of ocular accommodation on the test outcomes. In the latter method, of course, accommodation is essentially eliminated with a drug. In the former, accommodation is controlled with appropriately positioned fixation targets and "fogging lenses." Therefore, the section devoted to manifest retinoscopy will pay special attention to effective fixation targets and other aspects of the procedure that can have impact on the accuracy of test outcomes, while the section devoted to cycloplegic refraction will focus on the clinical application of cycloplegic drugs with young children.

Manifest Retinoscopy. The effectiveness of this procedure, assuming basic competency from the examiner, depends on how completely the patient's ocular accommodation is inhibited. This, of course, translates into the extent to which the patient can be induced to maintain fixation on some farpoint target through a lens-induced binocular blur. As such, the examiner's speed and the interest value of the fixation target are critical factors. Clearly, the longer the time required to complete the procedure and/or the weaker the interest value of the fixation target, the greater the likelihood that the patient will exercise some ocular accommodation or, in some other way, become less able, or less inclined, to co-operate fully in the activity.

What constitutes an effective fixation target and what procedural adaptations have been found to be useful in reducing the time required to complete a manifest retinoscopy?

Fixation Targets.   Because fixation on a point closer than 6 meters will stimulate accommodation, it is immediately evident that shorter-than-6-meter examination rooms should be equipped with appropriately positioned mirrors.

But more than fixation distance should be considered. Young children are very distractible, and there is much to distract them in a typical optometrist's examination room. Simply directing the child to "look at the chart across the room" is insufficient, even if the room is completely darkened. The retinoscope bulb, in itself, is a powerful distractor and will usually capture the child's attention. Interesting fixation targets are essential.

What are the characteristics of an "interesting" fixation target? It should be:

1. Visible. Use targets that are large, very easy to see.
2. Meaningful. Select things that the child can recognize, name, and discuss to some degree.
3. Sufficiently detailed so that the examiner can stimulate the patient's attention by posing questions, yet not so complex that it confuses the child or elicits accommodation.

Closed-loop cartoon films, comic-book slides, simple line-drawing slides, stuffed animals, and toys are useful. All of these have been found to be effective in helping children maintain fixation on some specified far point, particularly if the examiner is able to initiate a conversation relevant to the target while he conducts his retinoscopic examination.

For example, suppose you show the child a projected line drawing of a "gingerbread man." Such queries as, "What do you see?" "How many buttons on his tummy?" "Is he wearing shoes?" "Is he happy or sad?" "Is he sitting down or standing up?" are useful devices for engaging the child in the behavior you require from him.

Hand-held Lenses.   As already noted, it is important to carry out the procedure simply and rapidly. This implies very little dependency on such devices as a phoropter or even a trial frame. The former is too cumbersome and large. It may enhance speed, but it takes the child out of the examiner's direct view, thereby tending to introduce complications that erode the reliability of the test results. The latter tends to be unstable and uncomfortable, at best.

Some practitioners suggest the use of a pair of child's-size spectacles (e.g., Rx: +1.50D spheres, O.U.) that the youngster can wear during retinoscopy. This may be useful if the frames are comfortable, stay in place, and do not distract the child. Unfortunately, they often do not fit, are not comfortable, and do distract the child to the extent that instead of being a time-saver, they become a significant nuisance.

In most circumstances, the best all-purpose device for use with young children is a pair of trial lenses held in place by the examiner. This, in combination with being able to vary "working distances" and exploit the information derived thereby, will usually enable the examiner to complete the retinoscopy procedure within the limits of the child's ability to cooperate.

For example, in one hand, hold a pair of trial lenses (+1.50D or +2.00D— whichever you are accustomed to using) in front of the patient's eyes as she fixates the distance target. (Note: Remember, lenses must be placed before *both* eyes. There is no other way to prevent the child from exercising accommodation, short of cycloplegia, especially if the child is hyperopic [93].) Observe the retinoscopic reflex from your standard working distance. If something other than neutralization is observed, your options are obvious. Either substitute the lenses with a more suitable power, or change your position, moving closer to the child or away, as indicated. Changing positions will work very satisfactorily, within limits. Changing lenses becomes necessary only when a position change is insufficient to complete the retinoscopic examination, and even then taking measurements from different distances will reduce the number of lens changes you will have to make.

Cycloplegic Refraction. This procedure has certain distinct advantages, but it also has disadvantages. On the plus side, of course, is the control over accommodation that it provides. Fixation targets and distances are no longer important concerns. Hence, speed is not quite so critical a factor, although it does still count. On the other hand, cycloplegia is not without fault. An obvious one: it introduces potential danger into the situation. There is always the possibility that the child is sensitive to the cycloplegic agent, or that a latent galucoma will be made manifest. Granted, neither of these risks is high, but both do exist.

In addition, there are such concerns as determining the correct adjustment to be made for residual accommodation, and, perhaps just as important, the precluding of doing any nearpoint testing once the cycloplegic has taken effect.

In many cases, therefore, cycloplegic examination is not worth the time and effort. There are instances where it can be useful, however. As such, we will now consider a list of effective cycloplegic agents, their respective dosages, their special features, and those aspects of the examination that should be completed before the cycloplegic agent is administered (94).

Starting with the last topic on the list, the examiner should complete the following before instilling the cycloplegic agent (95):

1. Measure visual activity at all desired distances. The reason for this is self-evident.

2. Procure a thorough case history, paying particular attention to the child's medical history, especially his drug allergies. Do not overlook his emotional state

and its potential pertinence in light of the fact that certain emotionally disturbed patients will manifest psychomotor reactions to topical ocular drugs.

3. Examine the conjunctiva. Hyperemia is apt to increase systemic absorption of the drug through the conjunctiva.

4. Evaluate pupillary reflexes and make note of the normal pupil size under examination room illumination conditions.

5. Carry out a manifest refraction.

6. Assess accommodation function.

7. Assess binocular status.

8. Assess AC/A relationship.

9. Evaluate anterior chamber angle with a slit lamp.

10. Measure intraocular pressure.

Having done all this, and having observed no contraindicators, you may now select the appropriate drug. Bartlett cites the following characteristics as representative of a "clinically ideal cycloplegic" (96, p. 228):

1. Rapid onset
2. Full paralysis of accommodation
3. Sufficient duration to allow accurate assessment of refraction
4. Rapid recovery of accommodation
5. Dissociation of the cycloplegic effect from the mydriatic effect
6. Absence of local or systemic maleffects
7. Capacity for safe administration in the office by appropriate personnel

The most commonly used cycloplegic agents are the following:

Atropine sulphate solution   : 0.12% to 1.0%
Atropine sulphate ointment : 0.5% to 1.0%
Homatropine hydrobromide : 2.0% to 5.0%
Cyclopentolate (Cyclogyl)   : 0.2% to 2.0%
Tropicamide (Mydriacyl)   : 0.5% to 1.0%

For all practical purposes, atropine sulphate and cyclopentolate will meet the requirements of the optometrist (96). In fact, many authorities are inclined to take a very conservative position with regard to atropine sulphate, suggesting that it be used only with very young children who manifest strabismus. This, then, leaves cyclopentolate as the usual drug of choice. True, it is not as effective as atropine sulphate in inhibiting accommodation, but it is reasonably (and adequately) powerful and, in contrast to atropine, it is fast acting and relatively safe.

Dosage and Action. If the child is esotropic, use a 1.0% atropine sulphate ointment three times during the day before the examination. This is less than the classical dosage—three times a day for 3 days—but it is reported to be sufficient in most instances (97, p. 225).

You may administer one drop of 0.5% or 1.0% cyclopentolate solution, repeated in 5 or 10 minutes if needed. Children with fair complexions are apt to respond adequately to a single installation. Black children may require a slightly stronger dosage. Cyclopentolate will usually produce adequate cycloplegia within 45 to 90 minutes and will commence to lose effectiveness within 3 to 4 hours (98, p. 883).

Homatropine hydrobromide, a once-popular substitute for atropine, is no longer used very often because of the relatively poor cycloplegia it provides.

Tropicamide is a very fast acting mydriatic agent, but it does not inhibit accommodation sufficiently to satisfy the requirements for a cycloplegic examination.

Many examiners choose to enhance absorption of the cycloplegic by applying a topical anesthetic agent before instilling the cycloplegic drug (99). (Note: If a topical anesthetic agent is used in measuring intraocular pressure and if, as recommended, this is done before a cycloplegic agent is applied to the eye, then this discussion becomes superfluous. Clearly, there will be no need for additional anesthetic.) The drug most often selected: proparacaine hydrochloride 0.5%.

Adverse Drug Reactions. Adverse reactions to topically applied cycloplegic agents are usually either toxic or allergic (100). With atropine, allergic reactions may present as a contact dermatitis of the lids, manifesting erythema, pruritus, and edema. Papillary conjunctivitis and keratitis have also been noted. Allergic reactions to cyclopentolate are relatively mild and uncommon.

In regard to toxic reactions, atropine is capable of producing xerostomia, flushing of the face, hyperthermia, tachychardia, irritability, and delerium. These have often been paraphrased as "hot as a hare, red as a beet, dry as a bone, blind as a bat, mad as a wet hen." Hallucinations and ataxia have also been reported.

The toxic effects of cyclopentolate focus on the central nervous system, producing cerebellar dysfunction (e.g., dysarthria, ataxia, broad gait), hallucinations, confusion, disorientation, schizophrenia-like behavior, restlessness, apprehension, and anemia (101).

The best, but even then not foolproof, method for reducing the incidence of adverse drug reactions is to follow the preinstillation steps listed above. In addition, it is important to use as little of the drug as necessary, in its lowest concentration.

Dynamic Retinoscopy
Dynamic retinoscopy is used to measure the refractive status of the eye when it is fixating (accommodating) at nearpoint. The technique is especially useful with young children, in whom static retinoscopy is often not feasible. (Young children are rarely interested in fixating at distance when so much is going on right before their eyes.)

A number of ways have been proposed for carrying out dynamic retinoscopy. They are all similiar in that the patient is asked to fixate a nearpoint stimulus and keep it clear (i.e., exercise appropriate accommodation) while the examiner determines the lens power needed to "neutralize" the retinal reflex. Because the patient's eye and the plane of the retinoscope's mirror aperature are (theoretically) at conjugate points, no lens power adjustment for "working distance" is made. (Not all dynamic procedures provide this condition; see below.)

The procedures differ in how the neutral state is defined and in how one adjusts for at least some of the excess plus power (attributed to "lag of accommodation") that is measured under these circumstances. Sheard (102), for example, suggested beginning with the patient looking through his distance lens prescription—"with motion" is usually observed under these conditions—and adding plus lenses (O.U.) until "first (or "low") neutral" is observed. A standard deduction of 0.50D is then made (for lag of accommodation), and the remaining power represents the patient's proper nearpoint lens prescription. Tait (103), in contrast, advocated starting with excess plus power in place, reducing this until a "high-neutral" point is reached, and then adjusting for the lag of accommodation on the basis of a comparison between the patient's near and far phorias.

Others have proposed slightly different methods, but in essence, they are all very similar. All tend to overestimate plus (or underestimate minus) spherical power. Hence, if precise measures are required, the examiner must determine an adjustment that takes this into account. This is academic, however, when using dynamic retinoscopy with young children; precise measurements are not a great concern. The examiner's goal with young children is to determine whether or not they manifest sufficient refractive error to warrant lenses. This means that relatively low lens powers are not likely to be prescribed. Hence, the rule of thumb when determining how to use the information derived from dynamic retinoscopy, especially if (cycloplegic or noncycloplegic) static retinoscopy is impossible: If lenses are called for, then prescribe the power measured with dynamic retinoscopy. A 0.50D overcorrection will matter very little in such cases.

Book Retinoscopy

Book retinoscopy is a variation of dynamic retinoscopy. Like the latter, it involves the retinoscopic, evaluation as the patient fixates on a near-situated, accommodation-stimulating target. It differs from standard dynamic retinoscopy procedure in (a) where the fixation target is positioned, (b) what the examiner observes, and (c) how these observations are interpreted.

The term book retinoscopy first appeared in Gesell's report on the development of vision in young children (104) and since then in other publications (105,106). In its original form, the procedure consisted of three retinoscopic observations, one made from a distance of 15 feet, another from 7 feet, and the third from 20 inches, with the fixation target, in each instance, positioned adjacent to the examiner. The fixation target used at the 20-inch test distance (with children who could read) was a book; a picture book was used with younger children. Hence the name, book retinoscopy.

The goals of the procedure were to look for and record:

1. Relative brightness of the reflex, ranging from dull to bright
2. Color of the reflex, ranging from dull red to white

3. Speed, range, promptness, pick up and release motion (This refers to observations made as the child changed fixation from one point to another.)
4. Meridional differences

In discussing interpretation of these observations, Gesell suggested that "the evidence now available strongly indicates that the brightening and dulling of the retinal reflex is directly correlated with the activity of the higher nerve centers in the visual system" (104, pp. 184–85). He noted that the increased brightness characteristically occurred at the moment the child identified a target and went on to infer from this that the brightening could serve as an index of comprehension. The motion of the reflex was also perceived as signaling some "general state," probably best described as arousal. He observed that as "the child's eyes located the target, the reflex *brightened* and showed a *with* motion. When attention settled and held to the target, the motion became *against*. As the attention relaxed, there was a slow oscillation of *against*, to *with*, to *against*, until the attention withdrew entirely. The reflex then tended to revert to a basic dullness, which, in turn, disappeared with the next act of visual attention" (p. 177).

The color of the reflex was classified on a "five-step gradient": *dull red, dull pink, bright pink, white pink,* and *pink*. He speculated that color was related to "recognition and awareness" with the degree of "whiteness" being directly related to "cortical control," to the level of recognition and awareness.

Apell and Lowry (107) went on to publish a book retinoscopy "expecteds" for children from ages 21 months to 5 years, stating that the procedure produced results that changed in a predictable fashion as the children matured. They also presented book retinoscopy test outcomes that differentiated between "achievers" and "nonachievers," age 39 months and older, therein supporting Gesell's speculations regarding the link between "cortical control" and the degree of "whiteness" of the reflex observed during book retinoscopy.

Since then, research interest in the color of the reflex has waned, but there have been additional studies conducted relevant to reflex luminance changes.

Kruger, for example, published a number of papers relevant to differences in the brightness of the reflex in book retinoscopy (108,109,110,111). Initially, his goals were to

1. develop a photoelectric retinoscopy procedure that could record the luminance of the fundus reflex
2. determine whether the reflex does or does not change in luminance
3. provide preliminary data on the relationship between the luminance of the fundus reflex and different problem-solving tasks
4. investigate the cause of any luminance changes

Kruger produced an apparatus that was sensitive to luminance changes of less than 5 percent. (This is described in [109, p. 48].) He then went on to his other objectives, applying the apparatus with prepresbyopic adults as they engaged in various tasks under various conditions (e.g., solving mental arithmetic problems while under the influence of a cycloplegic as contrasted to noncycloplegic conditions; reading text of varying difficulty; reading lists of numerals as compared with solving addition problems). On the basis of these investigations, he concluded:

1. Relatively large changes in the luminance of the fundus reflex do occur during nearpoint visual activities.
2. A majority of trained clinicians are able to observe these luminance changes, especially if the magnitude of the changes is in excess of 10 percent.
3. Luminance of the fundus reflex increases in relation to the cognitive demands of the visual task. For example, the luminance of the fundus reflex was greater when the subject was engaged in solving addition problems than when he was simply reading numerals.
4. The observed increase in luminance of the fundus reflex is mediated by accommodation. Specifically, the increase in luminance is attributable to a decrease in accommodative lag.

Keller (112) also investigated the book retinoscopy procedure. He conducted a step-by-step analysis of the various phenomena noted by Gesell (i.e., brightness, color, etc.) and concluded that "it must be assumed that the observations of book retinoscopy are based entirely on the accommodative state of the eye being observed" (p. 487).

Bell Retinoscopy
The bell retinoscopy procedure was fist alluded to in the Gesell (104) study of vision development. The procedure calls for the examiner to be positioned 50 cm from the patient. The examiner's eye is aligned with the bridge of the patient's nose. A small metal cat-bell, suspended on a thin nylon thread, serves as fixation target; hence the name of the procedure. Initially, the examiner positions the bell against his forehead, so that is is 50 cm from the patient's eyes. It is then slowly brought closer to the patient. During all of this, the examiner monitors the retinoscopic reflex while the patient maintains' fixation on the approaching bell.
Although some early advocates of the procedure suggested that the color of the reflex also provided useful clinical data, the present consensus designates the main task of the examiner to be to record the distances (from the patient) at which the motion of the reflex changes: one measure to be taken as the bell approaches the patient: the other, as the bell is slowly moved back to its starting position.
A "normal response" has been described by Apell (113) as follows:

"A *with motion* should be seen at the start of the test, when the bell is 20 inches from the patient's eyes. It should change to an *against motion* when the bell is from 17 to 14 inches from the patient, and back to a *with motion* at 15 to 18 inches, as the bell is moved away from the patient. Usually, the change to an against motion occurs an inch closer to the patient than the shift from against to with" (p. 1025).

Apell also commented:

"The retinoscopic reflexes (even when normal) do not (necessarily) indicate the degree of flexibility or rigidity within the system. Probing with low plus spheres will help to determine the degree of flexibility. If, with plus lenses (usually + 0.50D spheres, O.U.), the test outcomes remain essentially the same (as they were without the lenses) but there is a smoother shift from one motion to the other, or a brighter reflex, or slight pupil dilation, then it is a sign of flexibility. However, if the shift to an against motion occurs before (at a distance greater than) 17 inches and the release is cut to 18 or 20 inches, or the reflex dulls, then rigidity is indicated" (113, p. 1025).

Apell described a variety of nonnormal responses and speculated on their relevance. Among these: (a) delayed shift to against motion—an indicator of "latent" need for additional plus; (b) always with motion—another indicator of a need for plus lenses for near: (c) always against motion—a myopic response: (d) astigmatic motion—perhaps an indication of astigmatism sponsored by convergence and accommodation; and (e) anisometropic motion—perhaps another version of a dynamically produced modification in refractive status.

Apell sums up his comments of the bell retinoscopy procedure by stating:

"Bell retinoscopy is a dynamic technique for investigating the individual's ability to align and focus his eyes under a natural seeing condition. It provides the examiner with insight into how this individual functions visually and provides a direction of probable optometric care" (p. 1027).

Thus far, no studies have been published regarding the clinical value of the procedure. It has not provoked critical comments in the literature, probably because it has never been widely used. Its advocates are apparently satisfied with its worth on the basis of their case-by-case experiences.

Monocular Estimate Method (MEM)

MEM was initially described by Haynes (114) (1960). It is a reliable (115) and valid (116) variation of the standard dynamic retinoscopy procedure. According to Beiber (117), its chief purpose is to "observe the child's spontaneous accommodative response to a detailed target presented at his customary working distance. The question being asked by the test is: 'Is the accommodative response equal to the accommodative stimulus?' In other words, is the visual system infocus, under-focused, or over-focused?" (p. 54).

MEM differs from standard dynamic retinoscopy in two ways. First, in the MEM, the testing distance is not the same for all patients; it is determined by the unique characteristics of the patient: his physical size or his preferred reading distance. In regard to the former, many clinicians choose to use the child's socalled "Harmon distance" as the testing distance (118). (Harmon distance refers to the distance from the child's elbow to his knuckle. Thus, testing may be done as close as 9 inches with small children.)

The second difference between MEM and standard dynamic retinoscopy: the examiner does not introduce lenses binocularly in an attempt to neutralize the retinoscopic reflex. Rather, he observes the reflex through the patient's habitual prescription (Plano, if the patient does not ordinarily wear glasses) and attempts to *estimate* the lens power that will neutralize the motion of that reflex. He then places a lens of this estimated power briefly before one eye and quickly assesses the accuracy of his estimate. The goal is to determine the patient's "natural" accommodative state without disrupting that state (see Figure 5.3).

The specific steps of the procedure (117, p. 55) are as follows:

1. Seat the patient comfortably.
2. Provide sufficient illumination to make possible the reading of small print when presented at nearpoint.
3. The examiner positions herself directly before the patient, but a trifle lower so that when the patient fixates the stimulus, his gaze is directed slightly downward, emulating a typical reading posture.
4. Direct the patient's attention to the fixation target. (The fixation target used most often is a 12 × 12 cm white card in which a centrally located 1.3-mm circular hole has been punched. The card contains printed words, or pictures, depending upon the patient's age and literacy. The card is held in a metal clip that attaches to the retinoscope in such a way that the retinoscope's light beam passes through the aperture in the card. This allows the examiner to make her observations from a position that is very close to the patient's visual axis.)

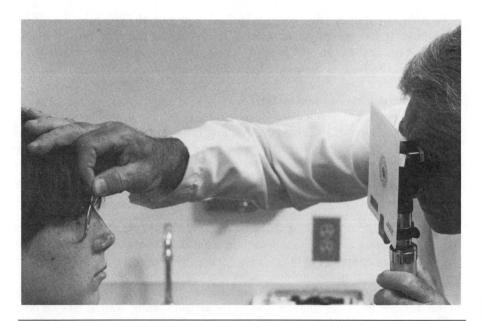

Figure 5.3 MEM retinoscopy.

5. The patient wears his habitual prescription. That is, if he usually wears glasses, he wears them during this test.

6. The examiner takes a position approximately 10 to 16 inches from the patient's eyes. Some optometrists prefer to use the Harmon distance (see above); others prefer to work from a set distance of their own choice.

7. The retinoscope beam is directed toward the bridge of the patient's nose and he is requested to read (or spell) the words on the target card; or, with nonreaders, to name the objects pictured on the card. As the patient does this, the retinoscope beam is moved quickly across the horizontal meridian of one eye, then the other. The examiner estimates the direction and approximate "power" of the reflex and, if desired, assesses the other meridians in a similar fashion.

8. A lens is placed in front of one eye that is equivalent in power to the estimate and the retinoscope reflex is reassessed. If this validates the estimate, the lens power is recorded. If it does not validate the estimate, the procedure is repeated with a more appropriate lens. For example, if the examiner initially, noted "with motion" of a moderate degree, she might hold a +0.50D sphere lens momentarily before one eye. Should this prove to be sufficient to neutralize the "with motion," she would record the test outcome as +0.50D. If, instead, the "with motion" persisted under this condition, she might select a +1.00D sphere lens for the next trial. If the retinoscope then revealed an "against motion," the examiner would probably record +0.75D as the test outcome and leave it at that, rather than prolong the test.

Most examiners are inclined to consider an MEM of +0.50D or +0.75D (115) as normal, attributing it to a lag of accommodation, a tendency for the accommodative mechanism to operate at less than maximum level. When the MEM shows a lag in excess of +1.00D, many optometrists consider prescribing some plus power, at least for near work.

In addition, over the past decade or so some optometrists have begun to measure MEM through contrived, provocative optical conditions; i.e., while the patient is looking through plus or minus lenses that are not warranted by refractive condition. Personal experience shows that patients do differ. In some, for example, the MEM outcome will remain unchanged despite relatively large changes in the optical conditions (e.g., patient shows 0.50D lag whether looking through own prescription, or through an additional +1.00D [O.U] and −1.00D [O.U.]. Others respond in an (optical bench) predictable manner. What these differences indicate has not yet been adequately defined, but they do exist and are worthy of investigation, particularly if one is at all influenced by Van Alphen's hypotheses (see above).

Chromoretinoscopy

This procedure is particularly relevant at this point in that its authors contend that it provides evidence for an alternative explanation for the lag of accommodation phenomenon (119,120). In essence, the technique involves measuring longitudinal chromatic aberration of the eye objectively, by combining retinoscopy with colored filters.

Specifically, they carried out static and dynamic retinoscopy measurements—the latter at 33 cm—through red and green filters (Kodak Wratten Filters Nos. 25 and 55) and compared these outcomes with the outcomes from standard (no filters) methods.

They found that red wavelengths are in focus on the retina during (farpoint) static retinoscopy and the green wavelengths during (nearpoint) dynamic retinoscopy. They based their explanation for the farpoint findings on the fact that the light provided by the retinoscope source, when reflected by the retina and filtered by the retinal blood vessels, has a dominant wave length very similar to what passes through the Kodak No. 25 (red) filter. They explained the nearpoint observations by proposing a "sparing of accommodation" phenomenon: that less accommodation is required to focus green wavelengths on the retina, thereby making it a reasonable occurrence for nearpoint fixation in an efficiently operating visual system.

Their original study (119) was conducted with adults. Later, they published the results of a study conducted with preschool-aged children (120). Here they reported the intriguing observation that although children age 4 years and above displayed the same characteristics as did the adults in their original report, children younger than 4 years did not show the ability to spare accommodation. In their cases, the red wavelengths were in focus on retina during both farpoint and nearpoint retinoscopy.

The implications of this observation have yet to be adequately examined. Obviously, it may have great clinical significance. Too little is now known, however, to warrant anything but interest and speculation.

Near Retinoscopy

Near retinoscopy, according to its author (121), is not a variation of dynamic retinoscopy. Rather, she maintains, it is a substitute for static retinoscopy. Her rationale: the fixation target, the retinoscope's light, when viewed monocularly in a darkened room, does not stimulate accommodation beyond that which is representative of the patient's dark-state accommodation, even when the light is positioned 20 inches from the patient's eye (122).

Mohindra has published reports that show an extraordinary high correlation between refraction as determined by this procedure and as determined by standard static retinoscopy procedures under both cycloplegic and manifest conditions ($r = .98$) (123). The procedure is conducted as follows:

1. Reduce room illumination as much as possible. Strive to obtain total darkness.

2. The examiner positions herself 20 inches from the patient. One of the patient's eyes is occluded, either by the examiner or by the patient himself or, in the case of infants, by the person holding the baby.

3. The patient is asked, or otherwise induced, to fixate the retinoscope light. (In the case of very young children, Mohindra advises that fixation will be enhanced

if the examiner produces interesting noises during the procedure. She also reports better success at eliciting sustained fixation from infants if the procedure is carried out while the child is being fed, speculating a "connection" between the sucking action and the palpebral muscles.)

4. Neutralize the retinal reflex in the two principal meridians with a lens bar or loose trial lenses.

5. Add an "adjustment factor" of $-1.25D$ to the lens power determined in step #4, above. Record this as the test outcome.

Mohindra initially justified the adjustment factor solely on the basis of empirical evidence. It appeared to be the predictable difference between findings obtained by near retinoscopy and findings obtained by static retinoscopy. Later, Owens and associates (122) proposed that the $-1.25D$ adjustment is derived by making a $-2.00D$ adjustment that takes into account the 20-inch working distance and then adding the $+0.75D$ on the basis of dark-state accommodation.

Recently, conflicting reports have appeared regarding the validity of this procedure. One team of investigators (124) carried out noncycloplegic near retinoscopy and standard cycloplegic retinoscopy on 311 children between the ages of 18 and 48 months. Their results indicated "little agreement between the two objective refraction methods." In contrast, another group (125) compared the two methods and concluded that "the two procedure produce essentially the same results." Why the conflicting conclusions? One explanation: Our experience with the near retinoscopy procedure has led us to believe that it yields reasonably valid information with young patients who are *not* hyperopic, but performs poorly with young hyperopes; we have observed as much as 5.00D underestimates of hyperopia when near retinoscopy results were compared with cycloplegic retinoscopy results. Hence, because the subjects of the latter study, cited above, were older, they were less apt to manifest latent hyperopia with noncycloplegic refraction than were the younger ones in the first study. This could very well explain the difference in conclusions.

Other procedures that might be useful and/or interesting:

Ophthalmoscopy. There may be times when the ophthalmoscope will be more effective than the retinoscope in obtaining an objective measure of the patient's refractive status (126). The procedure itself is self-evident: simply determine the lens power needed to obtain a focused view of the patient's fundus. Obviously, this provides a crude measure, but it is better than no measure at all. (In our view, it is a very rare situation where one was unable to obtain a measure with the retinoscope, yet was successful with the ophthalmoscope.)

Determining Tonic Accommodation with a Retinoscope. TA has become a topic of interest in recent years (see, for example, 127, 128, 129). It is as yet unclear just how these investigations will affect clinical thinking, but enough has been written to convince us that it should be mentioned here. Two procedures have recently been described for measuring TA with the retinoscope.

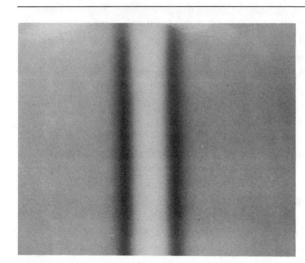

Figure 5.4
DOG target. (Photo
courtesy of C. Schor.)

One is near retinoscopy (see above). As documentation for this, the authors report high positive correlations between measures made with a laser optometer, an infrared optometer, and near retinoscopy (130). Unfortunately, their study did not include children. As noted above, the near retinoscopy procedure has not proven to be adequately valid with that age group—particularly with hyperopic children.

The other procedure employs a 0.2-cpd (cycles per degree) difference of Gaussian (DOG) fixation target (see Figure 5.4), which, when viewed in a dimly lit setting, "was found to be incapable of stimulating any reflex accommodation" (131, p. 437). TA is measured with Nott's dynamic retinoscopy procedure. This entails having the patient fixate the center of the DOG target (positioned at 40 cm) while the examiner, in lieu of using lenses, determines the distance from the patient where the retinoscope reveals "neutral" motion. The dioptric equivalent of the location of the retinoscope represents the patient's TA. For example, if the reflex is neutralized when the retinoscope is positioned 1 meter from the patient, then his TA is +1.00D.

SUBJECTIVE REFRACTION

Subjective refraction is, by definition, contraindicated with young children. The average child of 5 years or younger is much too influenced by distractors, and much too susceptible to language-sponsored confusion, to be viewed as a reliable reporter in a subjective examination. This leaves the examiner with no alternative but to measure the child's refractive status objectively, with a keratoscope and a retinoscope, and then assess the effect of the indicated lens prescription on visual acuity. (This last step, of course, is a form of subjective refraction. See Practical Suggestion 5-7.)

However, some more extensive subjective testing is possible with primary-grade children, and certainly a full-scale subjective procedure should be implemented with older children. There is no need to describe the standard subjective testing procedure here. But the potential value of certain binocular subjective refraction techniques is worth mentioning.

The central purpose of a binocular refraction is to obtain a prescription that balances the accommodative status of the two eyes. There are a variety of procedures for accomplishing this, two in particular that are useful with children age 5 and above. These are the Turville Infinity Balance (TIB) procedure and the AO Vectographic procedure. The former—the better of the two, in our opinion—uses a septum, positioned midway between the patient and the visual acuity chart, to control what each eye sees. The latter uses Polaroid filters, thereby making it sensitive to projection angle and room illumination. Hence our preference for the TIB. Both of these techniques have been fully described in journals as well as standard texts (see, for example, 132,133,134,135,136,137,138).

B. IS THE LENS PRESCRIPTION COMPATIBLE WITH THE VISUAL ACUITY MEASURES?

Once the patient's refractive status is determined, the optometrist faces two questions. First, does the patient demonstrate clear (20/20) acuity with the lens prescription derived from that assessment? Second, is the lens prescription compatible with the patient's visual acuity?

The first question is critical. If the patient's best corrected visual acuity is less than 20/20 in each eye, then some reasonable explanation must be established. It is not enough to simply record the data and go on. The reason for substandard visual acuity must be sought, identified if at all possible, and dealt with (see below for more discussion regarding this topic).

The second question is not so critical, but it is important. Prescribing lenses that are too strong is no more desirable than prescribing lenses that are too weak. The clinician strives to avoid both situations and, where possible, uses the subjective examination towards that end. But, as we have already observed, the subjective examinations of young children cannot be expected to yield reliable data. Thus, the optometrist has little to use to validate a lens prescription beyond its relationship with the patient's visual acuity.

Peters published data that are useful in this regard (139). It links visual acuity with refractive error (see Figure 5.5).

Figure 5.5 shows, for example, that a lens prescription of $-2.00D$, O.U., is not suspect for the patient with 20/200 uncorrected acuity, but should cause some doubts if the patient's unaided visual acuity is significantly better than that. Or, as another illustration, consider the myopic patient whose visual acuity through

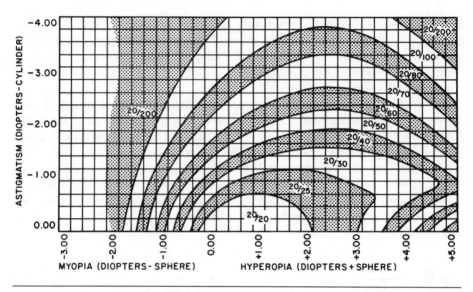

Figure 5.5 Relation between refractive error and visual acuity; age 5-15 (*N* = 2452) (from Peters HB. Relationship between refractive error and visual acuity at three age levels. AAAO 1961; 34 [8]:194).

his old lenses is 20/40 in each eye. What, according to the table, should the clinician do when he concludes that the patient needs an additional −1.50D spheres, O.U. in order to obtain 20/20 acuity in each eye? Obviously, he should recheck his data. That is simply too great a prescription change for the change in acuity.

In short, the information provided in Figure 5.5, though not helpful in determining a correct prescription, can be very helpful in alerting the optometrist to potential errors by revealing that the amount of lens power is not properly correlated with the amount of change in acuity derived from that power.

■
C. IS 20/20 VISUAL ACUITY ATTAINABLE IN EACH EYE?

Inevitably, some patients do not achieve 20/20 acuity in one or both eyes despite an accurate assessment of refractive status and provision of appropriate lenses. In such instances, the optometrist bears a responsibility for identifying the source of the acuity deficit or, at the least, establishing whether or not it is attributable to an active pathology. This process may ultimately require consultation with other professionals, but not until certain additional steps have been taken.

Ordinarily, a visual acuity deficit that does not respond to appropriate compensatory lenses stems from one of the following: (a) local or systemic pathology; (b) ocular structural deviation; (c) amblyopia caused by a refractive or binocular anomaly.

Therefore, unless the evidence indicates otherwise, the presence of an acuity loss that does not improve with proper lens application suggests that the optometrist should take the following actions, probably in the order shown here.

Consider the possibility of refractive amblyopia. The key indicators of refractive amblyopia are significant hyperopia and/or astigmatism combined with a history of delayed initial lens application. A so-called "critical period" has yet to be firmly established in humans but, acknowledging what is known about vision development in humans and nonhuman primates (140,141,142), it is safe to assume that such a phenomenon does exist. The child born with some impediment to clear eyesight faces the possibility of permanently reduced eyesight unless the impediment is removed, or in some way, neutralized, during the early stages of his life. How early is "early"? As already stated, presently that is moot, but one could reasonably argue that anything past the third birthday is no longer very early.

At this stage of the examination, the optometrist already has collected the pertinent information. He simply has to decide whether the patient's refractive status and case history could possibly constitute the basis for refractive amblyopia.

Consider the possibility of binocular misalignment. If the prescribed testing sequence of this book has been followed, the clinician will already have investigated this possibility. Binocular alignment was tested to some degree during the health assessment, when accuracy of fixation was determined by means of a stereoacuity test, a cover test, and perhaps some other instruments. It is appropriate to assume that the patient with relatively precise stereoacuity is not strabismic.

If stereoacuity was found to be substandard during the health assessment, it does not rule out the possibility of improved performance on the test once the refraction is completed. Refraction may have uncovered ametropia that could have affected performance on initial stereoacuity test. Obviously then, retesting will have to be done through the updated lens prescription.

Consider the possibility of malingering. See Chapter 3 for a discussion.

Reassess the patient's ocular health status, this time using the "secondary tests" that are not usually justified in an initial examination (also see [143,144]).

D. IS THERE A MARKED CHANGE IN REFRACTIVE STATUS?

Refractive status is changeable, but these changes are rarely precipitous. Therefore, when an abrupt change in refraction is noted, the optometrist has to consider all possible explanations and, ultimately, select one as being correct.

Abrupt changes in refraction are usually transient, most often in the direction of myopia (144). Listed below are the conditions that will come to mind when an abrupt change in a patient's refractive status is observed.

☐ Myopia

Diabetes Mellitus. This is the most common cause of transient myopia, the product of elevated blood sugar. Changes as great as 9 diopters have been reported. Adult patients are more vulnerable than children; fewer instances of diabetes-sponsored transient myopia have been reported among the younger group, but the possibility exists.

Drugs. Changes as great as 8 diopters have been reported in association with sulfa drugs. The myopia tends to decrease rapidly (ca. 5 days) but is apt to recur if the drug is reinstituted, even when there is a marked reduction in dosage. Diuretics such as Diamox or Hygroton, ACTH, corticosteroids, and acetylsalicylic acid have been known to cause transient myopia in some cases. Direct- and indirect-acting parasympathomimetics (miosis-producing) such as pilocarpine, neostigmine, phospholine iodide are also known to cause myopia.

Hysteria. When linked with ciliary muscle spasm, hysteria may be related to myopia.

Trauma. Trauma that causes lens damage, such as contusion or dislocation, may cause myopia. This may be permanent or transient, the former usually being due to traumatic mydriasis, lens opacities, and subluxation of the lens.

☐ Hyperopia

Drugs. Drugs, including antihistamines (e.g., Trimenton, Benadryl), systemic parasympatholytic agents (e.g., atropine sulfate, tincture of belladonna), topical parasympatholytic agents (e.g., atropine sulfate, tropicamide, cyclopentolate hydrochloride), and hypoglycemic agents that have been used to lower an elevated blood sugar have been linked to hyperopia.

Accommodative Paresis. Ocular trauma, ophthalmoplegia interna, and inflammation of the ciliary body can lead to hyperopia.

Ocular Trauma. Posterior dislocation of the lens, macular edema, and ciliary body contusion have been linked to hyperopia.

Orbital Tumor. Consider the possibility of orbital tumor with extraocular globe pressure and retinal striae when presented with a patient who has suddenly developed significant hyperopia.

Central Serous Retinopathy. This is another possible cause of sudden onset hyperopia in children.

■ PRACTICAL SUGGESTIONS

5-1. Line-drawing slides (e.g., snowman, bird, rabbit, ginger-bread man, etc.) are effective fixation targets for retinoscopy. They enable you to engage the child in conversation as you carry out the procedure (e.g., "Tell me when the bird turns red, . . . starts to fly, . . . etc.").

In lieu of this, a lighted spot located at distance can be used effectively with preschool children. Advise the child that the light is really emanating from a lighted "window," and that a dog, chicken, elephant, etc., is about to appear in the window. "Watch the window, and tell me *as soon as* you see the dog." The preschool child is likely to "see" the dog very quickly. Follow up on this with additional questions, such as "Is he a red dog or a blue dog?" "Is he a big dog or a small dog?" "Is the elephant there too?" (By this time, you should have completed retinoscopy.)

Another variation: Ask the child to tell you when the light turns a different color, starts to blink off and on, etc.

5-2. When conducting retinoscopy with a strabismic patient, it is advisable to occlude the eye not being examined so that you are not too far "off axis" with your retinoscope. In order to do this:

1. If retinoscopy is being done through a phoropter, simply position the instrument's occluder in front of the eye to be occluded.

2. If retinoscopy is being done with loose (hand-held) lenses, occlude the eye with the same hand that is holding the "fogging lens." For example, if you are measuring the refractive status of the patient's right eye, hold the fogging lens in your right hand, positioning that hand so that it also occludes the patient's left eye. Hold the retinoscope with left hand and take measures with your left eye. This enables you to to position your left eye in front of the patient's left eye, just to the left of the patient's right eye visual axis—the opposite of the standard procedure.

3. Switch hands, eyes, and position when ready to measure the refractive status of the other eye.

5-3. When doing "dry" static retinoscopy, try to make certain that the patient is not exercising accommodation. Place fogging lenses over *both* eyes, not just the one being observed with the retinoscope, and keep a watch on the patient's pupils as an indicator of accommodation. (This will probably require you to keep both eyes open while doing retinoscopy—a worthwhile skill to acquire.) Obviously, this is most important with uncorrected hyperopes.

5-4. Speed is very important when testing young children. You can make a fairly accurate assessment of refractive status by changing the distance between the retinoscope and the patient's eyes, and the power of the lenses placed before the patient's eyes. To facilitate this method of retinoscopy:

1. Prepare three or four sets of plus lenses (mounted in small plastic frames), powers ranging from about +2.00D to +8.00D, O.U.
2. Attach to your retinoscope a 1-meter length of string on which knots have been tied to indicate landmark distances; e.g., every 25 cm.
3. Make your first retinoscopic estimate without fogging lenses. Obviously, if you observe "against motion," you only have to shorten the retinoscopy distance, use the string to estimate the distance at which "neutral" was observed, and transform that into diopters.
4. If you observe "with motion," estimate the magnitude of that motion, place a set of the plus lenses in front of the patient's eyes, and again, alter retinoscopy distance until "neutral" is observed.
5. If the patient manifests hyperopic astigmatism, neutralize the least-power meridian first, then the other—as though you were going to write the lens prescription in terms of plus rather than minus cylinders. This places significantly less demand on your short-term memory.

5-5. Prepare your retinoscope for dynamic (Sheard, Tait, MEM, etc.) retinoscopy. On white paper, type two, 1-inch-long sequences of elite-size letters and numerals, single space, one above the other. Attach this (with transparent tape) to your retinoscope, just above the light source aperture. This makes an excellent target for the patient to fixate as you carry out the procedure. The patient's task: Read the letters and numerals, in sequence. If you need extra time, have the patient read them backward, or read every other one, etc., thus assuring you that he is accommodating, rather than simply looking in that direction.

5-6. If your patient is very young—and not willing to fixate upon a distance target—and, for whatever reason, you are prevented from employing a cycloplegic, then you will probably have to depend upon dynamic retinoscopy to determine the patient's refractive status. To determine a reasonable approximation of the amount of ametropia present under these conditions, do the following:

1. Position the retinoscope at 40 cm from the patient's eyes; encourage the patient to fixate on the retinoscope.

2. Place sufficient plus lens power before both eyes to elicit "against motion" with the retinoscope.

3. Reduce plus lens power in half-diopter steps until you reach a neutral point.

4. Subtract a +0.50D from the power determined in step 3.

5. Consider this to be the patient's lens prescription. (We acknowledge that this method may overestimate a patient's hyperopia, but not that much, keeping in mind that only fairly substantial powers will be prescribed; and, if an error is to be made, it should be in the direction of too much rather than too little plus.)

5-7. Subjective refraction takes on many forms, ranging from use of an astigmatic "clock dial," to cross-cylinder testing, etc. Clearly, this is not feasible with very young patients. However, that does not rule out subjective assessment. With that age group, simply placing the proposed lens powers in a child's trial frame (or holding them in front of the patient's eyes) and observing patient reaction may provide very useful data. (Note: The presence of a positive response from the child who displays 8 diopters of myopia—a smile, etc.,—when provided with −8.00D lenses, for example, is very reassuring to the clinician and provides evidence that confirms her objective measures. However, the absence of a positive response should not be interpreted as reason for not prescribing lenses. If retinoscopy revealed a significant refactive error, then prescribe it—regardless of the child's initial reactions. *The retinoscope, used correctly, does not misinform.*)

5-8. With children old enough to respond to some of the tests usually employed for subjective refraction:

1. Avoid asking the child to identify the "better" lens condition. "Better" is a relative term, and not well dealt with by young children.

2. Rather, if the goal is to balance the lens powers before the two eyes, introduce sufficient plus before both eyes to "blur" visual acuity to about 20/30, generate diplopia with about 6 diopters of vertical prism, and ask the child to identify the set of letters that is "worse"—"more blurred." Change lens powers to obtain equal blur in both eyes.

3. If the goal is to determine BVA, first identify the lens powers that provide the patient with 20/20 in each eye, then increase plus (or reduce minus) about 0.50D, O.U. Having done this, present *different* 20/20 letters (i.e., not the letters just read), and ask the patient to read them. If he can read them, add another +0.25 or 0.50D (O.U.) and repeat—once again, with a new set of letters. If he cannot read them, reduce the plus power in 0.25D steps (O.U.) until he can read them. This yields the BVA. There is no need—indeed, it is undesirable—to continue to reduce plus power simply because the child says that doing so makes the print look "better." (BVA is not analogous to *maximum visual acuity;* it refers to the maximum plus, or least minus, needed for the patient to obtain clear [20/20] eyesight without exerting accommodation.)

5-9. The standard method for documenting cycloplegia is significant blur at near-point—a subjective method. An objective method: Measure the child's refractive status (with retinoscope) as he fixates at distance and at near. If full cycloplegia has been obtained, no measurable differences should be observed.

■

REFERENCES

1. Goldschmidt E. Refraction in the newborn. Acta Ophthal 1969; 45:570.
2. Gonzales TJ. Conseraciones en torno a la refracción del racién nacido. Arch Soc Oftal Hisp-Amer 1965; 25:666.
3. Zonis S, Miller B. Refraction in the Israeli newborn. J Ped Ophthal 1974; 2:77.
4. Banks M. Infant refraction and accommodation. In: International Ophthal. Clinics. Electrophysiology and psychophysics: the use in ophthalmic diagnosis. Spring 1980; vol. 20, no. 1
5. Gleiss J, Pau H. Die entwicklung der refraktion vor der geburt. Klin Monatsbl Augenheilkd 1952; 121:440.
6. Graham MV, Gray OP. Refraction of premature babies' eyes. Br Med J 1963; 5343:1452.
7. Hosaka A. The ocular findings of premature infants, especially on the premature signs. Jap J Ophthal 1963; 7:77.
8. Scharf J, Zonis S, Zeltzer M. Refraction in Israeli premature babies. J Ped Ophthal 1975; 12:193.
9. Payne SM. Hypermetropia responsible for heterophoria, astigmatism and myopia. AAAO 1919; 2:30–39.
10. Dobson V, Fulton AB, Manning K, Salem D, Petersen RA. Cycloplegic refractions of premature infants. Am J Ophthal 1981; 91:490–95.
11. Nissenkorn I, Yassur Y, Mashkowski D, Sherf I, Ben-Sira I. Myopia in premature babies with and without retinopathy of prematurity. Br J Ophthal 1983; 67:170–73.
12. Fledelius HC. Ophthalmic changes from age of 10 to 18 years: a longitudinal study of sequels to low birth weight. II. visual acuity. Acta Ophthal 1981; 59:64–70.
13. Hirsch MJ. The refraction of children. In: Hirsch M, Wick R, eds. Vision of children. Philadelphia: Chilton Books, 1963.
14. Mehra KS, Khare BB, Vaithilingam E. Refraction in full-term babies. Br J Ophthal 1965; 49:276.
15. Santonastaso A. La refrazione oculare nei primi anni di vita. Assn di ottal, e clin ocul 1930; 58:852.
16. Dobson V, Fulton AB, Sebris SL. Cycloplegic refractions of infants and young children: The axis of astigmatism. Inv Ophthal Vis Sci 1984; 25(1):83–87.
17. Howland HC, Sayles N. Photorefractive measurements of astigmatism in infants and young children. Inv Ophthal Vis Sci 1984; 25:93–102.
18. Gwiazda J, Scheiman M, Mohindra I, Held R. Astigmatism in children: changes in axis and amount from birth to six years. Inv Ophthal Vis Sci 1984; 25:88–92.
19. Garber JM, Hughes J. High corneal astigmatis in the adult Navajo population.
20. Howland HC, Atkinson J, Braddock O, French J. Infant astigmatism measured by photorefraction. Science 1978; 202(20):331–32.

21. Mohindra I, Held R, Gwiazda J, Brill J. Astigmatism in infants. Science 1978; 202(2):329.

22. Ingram RM, Barr A. Changes in refraction between the ages of 1 and 3 1/2 years. Br J Ophthal 1979; 63:339.

23. Atkinson J, Braddock O, French J. Infant astigmatism: its disappearance with age. Vis Res 1980; 20:891.

24. Woodruff ME. Cross sectional studies of corneal and astigmatic characteristics of children between the twenty-fourth and seventy-second months of life. AAAO 1971; 48:650.

25. Cook RC, Glasscock RE. Refractive and ocular findings in the newborn. Am J Ophthal 1951; 34(10):1407.

26. Kempf GA et al. Refractive errors in the eyes of children as determined by retinoscopic examination with a cycloplegic. Washington, D.C.: Publ. Health Service Bulletin #182, 1928.

27. Sorsby A, Benjamin B, Davey JB, Sheridan M, Tanner JM. Emmetropia and its aberrations. London: Medical Research Council Special Report No. 293, 1957.

28. Goldschmidt E. On the etiology of myopia. Copenhagen: Munksgaard, 1968.

29. Hirsch MJ. Predictability of refraction at age 14 on the basis of testing at age 6: interim report on the Ojai Longitudinal Study of Refraction. Am J Optom 1964; 41:567–73.

30. Grosvenor TP. Primary care optometry: a clinical manual. Chicago: Professional Press, 1982.

31. Straub M. Archives d'Ophtalmologie (Paris) 1918–1919; 36:68.

32. Glickstein M, Millidot M. Retinoscopy and eyesize. Science 1970; 168(3931):605–606.

33. Millodot M, O'Leary D. The discrepancy between retinoscopic and subjective measurements: effect of age. AJOPO 1978; 55(5):309–16.

34. O'Leary D, Millodot M. The discrepancy between retinoscopic and subjective measurements: effect of light polarization. AJOPO 1978; 55(8):553–56.

35. Steiger A. Die entstehung der spharischen refractionen des manschlichen auges. Berlin: S. Karger, 1913.

36. Tron E. The optical bases of ametropia. Graefe's Arch 1934; 132:182.

37. Stenstrom S. Variations and correlations of the optical components of the eye. In: Sorsby A, ed. Modern trends in ophthalmology. 2nd ed. New York: Paul B. Hoeber, 1947.

38. Leary GA. The reconciliation of genetically determined myopia with environmentally induced myopia. AJOPO 1970; 47:702–709.

39. Sorsby A. Modern ophthalmology. Vol. 3. Washington, D.C.: Butterworth, 1964.

40. Stansbury FC. Pathogenesis of myopia. Arch Ophthal 1948; 39:273.

41. Grosvenor T. A review and a suggested classification system for myopia on the basis of age-related prevalence and age of onset. AJOPO 1987; 64(7):545–54.

42. Bullimore MA, Gilmartin B. Aspects of tonic accommodation in emmetropia and late-onset myopia. AJOPO 1987; 64(7):499–503.

43. Rosenfield M, Gilmartin B. Synkinesis of accommodation and vergence in late-onset myopia. AJOPO 1987; 64(12):929–37.

44. McBrien NA, Millodot M. The relationship between tonic accommodation and refractive error. Invest Ophthal Vis Sci 1987; 28:997–1004.

45. Borish IM. Clinical refraction. Chicago: Professional Press, 1970.

46. Bear JC, Richler A. Ocular refraction an inbreeding: a population study in Newfoundland. J Biosoc Science 1981; 13:391–99.

47. Bear JC, Richler A, Burke G. Nearwork and familial resemblances in ocular refraction: a population study in Newfoundland. Clinical Genetics 1981; 19:462–72.
48. Goldschmidt E. The importance of heredity and environment in the etiology of low myopia. Acta Ophthal 1981; 59:759.
49. Jablonski W. Zur vererbung der myopie. Klin Mbl Augenheilk 1922; 68:560–73.
50. Hoste A. Dei refraktionsverk altnisee bei ein—und zweieiigen zwillinger. Graefe, Arch fur Ophth 1941; 142:467–73.
51. Wixson RJ. The relative effects of heredity and environment upon the refractive errors of identical twins, and like-sex siblings. AJOPO 1958; 35:346–51.
52. Sorsby A. Sheridan M, Leary GM. Refraction and its components in twins. London: Privy Council, Medical Council Special Reports Series No. 303, 1962.
53. Knoblock WH, Leavenworth NH, Bouchard TJ, Eckert ED. Eye findings in twins reared apart. Ophthal Ped Genetics 1985; 5(1/2):59–66.
54. Rosner J, Aker J, Rosner J. A comparison of certain visual and cognitive characteristics in a cohort of triplets, two of whom are monozygotic. Presented at the 1987 annual meeting of the American Academy of Optometry.
55. Gardiner PA, James G. Association between maternal disease during pregnancy and myopia in the child. Br J Ophthal 1960; 44:172–78.
56. Birge HL. Myopia caused by prematurity. Trans Am Ophthal Soc 1955; No. 53:219–30.
57. Fletcher MC, Brandon S. Myopia of prematurity. Am J Ophthal 1955; 40:474–81.
58. Curtin BJ. Myopia: a review of its etiology, pathogenesis and treatment. Surv Ophthal 1970; 15(1):1–17.
59. Weekers R, Watillon M, Thomas-Decortis G. La myopie des prematures facteur de dissemblance dans la refraction des jumeaux monozygotes. Arch Ophthal (Paris) 1961; 21:217–26.
60. Perkins EJ. Glaucoma in the younger age groups. Arch Ophthal 1960; 64:882–91.
61. Gorin G. Developmental glaucoma. Am J Ophthal 1964; 58:572–80.
62. Moller HW. Excessive myopia and glaucoma. Acta Ophthal 1948; 26:185–93.
63. Gardiner PA. Dietary treatment of myopia in children. Lancet 1958; 1:1152–55.
64. Angle J, Wissmann DA. Age, reading and myopia. JAOPO 1978; 55(5):302–308.
65. Angle J, Wissmann DA. the epidemiology of myopia. Am J Epidemiology 1980; 111(2):220–36.
66. Jain IS, Jain S, Mohan K. The epidemiology of high myopia—changing trends. Ind J Ophthal 1983; 31(12):723–28.
67. Sato T. The causes and prevention of acquired myopia. Tokyo: Kanchara Shyppan, 1957.
68. Otsuka J, Kondo M. The experimental study of the influences of continuous contraction or relaxation of the ciliary muscle on the refraction. Acta Soc Ophthal Jap 1950; 54(Supp.):182.
69. Young F et al. Comparison of cycloplegic and non-cycloplegic refraction of Eskimos. AAAO 1971; 48(10):814.
70. Young F. The nature and control of myopia. AJOPO 1977; 48(4):451.
71. Young F. An estimate of the hereditary components of myopia. AAAO 1958; 35(7):333.
72. Young F. Leary GA. The inheritance of ocular components. AAAO 1972; 49:546.
73. Coleman DJ. Unified model for accommodative mechanism. Am J Ophthal 1970; 69(6):1063.
74. Young F. The effect of nearwork illumination level on monkey refraction. AAAO 1962; 39:60.

75. Young F et al. The transmission of refractive errors within Eskimo families. AAAO 1969; 46(9):675.
76. Van Alphen G. On emmetropia and ametropia. Supplement of Ophthalmologica 1961; 142:1–92.
77. Blank K, Enoch JM. Monocular spatial distortions induced by marked accommodation. Science 1973; 182(4110):393–95.
78. Miles PW. Errors in space perception due to accommodative retinal advance. AJOPO 1975; 52:600–603.
79. Enoch JM. Marked accommodation, retinal stretch, monocular space perception and retinal receptor orientation. AJOPO 1975; 52:376–93.
80. Wiesel TN, Raviola E. Myopia and eye enlargement after neonatal lid fusion in monkeys. Nature 1977; 226:66.
81. Rabin J, Van Sluyters RC, Malach R. Emmetropization: a vision dependent phenomenon. Inv Ophthal 1981; 20(4):561–64.
82. Smith EL III, Maguire GW, Watson JT. Axial length and refractive errors in kittens reared with an optically induced anisometropia. Inv Ophthal 1980; 19(10):1250–55.
83. Young FA. The development and control of myopia in human and subhuman primates. Contacto 1975; 19:16–31.
84. van Alphen GWHM. Choroidal stress and emmetropization. Vis Res 1986; 26(5):723–34.
85. McBrien NA, Millodot M. The effect of refractive error on the accommodative response gradient. Ophthal Physiol Opt 1986; 6(2):145–49.
86. Gilmartin B. A review of the role of sympathetic innervation of the ciliary muscle in ocular accommodation. Ophthal Physiol Opt 1986; 6(1):23–37.
87. Gilmartin B, Hogan RE. The role of the sympathetic nervous system in ocular accommodation and ametropia. Ophthal Physiol Opt 1985; 5(1):91–93.
88. Bullimore MA, Gilmartin B. Tonic accommodation, cognitive demand and ciliary muscle innervation. AJOPO 1987; 64(1):45–50.
89. Green PR. Mechanical considerations in myopia: relative effects of accommodation, convergence, intraocular pressure and the extraocular muscles. AJOPO 1980; 57(12):902–14.
90. Goode. Transaction Camb Phil Soc 1847; 8:493.
91. Placido. Peridico ophtal prat (Lisbon) 1880; 2(2):5–6, 44.
92. Sivak J. A simple photokeratoscope. AJOPO 1977; 54(4):241–43.
93. Bigsby WI, Gruber J, Rosner J. Static retinoscopy results with and without a fogging lens over the nontested eye. AJOPO 1984; 61(12);769–70.
94. Gray LG. Avoiding adverse effects of cycloplegics in infants and children. JAOA 1979; 50(4):465–70.
95. Bartlett JD. Administration of and adverse reactions to cycloplegic agents. AJOPO 1978; 55(4):227–33.
96. Robb R, Peterson RA. Cycloplegic refraction in children. J Pediatr Ophthal 1968; 5(2):110–14.
97. Amos DM. Cycloplegics for refraction. AJOPO 1978; 55(4)223–26.
98. Gettes BC. Choice of mydriatics and cycloplegics for diagnostic examination of children. In: Apt EL, ed. Diagnostic procedures in pediatric ophthalmology. Boston: Little, Brown, 1963.
99. Chang FW. The pharmacology of cycloplegics. AJOPO 1978; 55(4):219–22.
100. Hopkins G, Pharm B, Lyle WM. Potential systemic side effects of six common opthalmic drugs. JAOA 1977; 48(10):1241–45.

101. Yolton D, Kandel S, Yolton R. Diagnostic pharmaceutical agents: side effects encountered in a study of 15,000 applicants. JAOA 1980; 51(2):113–18.
102. Sheard C. Dynamic skiametry. Chicago: Cleveland Press, 1920.
103. Tait EF. A quantative system of dynamic skiametry. Am J Optom 1953; 30:113–29.
104. Gesell A, Ilg F, Bullis G. Vision—its development in infant and child. New York: Harper and Bros., 1949.
105. Pheiffer C. Book retinoscopy. AAAO 1955; 32(10):540.
106. Getman GN, Kephart NC. Book retinoscopy. OEP papers 1958; Series 2 (10–11).
107. Apell R, Lowry R. Preschool vision. St. Louis: A.O.A., 1959.
108. Kruger PB. Luminance changes of the fundus reflex. AAAO 1974; 52:847.
109. Kruger PB. The effect of accommodative changes on the brightness of the fundus reflex. JAOA 1976; 49(1):47.
110. Kruger PB. The role of accommodation in increasing the luminance of the fundus reflex during cognitive processing. JAOA 1977; 48(12):1943.
111. Kruger PB. Changes in fundus reflex luminance with increased cognitive processing. AJOPO 1977; 54(7):445.
112. Keller JT. An optical evaluation of book retinoscopy. JAOA 1977; 48(4):483.
113. Apell RJ. Clinical application of bell retinoscopy. JAOA 1975; 46(10):1023.
114. Haynes H. Clinical observations with dynamic retinoscopy. Opt Wkly October 27, 1960:2243, November 3, 1960:2306.
115. McKee G. The reliability of M.E.M. retinoscopy. Opt Monthly 1981; 72:30–31.
116. Rouse M, London R, Allen D. M.E.M. retinoscopy as a measure of accommodative response. AJOPO (in press).
117. Beiber JC. Why nearpoint retinoscopy with children? Opt Wkly 1974:54, 1974:78.
118. Harmon DB. Notes on a dynamic theory of vision. 3rd. ed. Published privately, 1958.
119. Bobier C, Sivak J. Chromoretinoscopy. Vis Res 1978; 18:247.
120. Sivak J, Bobier C. Accommodation and chromatic aberration in young children. Inv Ophthal 1978; 17(7):705–709.
121. Mohindra I. A technique for infant vision examination. AJOPO 1975; 52:867–70.
122. Owens D, Mohindra I, Held R. The effectiveness of a retinoscope beam as an accommodative stimulus. Inv Ophthal 1980; 19(8):942–49.
123. Mohindra I. Comparison of "near retinoscopy" and subjective refraction in adults. AJOPO 1977; 54(5):319–22.
124. Maino JH, Cibis GW, Cress P, Spellman CR, Shores RE. Noncycloplegic versus cycloplegic retinoscopy in preschool children. Annals Ophthal 1984; 16(9):880–82.
125. Borghi RA, Rouse MW. Comparison of refraction obtained by 'near retinoscopy' and retinoscopy under cycloplegia. AJOPO 1985; 62(3):169–72.
126. Richman JE, Garzia RP. Use of an ophthalmoscope for objective refraction of noncooperative patients. AJOPO 1983; 60(4):329–34.
127. Malmstrom FV, Randle RJ. Effect of a concurrent counting task on dynamic visual accommodation. AJOPO 1984; 61(9) :590–94.
128. Post RB, Johnson CA, Owens DA. Does performance of tasks affect the resting focus of accommodation? AJOPO 1985; 62(8):533–37.
129. Tan RKT. The effect of accommodation response on the dark focus. Clin Exper Optom 1986; 69(4):156–59.
130. Bullimore MA, Gilmartin B, Hogan RE. Objective and subjective measurement of tonic accommodation. Ophthal Physiol Opt 1986; 6(1):57–62.
131. Tsuetaki TK, Schor CM. Clinical method for measuring adaptation of tonic accommodation and vergence accommodation. AJOPO 1987; 64(6):437–49.

132. Morgan MW. The Turville infinity balance test. AAAO 1949; 26:231.
133. Brungardt TF. Use of Turville subjective technique in cases of ametropia and pseudoamblyopia—a case report. AAAO 1958; 35:37.
134. Eskridge JB. Rationale for binocular refraction. N Eng J Opt 1971; 22(6):160.
135. Grolman B. Binocular refraction—a new system. N Eng J Opt May 1966:118.
136. Eskridge JB. A binocular refraction procedure. AAAO 1973; 50:499.
137. Borish IM. Clinical refraction. Chicago: Professional Press, 1970.
138. Giles GH. Contemporary refraction—a critical survey of some current methods. Br J Phys Opt 1956; 13:190.
139. Peters HB. Relationship between refractive error and visual acuity at three age levels. AAAO 1961; 38(4):194.
140. Noorden GK von. Clinical observations on stimulus deprivation amblyopia (amblyopia exanopsia). Am J Ophthal 1968; 65:220.
141. Noorden GK von, Crawford MLJ. The sensitive period. Trans Ophthal Soc UK 1979; 99:442.
142. Vaegan, Taylor D. Critical period for deprivation amblyopia in children. Trans Ophthal Soc UK 1979; 99:432.
143. Sherman J, Richter S, Epstein A. The differential diagnosis of visual disorders in patients presenting with marked symptoms but no observable ocular abnormality. AJOPO 1980; 57(8):516.
144. Pau H. Differential diagnosis of eye diseases. Philadelphia: Saunders, 1976.

6

Question 6
What Is the Patient's
Binocular Status?

☐

This is another pivotal question. A binocular anomaly may signal an active local or systemic pathology, an ocular or neuromotor structural fault, a significant ametropia, or a functional disorder (1, p. 258). It is not something to be treated lightly.

On the other hand, ruling out a binocular anomaly is neither demanding nor complex. (Except, of course, with very young patients. With this group, the optometrist is often restricted to a few tests—described on pp. 230–235—and sometimes it is not even possible to administer these because of patient noncompliance.) If the patient displays continuous, clear, single, simultaneous binocular vision (henceforth referred to as *normal binocular vision*), in all directions of gaze at all fixation distances, it is reasonable to conclude that her binocular status is normal.

Translated into concrete terms, binocular status may be considered normal when there is evidence of:

1. Accurate binocular alignment in all positions of gaze at nearpoint and farpoint fixation
2. Immediate recovery of binocular alignment after it has been disrupted in some way
3. Clear (20/20) visual acuity (with lens correction, if so indicated) in each eye

In most instances, therefore, a few relatively simple tests are all that is needed, if no deviations are noted. Farpoint and nearpoint stereoacuity tests provide evidence regarding the accuracy of binocular alignment (2). The unilateral cover test administered as the patient assumes the various positions of gaze, at near and far, reveals the patient's ability to recover binocular alignment following a disruption. And, obviously, the visual acuity test lives up to its name.

But the situation becomes more complex when a deviation is noted or when the patient is too young to respond to stereoacuity and visual acuity tests. Testing strategies no longer follow a predetermined invariant sequence. Now the optometrist has to decide which additional tests will provide the information needed for determining diagnosis, treatment, and prognosis (3).

In brief, then, a few simple tests can rule out a binocular anomaly; more complex testing strategies are needed when an anomaly cannot be ruled out by these few simple tests.

In accord with that observation, this chapter is organized into four major sections: (1) a condensed discussion of binocular development as it is presently understood; when children typically begin to display binocular function and how that has been documented; (2) the detection of a binocular anomaly: basic tests of binocular status and their relative effectiveness with young children; (3) the differential diagnosis of three anomalies: strabismus, amblyopia, and nystagmus; (4) diagnostic methods that are appropriate for the very young strabismic patient.

The treatment of a binocular anomaly—guidelines for prognosis and referral, and a general overview of the various therapies presently in use—will be discussed later, in Chapters 9, 11, 12, and 13.

■

BINOCULAR DEVELOPMENT

What we know about the normal development of binocular function in humans derives from animal studies and investigations of young children. The former most often make use of monkeys and the fact that their visual systems resemble and perform much like the human visual system (4). The latter tend to compare the visual behaviors of children born with a binocular anomaly (e.g., strabismus) to children who appear to have normal binocular abilities (5). These two types of studies, in combination, provide what appears to be sufficient evidence for us to believe that the normal child is likely to function binocularly by about age 4 months—*if* he has not experienced some event or circumstance that altered the course of normal development.

From animal research, we know that the very young primate (monkey) binocular system is highly vulnerable to circumstances that disrupt binocular vision. Monkeys who were not allowed to use both eyes during their first months of life became stereoblind; their responses to random-dot stereograms were virtually identical to the stereo performance of clinically diagnosed stereoblind children, even if their binocular experiences were restricted for only a relatively short period of time and they were then restored to binocular viewing circumstances. In addition, subsequent cortical studies of these animals show that they did not develop binocular neurons in visual cortex to the extent that unhampered monkeys usually do (6,7,8). Similar evidence has been reported from studies employing cats (9).

From human subject research, we learn that stereopsis appears to be present in normal 4-month-old infants (10); that when children with aligned eyes were compared with strabismic children of the same age, the former displayed a capacity to appreciate stereopsis while the former did not (10,11,12); that no significant differences in pupil diameters under monocular versus binocular viewing conditions (binocular summation) were found until the end of the fourth month of life; and that by the end of the sixth month, the differences in pupil diameter under the two viewing conditions were adultlike in magnitude (13). We also know that stereopsis and various other binocular functions develop more or less in accord with the development of visual acuity, contrast sensitivity, and (perhaps) the tuning of high spatial frequency receptors, thereby suggesting that refractive anomalies such as anisometropia, which limit high-frequency spatial resolution and binocular integration, can present a major obstacle to the postnatal development of binocular vision (14).

THE DETECTION OF A BINOCULAR ANOMALY

The flow diagram shown in Figure 6.1 maps out an organized testing sequence for detecting, or ruling out, a binocular anomaly. Notice that although the diagram displays a number of junctures from which different branches originate, testing commences in all instances with a decision regarding the patient's stereoacuity. Adequate? Yes of no? (See A in Figure 6.1 flow diagram and below.)

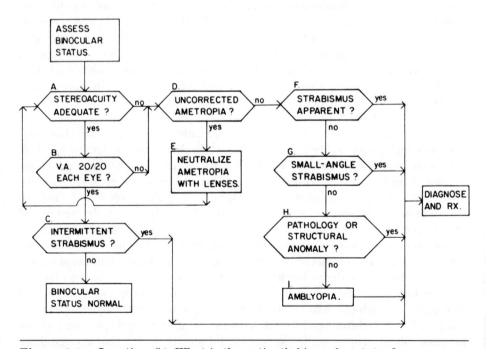

Figure 6.1   Question #6: What is the patient's binocular status?

■

A. STEREOACUITY ADEQUATE?

Stereoacuity is the quantitative expression of stereopsis. Central stereopsis is the binocular perception of three-dimensional space within the central zone of the visual field, or more precisely, the perception of the relative nearness and farness of object points within that central area obtained from disparate but fusible retinal images (15, p. 38). To measure an individual's stereoacuity, therefore, is to determine "the smallest amount of horizontal retinal image disparity that gives rise to a sensation of relative depth" (16, p. 966), with the measurement ordinarily expressed in seconds of arc.

Ogle (17) reported average adult nearpoint stereoacuity to be 20 seconds of arc. Parks (15), using commercially produced stereoacuity testing devices (Wirt stereotest at near; A.O. Vectograph slide at far), found that 24 seconds of arc at nearpoint and from 30 to 60 seconds of arc at farpoint "were average for the average adult with central single binocular vision" (p. 44). He also noted that individuals who lack central single binocular vision but do have peripheral fusion (see below) have an average stereoacuity of 200 seconds of arc at nearpoint (never better than 67 seconds of arc) and from 240 to 120 seconds of arc at farpoint.

It appears reasonable, therefore, to propose that stereoacuity of 50 seconds of arc, or better, at nearpoint and 100 seconds of arc, or better, at farpoint will not be achieved without accurate bifoveal alignment. Hence, in the context of the flow diagram, these constitute the criteria for making a decision regarding the adequacy of a patient's stereoacuity (with the exception of the Random-dot E stereotest; see pp. 191–194).

□ Stereoacuity in Young Children

As noted above, until very recently, it was assumed that young children did not have the capacity for refined binocular functions; that it was futile to seek a precise measure for such a complex function as stereopsis. Then, researchers such as Walk and Gibson (18), Bower et al (19), and Gordon and Younas (20) provided evidence that hinted at what has now become established as fact: very young children do appreciate stereopsis. Because this capacity is such a pivotal one in the diagnostic process, it behooves the optometrist to attempt to assess it in her very young patients as well as in her older, more easily tested ones. A valid suggestion! A worthy goal! But difficult to achieve.

Standard stereoacuity tests tend to be abstract, often involving visual illusions and requiring sophisticated discrimination and communication skills. Few stereoacuity tests are appropriate for 3- and 4-year-olds, and even fewer with children younger than that. This was clearly shown by Romano and colleagues (16) in their report of how children of different ages responded to the Titmus stereotest. (The Titmus stereotest is described below.) Their data indicate that exceptionally few

2-year-olds could demonstrate better than 3000 seconds of arc stereoacuity, but they then cautioned that this should not be interpreted as a lack of stereoscopic depth perception. They stated, " . . . on the contrary, he [the 2-year-old] almost certainly has stereoscopic depth perception, but we are unable to measure it with this test because of the nature of the test and the comprehension factor" (p. 970). Cooper and Feldman (21,22) report corroborative evidence, then go on to show that very young children can be tested successfully by employing an operant paradigm.

With this in mind, the next steps are to review the stereoacuity tests that are presently available and evaluate their appropriateness with children; determine what each requires of the patient and how those requirements match up with what young children are able to do.

□ Tests That Measure Stereoacuity

Most stereoacuity tests are designed to measure one's ability to detect small amounts of retinal image disparity within the context of a binocularly observed display. In turn, one's ability to detect small amounts of retinal image disparity under such conditions is affected by (a) the clarity of the retinal image in each eye and (b) the extent to which the nondisparate parts of the visual stimulus fall on corresponding retinal points in the two eyes. As such, performance on a stereoacuity test may be impaired by reduced visual acuity in one or both eyes, or by bifoveal misalignment. That, of course, is why the stereoacuity test is so useful at this point in the examination. If visual acuity is normal in each eye, then the only reasonable explanation for reduced stereoacuity is bifoveal misalignment.

FARPOINT TESTS

(See, also, Table 6.5.)

Howard-Dohlman Test (23)

This is the "grand-daddy" of present-day stereoacuity tests. It employs a device (Depth Perception Apparatus, Lafayette Instrument Co. #1702) that requires the patient, viewing from a distance of 6 meters, to position a black vertical rod directly alongside a second black vertical rod so that the two rods appear to be equidistant from him. The patient views the rods through an aperture that obstructs peripheral cues. All that is visible to him is the central portion of each vertical rod against a blank white background. Patient performance is measured in terms of the accuracy of rod placement.

To administer the test follow this procedure:

1. Position the rods so that they are not equidistant from the viewing aperture. One rod should be set at a 6-meter distance; the other, somewhat closer or farther than that.

2. Instruct the patient to adjust the position of the second rod, by manipulating a string, so that the two appear to be directly alongside each other, equidistant from him. (Note: With younger children, it is advisable to demonstrate, concretely, what "directly alongside" means and to test their understanding of that phrase. This may be accomplished by having the child initially stand directly adjacent to the rods rather than 20 feet away. Once he has demonstrated that he understands the concept, the test should proceed in standard fashion.)

3. Instruct the patient, if necessary, that he is not to move his head from side to side. Such movements would produce lateral motion parallax, thereby providing sufficient monocular cues to invalidate the test as a measure of bifoveal alignment. Young children are not apt to attempt this, but it is possible and therefore worth keeping in mind.

4. Assess patient performance in one of the two following ways. (a) Identify the minimum error that defines 75 percent of 20 patient trials. For example, if the patient's responses ranged from an error of 10 cm to 0.5 cm, with 75 percent of these falling in the 7.0 cm to 0.5 cm range, then his "score" would be 7.0 cm (24, p. 274). (b) Calculate the "average" error, as determined from three or four trials (25, p. 51).

Patient performance may then be converted from centimeters of error into seconds of arc. Table 6.1 (25, p. 52) shows the stereoacuity equivalents for alignment errors ranging from 0.5 cm to 50 cm, assuming a patient inter-pupillary distance (I.P.D.) of 60 mm. For example, an error of 10 cm, as determined by either of the methods described above, translates into a stereoacuity of 33 seconds, which, in turn, indicates that the patient is sensitive to retinal image disparities as small as 33 seconds of arc. Also shown in that table is the formula for converting centimeters of error into seconds of arc, thereby allowing for I.P.D.s other than 60 mm. For clinical purposes, however, the table is sufficient. The error introduced by I.P.D. variance is not all that significant.

Clinical Effectiveness. The Howard-Dohlman test is useful with children as young as age 5 years.

Positive Features. The child may respond without speaking. What the test requires can be illustrated with concrete materials as well as with words.

Negative Features. A certain amount of pretraining is usually necessary, especially with young children, and the apparatus occupies a significant amount of space.

A.O. Vectographic Stereotest
This test is incorporated into an A.O. Projecto-chart slide. It is available in two forms: one for children; the other for adults. Both are useful. School-aged children are usually able to respond to the adult slide version and, between the two, the adult test tends to generate less ambiguous data.

$$ETA = I.P.D. \ (x)/d^2 \times 206,000$$

Eta:	symbol of stereoacuity in seconds of arc
I.P.D.:	interpupillary distance in mm
x:	alignment error in mm
D:	testing distance from patient to rods in mm

Alignment Error (mm)	Stereoacuity
5	2″
10	3″
20	7″
30	10″
40	13″
50	16″
60	20″
80	26″
100	33″
200	66″
300	99″
400	132″
500	165″

From Griffin JR. Binocular anomalies. Chicago: Professional Press, 1976, p. 52.

Table 6.1 Howard-Dolman Test for Stereopsis. Performed at 6 meters. Assume I.P.D. of 60mm. Stereoacuities were determined by the above formula.

The vectographic slide is constructed so as to control what each eye sees. This is accomplished with polarizing filters that are positioned orthogonally, the one at axis 45°, the other at axis 135°. When a pair of images are projected through such filters, they both appear the same to a normal, naked eye. But when the binocular patient looks at the pair of projected images through compatible filters (i.e., one set at 45°, the other at 135°), each image is visible to one eye only, even though the general, unfiltered visual environment surrounding the projected images is visible to both eyes simultaneously. This allows for the presentation of disparate images within a binocularly perceived field, which, under appropriately controlled conditions, makes stereoacuity testing possible. (Note: This setup requires a projection screen that does not depolarize light. An ordinary beaded screen will not do. An aluminum screen, or one made from a polyvinyl sheet, works well.)

Adult. The adult version of the AO vectographic stereotest comprises four lines of rings, five rings in each line. To the naked eye, four of the five rings in each line appear to be single, clear images. The remaining one looks different—out of focus, the result of two superimposed rings that are out of register. This is most evident in the top line and less so in each subsequent one. Figure 6.2. portrays the array of rings as seen by the naked eye.

When one looks at the out-of-register rings in each line through compatible polarizing filters, one notes that only one ring of the pair is visible to each eye: the left ring to the right eye, and vice versa. That is, the rings are positioned in "crossed disparity." Because the degree of disparity is slight, 4 minutes of arc in the top row when the chart is accurately calibrated, and because, also, the visual environment surrounding the display is not affected by the polarizing filters, a binocular patient wearing filters automatically fuses the two disparate, out-of-register, rings into a single image. This causes that ring to appear to be floating forward, to look as though it were displaced off the screen in the direction of the patient.

The second line of rings resembles the top line except that the disparate rings are not as much out of register as they are in the top line. Here the disparity of the overlapping rings is equivalent to 3 minutes of arc. The third line presents 2 minutes of arc disparity and the bottom line a disparity of 1 minute of arc.

To administer the test, follow these steps:

1. Present the full array of rings to the patient. The patient looks through habitual Rx and polarizing filters.
2. Direct the patient to: "Look at the top line of circles. Which one of these circles *looks as though* it is floating off the screen? The first, second, third, fourth, or fifth?" (Point to each as you designate it, if needed.) (Also, see Practical Suggestion 6-1.)
3. Repeat with remaining three rows, if justified.

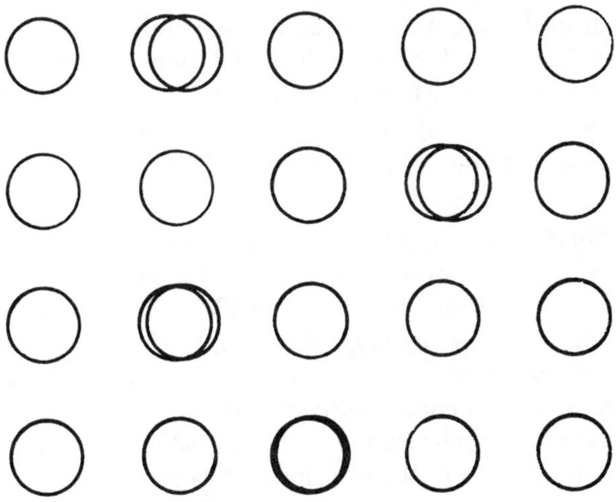

Figure 6.2
A.O. Co. adult farpoint vectographic stereotest.

4. If patient is confused, (a) show only one line of rings at a time, masking the others; (b) if this also confuses, show only two rings at a time—a disparate one alongside a nondisparate one. This reduces the patient's instructions to: "Which ring looks as though it is closer to you, *the one on this side* [touch the patient's hand, or point], or the one on this side [touch the other hand]?"

If confusion persists, shorten the viewing distance by positioning the patient halfway between the examining chair and the screen and repeat the test from this location. (Keep in mind that this will affect the relative disparity of the rings. Reducing the viewing distance by 50 percent doubles the relative disparity.)

If the patient now responds appropriately, return him to the original viewing position and repeat steps 1, 2, and 3, above.

Stereoacuity is measured in terms of threshold. The patient who can correctly identify the ring that appears to be floating forward in the bottom line is said to display a stereoacuity of 1 minute of arc. If he cannot get beyond the third line, stereoacuity is recorded as 2 minutes of arc, and so on.

Clinical Effectiveness.   The adult stereotest is useful with children as young as age 5 years. It is apt to confuse children younger than that.

Positive Features.   This test requires very little equipment beyond what is usually on hand in an optometric office. It offers a satisfactory range of disparities for farpoint testing. The stimulus presentation can be altered in order to reduce distractions. This not only simplifies the visual display, it also enables the child to respond with far fewer spoken words.

Negative Features.   The visual effect of fusing crossed disparity stimuli, the "float" of the ring, is an abstraction. It cannot be "proven" concretely. In addition, the visual stimuli, especially those with the greatest disparity, provide monocular cues. In other words, a monocular person is likely to see "something different" about the target ring in the top line of the array; even though it does not appear to float forward, it will be displaced laterally. This will be evident to the monocular person, enough to make it unique, and is therefore likely to be singled out by the child who, though not binocular, seeks to meet the examiner's expectations by giving some response to the situation.

Child.   The child version of AO vectographic stereotest differs from the adult slide in one significant way. Instead of presenting a matrix of twenty circles, four lines, five circles per line, the child is shown an array made up of five geometric designs: a star, triangle, plus sign, circle, and square. Each design represents a different degree of disparity, ranging from 4 to 0 minutes of arc. Because all are presented in crossed disparity, the designs will appear, to the binocular viewer wearing appropriate filters, to be floating forward different amounts.

To administer the test, follow this procedure:

1. Present the array of geometric designs to the patient. Have the patient look through habitual Rx and polarizing filters.

2. Direct the patient to: "Look at the designs. Which one *looks* closer, as though it were floating off the screen? The star, triangle, plus sign, circle, or square?" (Point to each as you name it, if needed.)

3. If the patient responds appropriately to this first request, repeat with the four remaining designs, saying: "Which one comes next, the triangle, plus sign, circle or square?" Continue until each design has been ranked in respect to relative disparity.

4. If the patient is confused, (a) show only two designs at a time, the star and square, for example; or (b) if confusion persists, shorten the viewing distance by positioning the patient closer to the screen. (As already pointed out, this will alter the relative disparity of the paired stimuli.) If this clears up the confusion, return the patient to the original viewing position and repeat steps 1, 2, and 3, above.

5. Stereoacuity is measured in terms of threshold. The patient who can identify the relative position of all designs is said to display 1 minute of arc stereoacuity, and so on.

Clinical Effectiveness. The child slide stereotest is usually too demanding for children age 4 years and younger. In practical terms, therefore, it is not too different from the adult slide.

Positive Features. The child does not have to be able to use ordinal numbers: he simply has to name the shapes, and even this can be avoided by constructing an appropriate key card. Pointing would then be adequate. Because the geometric designs are of unequal size and are not arranged in rows and columns, there are none of the monocular cues that the adult slide provides.

Negative Features. Just as with the adult slide, the "float" cannot be proven concretely; it is an abstraction, an illusion, and therefore difficult for preschool-aged children to grasp.

NEARPOINT TESTS

(See, also, Table 6.6)

Frisby Stereotest

This is a relatively new test (26). It comprises three (17-cm) square, clear plastic test plates of different thickness: 6mm, 3mm, and 1mm. One surface of each plate is sectioned into four 6 × 6-cm squares. Each square contains a randomly arranged array of blue triangular shapes that vary in size and orientation. No single square is distinctive; each looks much like the other three (see Figure 6.3).

On the reverse surface of each test plate is a small circular pattern (3.5cm in diameter) made up of the same kind of triangular shapes. The circle is positioned in the center of one of the above-mentioned squares. The effect of this: An in-

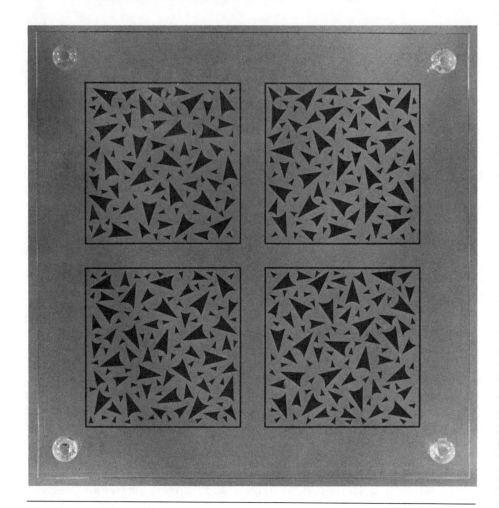

Figure 6.3 Frisby stereotest.

dividual with normal binocular vision, looking directly at the front surface of the 6-mm test plate, sees four squares containing randomly arranged shapes with one square appearing to have a (3.5-cm) circular indention, the product of juxtaposing the visual stimuli on front and rear surfaces of the plate. In contrast, the individual with a deviation that disrupts binocular function will not perceive the indention; all four squares will look the same.

The test, then, is simply one of identifying, pointing to, the square that contains this circular indention, with the relative difficulty of the task determined by plate thickness in combination with viewing distance. The thicker the test plate and/or the shorter the viewing distance, the easier the detection task. Table 6.2 shows the disparities created by the three test plate thicknesses at different (30- to 80-cm) viewing distances.

| Viewing Distance | Plate Thickness | | |
cm	6mm	3mm	1mm
30	600	300	100
40	340	170	55
50	215	110	35
60	150	75	25
70	110	55	20
80	85	40	15

Table 6.2   Frisby Stereotest Disparities

The test requires no special filters. The test plates are designed so that they may be presented in any orientation: there is no specific "top" or "bottom." Hence, the validity of a child's response may be confirmed by rotating the test plate (out of the child's view), then presenting it again, thereby ruling out "position preference" responses.

Finally, the test plate may be reversed so that instead of seeing an indentation, the circular pattern will appear to project toward the patient instead of away from him.

To administer the test, follow these steps:

1. Position the 6-mm test plate 40 cm from the patient. (The test includes a tape for measuring this exactly.)

2. Orient the test plate so that the front surface, the one closest to the patient, is perpendicular to the patient's visual axes.

3. Eliminate background confusion by placing a sheet of white paper against the back surface of the test plate. (The test envelope may be used for this purpose.)

4. Keep reflections from the test plate front surface to a minimum.

5. Direct the patient to "find, or touch, the hidden *ball*" or "circle" or "hole." (Note: The patient should be prevented from making side-to-side head movements. Such movements would introduce motion parallax, thereby invalidating the test. Generally, young children do not activate such movements, but it is a possibility.)

6. If the patient does not understand the task, (a) place his finger on the square that contains the "hidden circle" and have him look at that square. Then reorient the test plate (out of the patient's view) and repeat step 5. (b) Tilt the test plate back and forth, so that it is not perpendicular to the patient's visual axes. This will make the identification task easier, no longer dependent solely on bifoveal alignment. If this clears up the confusion, repeat steps 1 through 5, listed above.

7. Now reorient the test plate and repeat steps 1 through 5 again.

8. Consider three successive correct responses to a specific condition to be evidence of the patient's ability to correctly identify the "hidden circle." Once this is accomplished, substitute the 6-mm test plate with the 3-mm test place. (Note: Keep guessing at a minimum by [a] reorienting the test plate; [b] watching

the patient as he makes his decisions. It is not difficult to differentiate between random, albeit lucky, pointing and a considered-decision process.)

9. After three consecutive correct responses with the 3-mm test plate, either relocate the plate to a 60- and/or 80-cm test distance or retest at 40 cm with the 1-mm test plate.

10. Threshold is determined by identifying the test plate/test distance that marks the end of valid judgments. This is not critical for clinical use. In general, testing may cease and performance judged to be indicative of a normal binocular status when the patient displays 50 seconds of arc stereoacuity. This may be accomplished with the 3-mm test plate positioned at a 70-cm distance, or with the 1-mm test plate at somewhere around a 40-cm distance.

Clinical Effectiveness. The Frisby stereotest is applicable with children as young as age 3 years and it may be simplified further for younger children (27) (see Practical Suggestion 6-1).

Positive Features. The child need not look through, and be distracted by, filters. A simple motor response suffices; the child need not speak. Monocular cues are not apparent if the plate is properly lighted and positioned, and if the child does not exploit motion parallax.

Negative Features. The "hidden circle" or "hole" concept is in abstraction; even though it is the product of a true-distance condition, it remains an illusion. In addition, the four-alternatives format is often confusing for young children.

Verhoeff Stereopter (A.O. Co.)

This is a compact device, designed to be held by the examiner. In one aspect, it resembles the Howard-Dohlman test. The patient views an arrangement of three thin, black, vertical rods against a plain white background and identifies the one rod that is not on the same plane as the other two (see Figure 6.4). The relative positions of the rods may be altered by the examiner; eight different test settings are possible.

Stereoacuity is measured by determining the maximum distance from which the patient is able to make accurate judgments. This is then converted into a disparity detection threshold index, expressed in minutes or seconds of arc. Table 6.3 shows the stereoacuity equivalents for test distances ranging from 10 cm to 300 cm, assuming an I.P.D. of 60mm.

Clinical Effectiveness. This test is useful with children as young as age 5 years.

Positive Features. Like the Howard-Dohlman test, the patient's judgment is based on a concrete condition rather than a visual illusion produced by filters. The child need not speak; she simply has to point to a key card (prepared by the examiner) that shows three vertical lines arranged the way the rods appear in the Verhoeff Stereopter.

Figure 6.4
Verhoeff Stereopter.

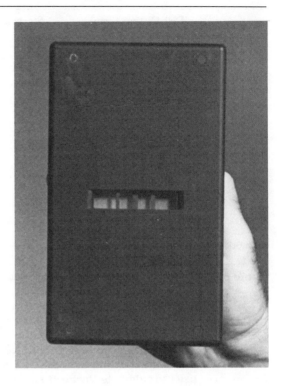

Negative Features. Unless the display is positioned precisely perpendicular to the patient's visual axes, and evenly illuminated, other depth cues in addition to disparity become available to the patient, thereby neutralizing its validity as a test of bifoveal alignment.

Hering Falling Bead Test
This test (28) is older than the Howard-Dohlman. It never gained wide acceptance and, at present, is virtually extinct. It is included here for two reasons. First, it has historical salience. Second, it was a worthy, albeit crude, attempt to introduce a time component into a measure of stereoacuity. The test was designed to investigate the patient's ability to make depth judgments quickly. The patient looks into a short black tube. A wire, inscribed with a "fixation mark" is attached to, and extends beyond, the far end of the tube. The patient observes as the examiner drops beads at various distances in front of and beyond the fixation mark, and reports what he perceives; that is, that the beads are "closer" or "beyond" the fixation mark.

Clinical Effectiveness. As already noted, the test is no longer in use. However, the concept of measuring stereoacuity under time-controlled conditions does have some merit.

Test Distance (cm)	Stereoacuity (seconds of arc)
10	3090″
20	772″
30	343″
50	124″
60	86″
80	48″
100	31″
110	26″
130	18″
150	14″
200	8″
300	3″

From Griffin JR. Binocular anomalies. Chicago: Professional Press, 1976, p. 53.

Table 6.3   Verhoeff Stereoptor Testing Distance and Corresponding Stereoacuities. All eight targets must be responded to correctly. The following stereothreshold values are calculated for an interpupillary distance of 60 mm. The eta values (stereoacuity) are calculated using an X value of 2.5mm. This is the displacement of one strip from the plane of the other two strips. The same formula as applied with the Howard-Dolman Test is used to calculate Verhoeff stereoacuities.

Titmus Stereotest

This test is based on the use of polarizing filters and contour stereograms (see Figure 6.5). It contains three subtests.

First, the Housefly subtest. To the binocular individual viewing the stimulus through compatible filters, it appears as a mamouth insect (see Figure 6.5) whose body and wings project an inch or so forward, off the page. Many optometrists consider this to be the best device for testing young children because of the "startling" effect of the super-sized fly.

To administer the test, use the following procedure:

1. The patient looks at the stereogram through polarizing filters. Testing distance is not critical. The disparity represented by the stimulus is approximately 3000 seconds of arc when viewing distance is 40 cm. Hence, shortening or extending the test distance somewhat will have very little effect on the relative demand of the test.

2. Direct the patient to "pinch" the fly's wings. Take note of where she initially places her finger as she responds. She should locate the wing about an inch or so off the page, closer to her.

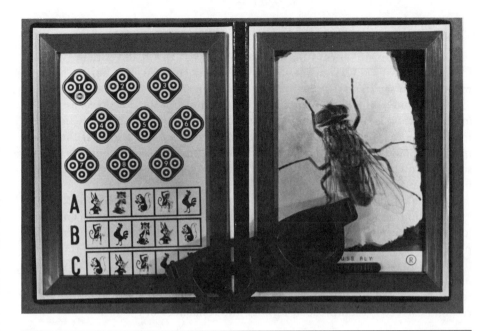

Figure 6.5   Titmus stereotest.

3. Because young patients' responses often lack preciseness, it may be useful to retest the child with the stimulus in an uncrossed-disparity position. To do this, turn the page upside down. The wings of the fly should now appear to be beyond the plane of the page and the child's "pinch" should reveal that phenomenon. (Also, see Practical Suggestion 6-1.)

Clinical Effectiveness.   This test is often recommended for children as young as age 2, but for all practical purposes it is not very satisfactory with children younger than age 3.

Positive Features.   The stimulus is eye-catching; distractors are kept to a minimum.

Negative Features.   It is a test of gross stereopsis (3000 seconds arc). Precise bifoveal alignment is not prerequisite to perceiving the stereo effect of the fly. In addition, the responses of young children are often ambiguous and difficult to interpret.

The second, the Animals subtest, consists of three rows of drawings of animals, five animals in each row (see Figure 6.5). The test is constructed so that when the drawings are viewed by a binocular person wearing compatible filters, one animal in each row appears to project forward, while the others remain flat on the page. Each row represents a different disparity, ranging from 400 seconds arc in row A to 100 seconds in row C.

To administer the test, follow these steps:

1. Hold test plate 40 cm from the patient's eyes. Direct the patient (wearing filter spectacles) to "Look at row A." (With young children, it is best to point to row A as you say this.)

2. Continue with "Show (or tell) me which animal in this row looks as though (or looks like) it is sticking out (or coming closer to you)—the rabbit, cat, squirrel, monkey, or rooster?" Point to each animal as you name it. (Note: If there is a question about the patient's familiarity with the designations of the animals, simply say, "This one, or this one, or . . ." and so on, as you point to each of the animals in the row.)

3. If the child responds appropriately, proceed through rows B and C.

4. If child appears to understand the demands of the test but is unable to identify the correct stimulus in row A, shorten the test distance. If this improves performance, take note of that distance. Then return the test plate to the 40-cm distance and determine whether the child is now able to respond correctly to row A. If not, then her stereoacuity may be calculated on the basis of the reduced test distance you noted previously. If, on the other hand, she is now able to respond correctly, then proceed through the remainder of the test.

Clinical Effectiveness. This test is generally useful with children as young as age 4.

Positive Features. It provides very few monocular cues, despite the use of contour stereograms.

Negative Features. It is limited to documenting a disparity detection threshold of 100 seconds of arc when positioned 40 cm from patient. The drawings are too small to be used for extended distance testing.

The third, the Circles subtest, is made up of nine rotated squares, each of which contains four circles (see Figure 6.5). One circle in each cluster is made up of a disparate stimulus. Hence, when it is viewed by a binocular person wearing polarizing filters, that circle will appear to be floating forward. A different amount of disparity is represented in each of the squares, ranging from 800 seconds to 40 seconds of arc.

To administer the test, do the following:

1. Hold test plate 40 cm from the patient's eyes. The patient wears polarizing filter spectacles.

2. Direct the patient to "Look at the four circles [or rings] in square [or box] number one [point to it as you name it]. Which ring looks as though it comes forward [or pops out, or sticks out] . . . the one on the top, bottom, left, or right?" (If directional labels cause confusion, see Practical Suggestions 1-22 and 1-23.)

3. Proceed in this manner until the threshold is measured.

Clinical Effectiveness.   This subtest is usually applicable with children age 5 and older.

Positive Features.   It provides a full range of disparity conditions.

Negative Features.   Monocular (lateral displacement) cues are fairly obvious in the first four of five items. Hence, a stereoacuity measure of 100 seconds of arc, as derived from this test, may not be valid. In addition, the communication requirements of the test often confuse young children, who then respond inappropriately because of that factor rather than because of reduced stereoacuity (5).

A.O. Co. Vectographic Stereotest
This test resembles the A.O. adult farpoint stereoacuity test. It consists of ten rows of circles, five circles in each row. When these are viewed, binocularly, through compatible polarizing filters, one circle in each row appears to project forward, the result of a crossed-disparity orientation. The patient's task: identify the circle in each row that projects forward. The ten rows represent ten levels of difficulty, ten disparities ranging from 600 to 12 seconds of arc when positioned 40 cm from the viewer's eyes.
   To administer the test, follow these steps:

   1. Hold test plate 40 cm from the patient's eyes. The patient wears filter spectacles.
   2. Direct the patient to "Look at the five circles [or rings] in row 1. [If necessary, point to that row as you name it.] Which ring looks as though it comes forward . . . [or pops out] . . . the first, second, third, fourth, or fifth?" (Note: If needed, move your finger from [the patient's] left to right as you designate the circles, so as to give a different spatial location to each one. Obviously, this may not be needed with older children, but it is useful, often necessary, with 5- and 6-year-olds.)
   3. Proceed in this manner until the threshold is measured.

Clinical Effectiveness.   This test is usually applicable with children age 5 and above. Certain kindergarten-aged children, however, will not be able to deal with the response requirements of the test; i.e., naming the position of the circle that stands forward. And, in this format, pointing to the circle is not always helpful because of the proximity of the adjacent circles.

Positive Features.   The test provides a wide range of disparity conditions.

Negative Features.   Monocular (lateral displacement) cues are fairly obvious in the first five rows. Hence, a stereoacuity measure of 120 seconds of arc, as derived from this test, may not be valid. As already noted, the communication requirements of this test are often beyond the capacities of the 5-year-old.

Lang Stereotest

This recently developed test (29) makes use of a technique called panography. Two similar pictures are viewed through cylindrical elements; the pictures and cylindrical elements are constructed so that each eye sees but one of the pictures. If the patient is binocular, the pictures are fused into a single stereoscopic image; in this case, a cat, a car, and a star, with the former representing 1200 seconds of disparity; the latter two: 600 seconds.)

To administer the test, use this procedure:

1. Hold the (9.5 × 14.5-cm) test card 40 cm from the patient's eyes. No filter lenses are required.

2. Direct the patient's attention to the pictures and ask that he "Tell [or show] me which of these looks the closest to you."

Clinical Effectiveness.   The Lang test is appropriate as a screening test for children 4 years of age.

Positive Features.   Requires no filter glasses and presents easily recognizable and named figures.

Negative Features.   Disparity is fixed and relatively gross. To reduce the disparity of the stimuli, the distance has to be increased to the point where it goes beyond reasonable limits. Therefore, the test does not ordinarily measure stereoacuity threshold; it functions as a screening test.

Randot Stereotest

The Randot stereotest consists partly of items made up of random-dot patterns and partly of standard contour stimuli that are presented in a way that suggests they are derived from random-dot patterns. The first section of this three-part test—Randot Forms—is representative of the former.

The Forms subtest is divided into two segments. Both consist of four rectangular random-dot arrays in which (in each of the two segments) all but one of the rectangles presents a design of some sort to the binocular patient. In one segment—the uppermost—500 seconds arc stereoacuity is required to perceive the designs; in the lower segment, 250 seconds arc stereoacuity is called for. As such, this portion of the test is not intended to measure refined stereopsis; rather, it serves more as a screening test—especially for children who have yet to develop the communication skills needed for the other two sections of the test.

To administer the test, do the following:

1. Hold the test plate 40 cm from the patient's eyes. The patient wears polaroid filters.

2. Direct the child's attention to the upper four rectangles and assess his ability to perceive and name the designs. This may be done in a number of different ways; probably the most effective: "Show me the *star*; . . . the *ball*; . . . . etc."

Or, as a variation: "What do you call this?" (while pointing to one of the rectangles). Alternatively, ask "Which of these [point to the four rectangles] does *not* have a design?" (We do not recommend this method with young children. The concept of "does not have" is confusing.)

3. Follow the same procedure in administering the lower (more difficult) segment of this subtest, wherein the designs are a block, a triangle, and a cross; the fourth rectangle contains "nothing" but random dots.

Clinical Effectiveness. This subtest is applicable with children as young as 4. It may very well elicit valid responses from a 3-year-old, but many children of this age are confounded by the abstract nature of the task.

Positive Features. No monocular cues. Stimuli are generally familiar to preschool-aged children.

Negative Features. It is not a test of refined stereopsis. As such, precise bifoveal alignment is not needed to respond accurately. Hence, it serves more as a screening test than to determine threshold.

The Animals subtest is identical to the animal subtest in the Titmus stereotest. There is no need to repeat that material here (see p. 187).

The Circles subtest is very similar to the Circle subtest in the Titmus stereotest, except that it offers ten levels of difficulty, each presented in a three-alternative array, and tests a range of stereoacuity from 400 seconds to 20 seconds arc.

To administer the test, use this procedure:

1. Hold the test plate 40 cm from the patient's eyes, direct her attention to the first rectangle and ask: "Which of these three circles looks as though it is closer to you—the one on *this* side [point], the one on *that* side [point], or the one in the *middle* [point]?" (or "Which circle sticks out?"), etc.

2. Continue in this fashion through the other rectangles until the threshold is reached.

Clinical Effectiveness. This subtest is usually applicable with children age 5 and above.

Positive Features. No monocular cues; provides a broad range of disparities—from 200 to 20 seconds of arc.

Negative Features. Places significant communication demands on the patient; demands that are usually beyond the capacities of a 4-year-old.

Random-dot E Stereotest
The Random-dot E stereotest is based on the work of Julesz (30). It consists of two 8 × 10-cm, acetate-covered, random-dot, vectographic stereograms, a pair of compatible polarized filters, and a demonstrator (Demo). This latter is con-

structed of heavy-weight paper and printed to simulate a random-dot stereogram. Centered on the Demo is a large (4.8-cm square) embossed E that is used to familiarize the patient with what he is to look for in the random-dot stereograms (see Figure 6.6).

One of the stereograms is blank; it presents an array of randomly organized dots that looks more or less the same to the naked eye and through the polarized filters. (See Practical Suggestion 6-1.) The other stereogram appears blank to the naked eye, but reveals a "floating" E, similar in size to the one in the Demo, when viewed through the filters by someone who is binocular.

To administer the test, follow these steps:

1. Show the Demo to the patient and say (if patient is preschool), "This is an E," or simply, "Look at this E." Then set the Demo aside, (Do not overexplain the features of an E—its orientation, etc. Not only is this irrelevant, it may also be confusing.)

2. The patient looks through polarizing filters as you hold the two random-dot stereograms (one in your right hand, the other in your left) 1.5 meters from her eyes. (This is a departure from the published standard procedure for this test. It calls for 0.5- and 1.0-meter testing distances. We recommend the 1.5-meter testing distance because we, and others, have found it to be significantly more sensitive

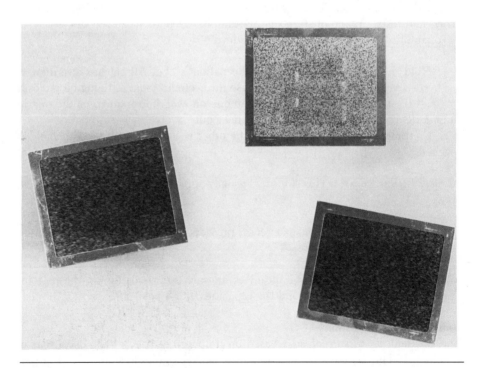

Figure 6.6   The Random-dot E stereotest.

Distance	Disparity	Distance	Disparity	Distance	Disparity
50 cm	504″	2 ft.	413″	9 ft.	92″
100 cm	252″	3 ft.	275″	10 ft.	83″
150 cm	168″	4 ft.	206″	11 ft.	75″
200 cm	126″	5 ft.	165″	12 ft.	69″
300 cm	84″	6 ft.	138″	13 ft.	63″
400 cm	63″	7 ft.	118″	14 ft.	60″
500 cm	50″	8 ft.	103″	15 ft.	55″
				16 ft.	52″

From: Test instructions.

Table 6.4   RDE Disparities as a Function of Distance

to visual acuity deficits and binocular anomalies, even small-angle deviations [31,32,33,34]).

3. If you have doubts about the child's ability to comprehend the task, do a few preliminary trials at 33 to 40 cm. This will not test stereoacuity very precisely (see Table 6.4 for stereoacuity values at different test distances), but it will test the child's understanding of the task. Then, if she responds appropriately at the shorter test distance, continue the test at 1.5 meters (see Practical Suggestion 1-31). (Note: Make sure that the examination area is adequately illuminated. In most cases, it is advisable to hold the stereograms a bit below the patient's eye level, tilted so that they are perpendicular to her visual axes. This tends to provide adequate light and reduces annoying reflections from the acetate material that covers the stereograms.)

4. Have the patient "Point to the E" (see Figure 6.7). Once the patient has responded, place both stereograms behind your back (ostensibly to alter their

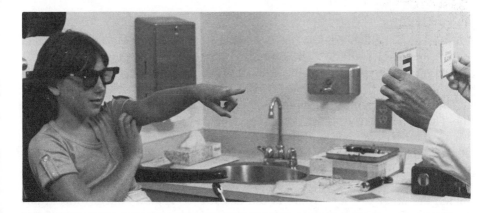

Figure 6.7   Administering the RDE stereotest.

respective positions), then show them again at the 1.5-meter distance and repeat the request, "Point to the E."

5. Repeat the above procedure until you are convinced about her ability to discriminate the "E" at that test distance, or—if you are not secure in making this judgment—until she has (a) achieved four successive correct responses or (b) had six trials—whichever of these two occurs first. Four successive correct responses within six trials probably constitute a "pass"; less than that, a "fail" (see Practical Suggestion 1-37). Also, vary the location of the "E" in an apparently random manner. A typical presentation sequence is Trial #1: E in right hand; #2: E in right hand; #3: E in left hand; #4: E in right hand; #5: E in left hand; #6: E in left hand.

6. Record the outcome as a "pass" or "fail." This is preferable to recording stereoacuity. The latter will be misleading because, as noted above, the Random-dot E stereotest, when administered at 1.5 meters, is remarkably difficult to pass unless the patient has normal binocular vision and her visual acuity is relatively good.

Clinical Effectiveness.   The Random-dot E stereotest has been found to be useful with children as young as age 3 (33).

Positive Features.   The child is asked to make a single, nonverbal response. Once the child has been indoctrinated to this basic requirement, there is nothing else for her to understand in order to respond to the test. She need not recognize the stimulus as the letter E.

Negative Features.   Polarizing filters are required; these may distract the young child. Also, if a quantification of stereoacuity is needed, rather than a simple "pass" or "fail"—because of some job prerequisite, perhaps—this test will not provide a valid measure. In order to demonstrate 50 seconds arc stereoacuity, the patient must be able to discriminate the E at a distance in excess of 16 feet!

TNO Stereotest
This test also employs random-dot stereograms, but it uses color filters instead of polarizing materials (35,35). There are three subtests: a screening test, a suppression test, and a graded stereoacuity test. Only the first and the last will be discussed here.

The screening subtest consists of three test plates (pages). Plate 1 resembles the Titmus Housefly subtest. One large butterfly is visible to all viewers (see Figure 6.8). The same plate contains a second butterfly, but it is visible only when viewed binocularly through compatible color (red/green) filters. Plate 2 consists of four different sized circles (or "discs" or "balls"). Two of these, the largest and the next-to-smallest, are visible only when viewed binocularly through the color filters; the other two are visible to the naked eye. Plate 3 contains a centrally located plus sign (visible without filters) surrounded by four other geometric forms

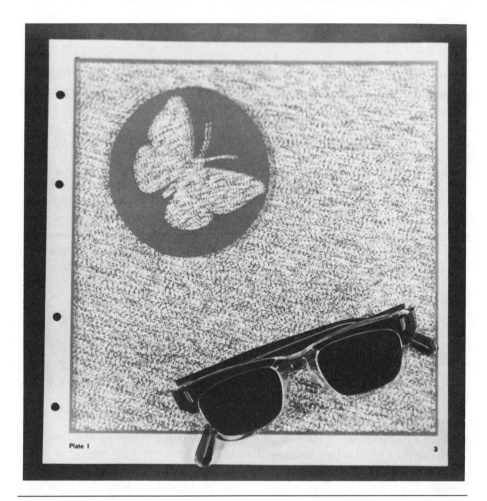

Figure 6.8   TNO stereotest plate I.

(disc, square, triangle, and diamond) that cannot be seen unless viewed binocularly through compatible red/green filters. All three screening plates present disparities of about 2000 seconds of arc when positioned 40 cm from the patient.

To administer the test:

Plate 1: Ask the child to "Touch the butterflies," or "Tell me how many butterflies you see."

Plate 2: "How many balls do you see?"

Plate 3: "Show me a . . . circle, . . . a square, . . . etc.," or, if a key card is used, "show me one that looks like this, etc." In all instances, successful performance indicates an ability to detect gross disparity—about 2000 seconds of arc.

Clinical Effectiveness. These screening plates are useful with children as young as 2 1/2 to 3 years of age.

Positive Features. Communication requirements of the test are relatively undemanding. Red/green filters are not as sensitive to head tilt as are the polarizing filters.

Negative Features. The test is crude. In addition, the test overtests, if all three plates are used.

The quantitative plates subtest consists of twelve items distributed on three plates (i.e., page). To the naked eye, each plate contains four 7.2-cm squares, all similar in appearance; all contain red/green random dot arrays. To a binocular viewer, looking through appropriate red/green filters, each of the squares contains a circle (or disc) from which a 60-degree wedge has been deleted. The stereograms vary in two ways: (a) the orientation of the missing wedge; (b) the degree of disparity between the wedge and the main body of the disc, this ranging from 480 to 15 seconds of arc when the viewing distance is 40 cm.

To administer the test, do the following:

1. Hold the test booklet 40 cm from the patient's eyes. The patient wears appropriate red/green filter spectacles.
2. Direct the patient's attention to item #1 and ask: "Where is the wedge in this circle: at the top, left, bottom, or right?" (See Practical Suggestions 1-22 and 6-1.) Proceed through the items until the threshold is obtained.

Clinical Effectiveness. This subtest is very demanding for young children. It is rarely useful with children younger than age 6.

Positive Features. It offers a broad range of disparities, thereby providing a refined measure of stereoacuity.

Negative Features. The communication demands of the subtest are high. Children not yet in first grade tend to be confused by this.

SOME COMMENTS REGARDING THE DIFFERENCE BETWEEN RANDOM-DOT AND CONTOUR STEREOGRAMS

The A.O. vectograph and the Titmus stereotests are made up of line, or contour, stereograms. The Randot, RDE, and TNO employ random-dot stereograms.

Patient performance will often differ on these two types of tests, and at least two explanations have been proposed. An obvious explanation, already discussed: cues other than disparity are available in a contour stereogram, thereby reducing the relative difficulty of the test for some patients (37). Because the stimuli in such tests are usually organized symmetrically, a small lateral displacement of one stimulus within the array is apparent to the monocular viewer. This is not true of most tests using random-dot stereograms. Properly constructed, they provide no useful monocular cues.

A second explanation for differences in patient performance on a test using line stereograms and one using random-dot stimuli has been proposed by Carmon and Bechtoldt (38), subsequently corroborated by Benton and Hacaen (39), and again by Hamsher (40). They all report that patients with disease of the right cerebral hemisphere display difficulty with tests of global stereopsis—tests that use random-dot stereograms—yet do not reveal similar deficiencies in tests of local stereopsis—those that use line or contour stereograms. This hypothesis requires more study before it can be accepted as fact, but the data are sufficiently interesting to warrant mention.

INFORMAL MEASURES OF STEREOPSIS

(See, also, Table 6.7.)

A standardized method of measurement is almost always preferred over an informal method, all else being equal. There are occasions, however, when a standard procedure is not applicable, particularly when it comes to the assessment of a young person's stereoacuity. The child may not understand the test: or he may already be so familiar with the test that he balks at another administering or, worse yet, responds on the basis of what he recalls rather than what he sees. In these instances, it is helpful to have alternative procedures available, even if they are nonstandard.

The procedures listed below are examples of alternative procedures for estimating a child's binocular status. They are organized according to the instrument to be used: Brewster stereoscope, Wheatstone stereoscope, anaglyph plates, vectograph plates. The list is not exhaustive, but it is sufficient to illustrate the wide variety of methods available for informally assessing stereoacuity.

Brewster Stereoscope

Keystone Visual Skills Test #7 (DB-6D). This is a farpoint stereopsis screening test cited earlier (see Chapter 1). It is based upon the same concept that underlies so many of the other tests already described. It presents rows of stimuli (geometric designs) to both eyes, wherein one form in each row is designed to stimulate disparate retinal points while the others in that row do not. The patient's task: identify the form that stands forth, the form produced by disparate stimuli.

Nearpoint Stereopsis Test (Keystone #5111). This is very similar to the just-described farpoint test. In this instance, however, the test is designed for the nearpoint setting on the Keystone Telebinocular.

Gross Stereopsis Test (Keystone Peek-A-Boo Series). Here, the format is a clown with four balloons, each of which presents a different disparity. To the binocular viewer, one balloon looks "closest," another "farthest away," and so on. Figure 6.9 shows this stereogram.

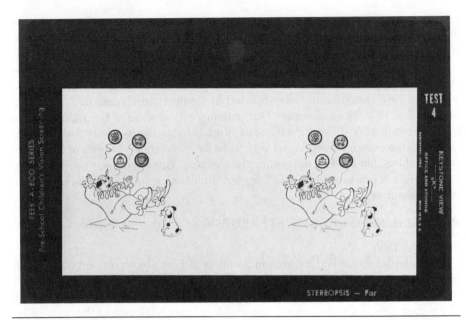

Figure 6.9   Keystone View clown stereotest.

Etc.   There is an abundance of third-degree fusion targets designed for the Brewster stereoscope. Most of them were manufactured in the years preceding the advent of anaglyph and polarizing filters, but they continue to be available (e.g., from Keystone View Co., Bernell Corp.). Most desirable for use with children are those that provide uncomplicated stimuli—uncomplicated in terms of visual array and language demands.

Wheatstone Stereoscope
Any central-stereopsis (third-degree fusion) target that is designed for a major amblyoscope (e.g., synoptophore) will do, although some are more suitable than others. Simpler targets are best for children, particularly those that minimize the need for complex oral responses. Because of the capacities of the Wheatstone stereoscope, the same targets may be used at simulated nearpoint and farpoint distances.

Anaglyph Plates
Keystone Basic Binocular Test (Keystone #6130).   This series is very useful, but it also has drawbacks. On the plus side, it employs pictures that are interesting to children and, in many instances, the child may respond by pointing instead of speaking. On the negative side: Most of the plates test peripheral, not central, stereopsis (see Diagnosis of Strabismus, below).

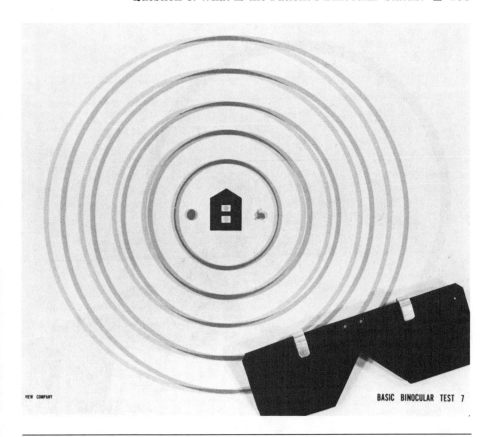

Figure 6.10   Keystone Basic Binocular Test #7.

Of particular value in this series are tests #7 and #9 (see Figures 6.10 and 6.11.) The former presents to the binocular viewer a series of concentric rings that appear to be located on different planes. Gross stereopsis may be probed by determining the child's perception of the relative position of the largest and smallest rings. If peripheral binocularity is intact, one of these will appear distinctly closer to the viewer. This, of course, depends upon the orientation of the color filters.

Test plate #7 may also be used to investigate more refined disparity detection skills. In the center of that test plate is a black "house" bracketed by an anaglyphic ball on one side and an anaglyphic rabbit on the other. The binocular viewer, looking through compatible redgreen filters, will perceive the house to be flat on the plate, with one anaglyph target floating forward (in front of the house, closer to the viewer) and the other behind the house, farther away. Test plate #9 is less complex. It consists of (disparate) red and green ducks within a black circle. The individual with normal binocular vision will see the duck "in front of" or "behind"

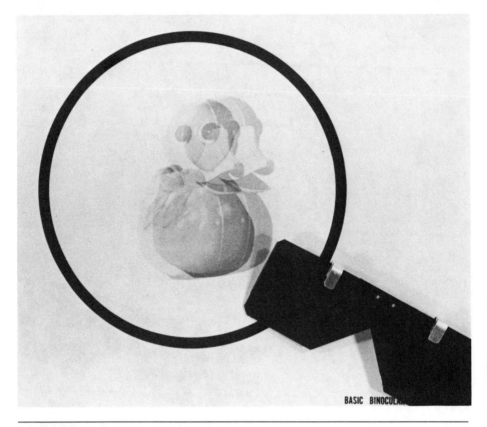

Figure 6.11   Keystone Basic Binocular Test #9.

the circle, depending on the position of the red and green filters in relation to his eyes.

Vectographic Plates
Vectograms (StereoOptical Co.).   There are a number of useful stereograms in this set. They vary in (a) the pictorial nature of the stimuli (i.e., nursery rhyme figures; a clown with blocks [see Figure 6.12]; a view of a large city from the air); (b) the number of different disparities presented within a single display (e.g., great variance in disparities presented in the aerial scene, fewer in the nursery rhyme figures); and (c) the variability of the disparity (i.e., some are single vectograms in which disparities are fixed; some are pairs of vectograms, wherein disparities may be changed by changing the relationship between the two vectograms).

Orthofusor (B&L).   These are very similar in design to the vectograms just described. They differ in that (a) they are smaller in size; (b) they are all variable

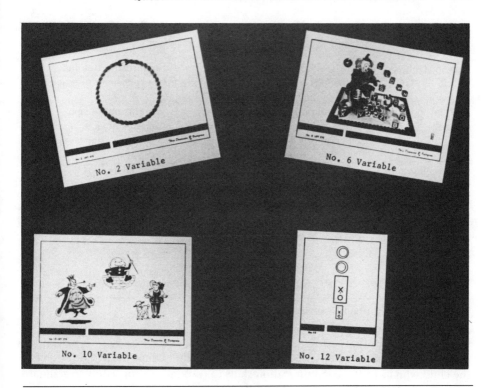

Figure 6.12   Vectograms #2, 6, 10, and 12.

disparity stereograms; (c) the pictorial nature of the stimuli tends to be too complex for young children.

Two Pencil Alignment Test.   This test requires nothing more in the way of equipment than two sharpened pencils, each about 6 inches long. The examiner holds one pencil, oriented horizontally, about 50 cm in front of the patient, gives the second pencil to the patient, and says: "Hold your pencil like this (horizontally) and touch my pencil point with your pencil point." According to Reinecke (41), the patient with normal stereoacuity will be able to bring his pencil point, accurately and repeatedly, to within 1 cm of the examiner's pencil point. He also suggests that the examiner stay well behind the pencil he is holding so that background (from the patient's perspective) is not fused, thereby making the patient's performance a true test of his ability to detect relative position and depth. The test may be used in any position of gaze.

□ **Summary**

Tables 6.5, 6.6, and 6.7 list all the tests described above. Clearly, there is no shortage of useful stereoacuity tests, *as long as the patient is at least 3 years old*.

Test	Age	Positive Features	Negative Features
Howard-Dohlman*	5	Response is nonverbal Presents concrete displays rather than illusions	Requires pretraining Occupies a lot of space
A.O. vectographic (adult)**	5	Requires little space, equipment Tests a satisfactory range of disparities at farpoint	Presents an illusion Contains obvious monocular cues at easier levels of the test
A.O. vectographic (child)†	5	Child names shapes rather than ordinal positions Very few monocular cues	Presents an illusion All stimuli but one are disparate; hence, child must understand concept of relative comparisons

*See p. 176.
**See p. 178.
†See p. 180.

Table 6.5　Distance Stereoacuity Tests

(For additional comparisons, see [42,43,44,45].) What about the child not yet 3, the child who lacks the communication skills to respond appropriately to standard stereoacuity tests? How may his binocular status be assessed?

One option would be to compare monocular and binocular VEPs (46). The VEP technology has been used long enough, for enough different purposes at enough different sites, to assume its validity. Surely it can only be a matter of time before such devices become practical for general office installation.

A second option—it, too, limited presently to experimental sites but showing promise—is the use of anaglyphic dynamic random-dot displays on a cathode ray tube (47).

If these two methods are not feasible, and if a way to simplify the test cannot be devised, then the optometrist has no choice but (a) to recognize that single binocular vision develops on the basis of straight eyes and similar, clear images stimulating each retina and that, (b) therefore, a reasonable and valid inference may be drawn on the basis of objective observations (e.g., position of corneal reflexes, cover tests, assessment of ocular motilities, refractive status) in conjunction with visual acuity, measured as accurately as possible. These are all powerful tests. They provide much information. Their value should not be minimized because of their simplicity.

□ If Stereoacuity Adequate? = No

Substandard stereoacuity suggests a number of possible clinical deficits, all of which may have to be ruled out. But, the ruling-out process is most efficiently accomplished if the tests are ordered heuristically. For this reason, the next step in the detection process is to make certain that faulty stereoacuity is not due to uncorrected ametropia (see D on Figure 6.1 flow diagram and below).

□ If Stereoacuity Adequate? = Yes

High-grade stereoacuity in at least one position of gaze and/or one fixation distance rules out constant strabismus, but it does not preclude a mild, unilateral amblyopia (or a strabismus that manifests in other positions of gaze or at fixation distances other than the standard ones used for testing. Some of these conditions are cited in Chapter 4, p. 126). Hence, the next step is to determine the (best corrected) visual acuity in each eye (see B on Figure 6.1 flow diagram and below).

■
_____

B. VISUAL ACUITY (BEST CORRECTED) 20/20 IN EACH EYE?

A full discussion regarding the development of visual acuity, and various ways to test it, appears in Chapter 3.

□ If No

Make certain that the reduced visual acuity is not due to uncorrected ametropia. Measure refractive status, if it has not yet been done, or retest it if there is a reasonable doubt as to its validity (see D on Figure 6.1 flow diagram and below).

□ If Yes

This indicates that the patient presents neither constant strabismus nor amblyopia. All that remains, then, is to rule out intermittent strabismus (see C on Figure 6.1 flow diagram and below).

Test	Age	Positive Features	Negative Features
Titmus circles (see p. 188)	5	Provides a full range of disparity conditions	Stereoacuity of 100 seconds arc may be obtained on the basis of monocular cues; young children's responses are often ambiguous, difficult to interpret; requires filters
A.O. vectographic (see p. 189)	5	Provides a full range of disparity conditions	Stereoacuity of 120 seconds arc may be obtained on the basis of monocular cues; young children's responses are often ambiguous, difficult to interpret; requires filters
Verhoeff stereopter (see p. 184)	5	Presents concrete display rather than illusion; responses need not be verbal; does not require filters	All stimuli are on different planes; hence, child must understand concept of relative comparisons
Randot circles (see p. 191)	5	Provides a full range of disparity conditions	Stereoacuity of 100 seconds arc may be obtained on the basis of monocular cues; young children's responses are often ambiguous, difficult to interpret; requires filters
TNO Qualitative plates (see p. 196)	5	No monocular cues; provides a full range of disparity conditions	Young children's responses are often ambiguous, difficult to interpret; requires filters
Titmus animals (see p. 187)	4	Very few monocular cues; responses need not be verbal, and even those are not demanding	Does not test beyond 100 seconds arc under standard conditions; requires filters
Randot animals (see p. 191)	4	Very few monocular cues; responses need not be verbal, and even those are not demanding	Does not test beyond 100 seconds arc under standard conditions; requires filters
Lang (see p. 190)	4	Stimuli are very familiar to young children; child need not respond verbally; does not require filters	Tests only crude levels of stereoacuity
Frisby (see p. 181)	3	Does not use filters; presents concrete display rather than illusion; very few monocular cues if stimulus is held correctly and child is not allowed to exploit motion parallax	Test is somewhat awkward to hold correctly; concept of embedded "ball" may be confusing; four alternatives may go beyond the abilities of many 3- to 4-year-old children

Test			
Titmus fly (see p. 186)	3	Stimulus is eyecatching; presents few distractors	Measures gross stereopsis only; young children's responses are often ambiguous, difficult to interpret; requires filters
Randot Forms (see p. 190)	3	Stimuli are very familiar to young children; child need not respond verbally; no monocular cues	Tests only crude levels of stereoacuity; requires filters
Random-dot E (see p. 191)	3	Extremely valid when administered at 1.5 meters; responses need not be verbal; easy to manipulate; no monocular cues; presents only two alternatives	Requires filters; does not allow for precise measure of stereoacuity even though it is extremely difficult to pass at 1.5 meters (165 seconds arc)
TNO Screening (see p. 194)	3	Responses need not be verbal; easy to manipulate; no monocular cues	Requires use of filter glasses; measures crude stereoacuity only
Modified Frisby (see p. 254)	1	Same as standard Frisby (see above); easy to manipulate; presents only two alternatives	Tests only crude levels of stereoacuity

Table 6.6 Near Stereoacuity Tests

Device	Targets
Two pencils (see p. 201)	Pencils
Brewster stereoscope (see p. 197)	Keystone Visual Skill Test (Card DB-6D: farpoint) (Card 5111: nearpoint) Keystone Peek-A-Boo Series Bernell Biopter Screening Test Any stereogram that provides the illusion of depth
Wheatstone stereoscope (e.g., synoptophore) (see p. 198)	Any stereogram that provides the illusion of depth
Red/green plates (see p. 198)	Keystone Basic Binocular Tests Any stereogram that provides the illusion of depth
Vectographic plates (see p. 199)	Stereo-Optical vectograms Bausch & Lomb Orthofusor

Any of the devices listed here may be used to assess a child's ability to perceive depth; i.e., align both eyes accurately. Each, in its own way, presents disparate stimuli to each eye in the context of a binocularly fused field.

Table 6.7   Informal Assessment of Stereopsis

■

C. EVIDENCE OF INTERMITTENT STRABISMUS?

The term *strabismus* refers to the condition of bifoveal misalignment. The term *intermittent strabismus* refers to a condition in which strabismus does manifest, but not constantly. At times the patient's binocular status is normal; other times he displays strabismus. As such, it would be just as accurate to identify intermittent strabismus as "intermittent normal binocularity," so long as "binocular" met the conditions defined on page 175: i.e., the patient displayed adequate stereoacuity. (We recognize that in defining all intermittently binocular patients as intermittent strabismics, we are ignoring such labels as periodic strabismus, cyclic strabismus, etc. We do this intentionally in order to stress the fundamental principle that we will employ when discussing treatment; namely, that the patient who is able to display adequate stereoacuity—at least sometimes, under some circumstances— offers a different condition, in terms of treatment options, than the patient who can never display adequate stereoacuity, even though his eyes may appear to "look straight" at times, and misaligned at others. For additional discussion regarding this point, see p. 221.)

Evidence of intermittent strabismus is often noted in the case history, during unilateral and alternating cover tests, during nearpoint of convergence test, when testing ocular motilities, and/or during the late stages of a vision evaluation, as the patient fatigues.

In the case history, the patient (or his parent) is apt to report that signs and symptoms of strabismus occur only under certain conditions: at certain times of the day, or when he is looking at a specific distance or in a specific direction.

When administering the unilateral (see p. 218) and alternating (see p. 218) cover tests, intermittent strabismus may be more apparent if the occluder is held in place a little longer than usual, and if both detailed and nondetailed targets are used at far and/or near. Indeed, some patients with "convergence excess" manifest the condition only when fixating at a target held very close to their eyes—e.g., within 20 cm. Hence, it may be informative to conduct a cover test while the patient fixates at a target as close as that. Similarly, some patients with "divergence excess" manifest the condition only when in an inattentive state; e.g., when "daydreaming." Hence, it may also be useful to administer a cover test while the patient fixates on a poorly defined target that is well beyond the standard 6-meter test distance; out a window at a utility pole, for example, or down a long corridor at a light switch plate.

In the late stages of an examination, stay alert to the possibilities of intermittent strabismus by observing the patient carefully and, where there is any suspicion at all, by readministering the cover and nearpoint of convergence tests.

□ If Evidence of Intermittent Strabismus? = Yes

Initiate strabismus diagnostic procedures (see below).

□ If Evidence of Intermittent Strabismus = No

The optometrist may conclude, with reasonable certainty, that no anomaly exists, that the patient's binocular status is normal. Although there is always the chance of omission through oversimplification, it is appropriate to stop investigating binocular status at this point and proceed to the next basic question of the examination (see Chapter 7).

___■_____

D. UNCORRECTED AMETROPIA?

If refractive status has already been determined, then no further testing is needed to answer this question—unless there is uncertainty about the validity of the recorded refraction outcomes. If refraction has not yet been done, now is the time. It is illogical to go further without that information.

Mention should be made here about the special value of cycloplegic refraction and binocular refraction procedures for determining refractive status in cases of nonstrabismic anisometropia with related intractable visual acuity deficits. The first is self-evident. In respect to the latter, subjective testing is much more valid and decisive under binocular refraction testing conditions in such cases, so long as the patient is able to perceive the right eye and left eye stimuli simultaneously. Obviously, the benefit of this testing setup is that it enables the better eye to control the fixation process for the partner eye, thereby causing the poorer eye to align fairly accurately (in the absence of strabismus) and steadily. This, in turn, optimizes the visual acuity potential of the poorer eye.

☐ If Uncorrected Ametropia? = Yes

Determine the ametropia and repeat the testing sequence with compensatory lenses in place (see E on Figure 6.1 flow diagram).

☐ If Uncorrected Ametropia = No

Look for evidence of strabismus (see F on Figure 6.1 flow diagram and below).

F. STRABISMUS APPARENT?

If stereoacuity is adequate, then the likelihood of (constant) strabismus is negligible. If stereoacuity is not adequate, then strabismus is indeed suspect and more testing is necessary.

☐ If Strabismus Apparent? = Yes

Terminate the detection process: initiate diagnostic process (see below). This does not imply the absence of other contributing factors, as yet undetected. Rather, it acknowledges that once a binocular anomaly is detected, the sequence of testing should be organized in a way that takes that knowledge into account.

☐ If Strabismus Apparent = No

Reflect for a moment; what has been determined to this point? Only that the patient displays substandard stereoacuity that is not explained by an apparent strabismus or uncorrected ametropia. Other possible explanations for the reduced stereoacuity must be considered. First among these is small-angle strabismus (see G on Figure 6.1 flow diagram and below).

■

G. EVIDENCE OF SMALL-ANGLE STRABISMUS?

The topic of small-angle strabismus has a short but very active and diverse history in the literature. Some authors prefer to apply the term solely on the basis of the magnitude of the deviation, proposing that anything less than 5 degrees represent, a small-angle, or "micro," strabismus (48). Others argue that the term should be applied only when a cluster of specific clinical signs are noted (see historical review in [24, pp. 303-305]).

The view represented here is that small-angle strabismus is a binocular deviation too small to be detected by standard direct observation methods. Small-angle strabismus is often inferred rather than observed. The unilateral cover test does not reveal it. (Although if the test is repeated with greater than usual care once a small-angle strabismus is suspected, a slight previously unnoticed "flick" may be seen.)

□ Characteristics of Small-Angle Strabismus

Small-angle strabismus is characterized by a triad of clinical signs that have been identified as the "monofixation syndrome" (15):

1. Reduced stereoacuity. Rarely is it better than 100 seconds of arc at near when measured with line/contour stereograms such as the Titmus stereotest; it is usually worse than this when random-dot stereogram testing is done; for example, patients with small-angle strabismus rarely, if ever, pass the Random-dot E stereotest when it is administered at 1.5 meters.

2. Mild, unilateral amblyopia; one eye capable of 20/20 or better, while the best (corrected) distance visual acuity in the other eye is no better than 20/25 and usually no worse than 20/40. A moderate anisometropia is often noted.

3. A small (about 3 degrees) facultative central scotoma (suppression area) within the visual field of one eye.

None of these is sufficient evidence by itself to support an inference of bifoveal misalignment. But, when they are all present, the opposite is true.

Now another glance at the flow diagram (Figure 6.1). What has already been determined in regard to these three characteristics of small-angle strabismus:

reduced stereoacuity, mild unilateral amblyopia, and a small unilateral facultative central scotoma? Stereoacuity and visual acuity have already been measured. If only one of these two conforms with the triad noted above—and it is impossible to reach this location in the flow diagram unless at least one of the two is deficient— then small-angle strabismus is ruled out. If both of these conform with the characteristics listed above, then a test for the presence of a unilateral facultative central scotoma is now called for.

☐ Tests for Facultative Scotoma

There are a number of ways to test for a small central facultative unilateral scotoma (49). The two tests described here are among the least complex and therefore are desirable for use with children (15,24,25,50,51,52).

COMPARISON OF RESPONSES TO THE WORTH 4-DOT TEST, WHEN IT IS ADMINISTERED AT NEARPOINT AND FARPOINT

The Worth 4-dot test consists of a light stimulus made up of four illuminated spots: two green, one red, one white.

The apparatus that is most often used for farpoint testing (at 6 meters) projects a small (1.25°) image onto the retina. The nearpoint apparatus, when held at 33 cm, projects a larger (approximately 6°) image onto the retina (see Figure 6.13). When the dots are viewed through anaglyphic filters, the patient with binocular fusion will report four dots; two green, one red and one "mixed red/green." The patient who lacks binocular fusion will report either two dots or three dots or five dots, depending upon the motor and sensory states of the eyes. A response of two dots or three dots from a patient who has two functioning eyes indicates *suppression*, a cortical ignoring of visual sensations from one retina that occurs only when both eyes are open.

The patient with a small facultative central scotoma, therefore, will report either two or three dots when the Worth 4-dot farpoint test apparatus is shown from 6 meters, if the *facultative scotoma is larger than 1.25°*. If this patient then views the same test apparatus from a 1-meter distance, from where it projects a much larger (7.5°) image onto the retina, he may report seeing all four dots, *if his facultative central scotoma is smaller than 7.5°*, and if his eyes are sufficiently aligned to allow some degree of fusion.

Hence, one method for eliciting evidence of a small, central unilateral facultative scotoma is to present the Worth 4-dot farpoint test apparatus from a 6-meter distance and then reduce the distance or, the opposite: present the Worth 4-dot nearpoint apparatus at 33 cm and then extend the distance. In either case, the distance at which the suppression manifests implies the size of the facultative scotoma.

Figure 6.13
Nearpoint Worth 4-dot
test.

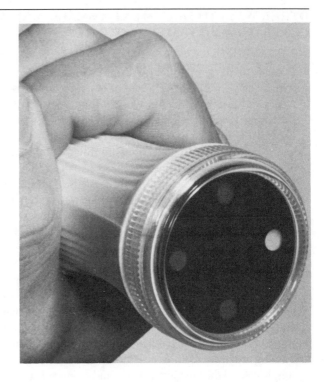

4 BASE-OUT PRISM TEST

This test requires a 4-diopter prism and a small, well-defined, farpoint fixation target. To administer:

1. As the patient fixates the stimulus, place the 4-diopter prism, base out, before one of her eyes (e.g., the left). If no movement is noted in that eye, it suggests that the patient did not observe the effect of the prism, which, in turn, implies a suppression scotoma in that eye. If, on the contrary, that eye (i.e., the left) is seen to shift in the direction of the apex of the prism (to the right, in this example), ostensibly to refixate the target, it indicates the absence of foveal suppression in that eye. If the opposite (right) eye is seen to make a slow, fusional adduction movement, it implies that it had first made a movement yoked with the eye behind the prism and is now manifesting a normal fusional reflex. Hence, it implies the absence of a foveal suppression in *that* eye.

2. To double check, repeat test with prism placed in front of the other eye. If the 4 base-out prism test and/or the Worth 4-dot test viewed at different distances reveal(s) a small facultative central scotoma, interpret it for what is appears to be; and when this is seen in conjunction with reduced stereoacuity and reduced visual acuity in one eye, assume the presence of small-angle strabismus.

OTHER WAYS TO DOCUMENT A SMALL, UNILATERAL, CENTRAL FACULTATIVE SCOTOMA

- Draw a small (approximately 3-mm diameter) circle on a sheet of white paper with a red pencil. Place this sheet of paper on a sheet of red plastic. The patient wears red green filter glasses, positioned so that the eye suspected of having the suppression area cannot see the drawn red circle. (This describes a now-unavailable instrument: the Brock Posture Board.) Have the patient hold a small white light source (e.g., a transilluminator bulb) against the back of the sheet of red plastic. Under these conditions, the red light produced by the transil-lumintor bulb will be visible only to the suspected eye when the red green filters are in place. Direct the patient to position the red light within the red circle, first while not wearing the filters, then with the filters in place. (The first trial is to make certain that he is able to perform the required behavior. Clearly, it is not a test for suppression under these circumstances; a monocular individual could perform this task. The second trial does test for suppression.) If the patient has a small central facultative scotoma in the eye stimulated by light source, it (the red light) will disappear from view—be suppressed—when he attempts to place it within the red circle and will reappear as he moves it away. (Obviously, it will also be apparent if his other eye is occluded.)
- Use the *suppression control marks* that are on most vectographic tests and training devices. If they are too large to be suppressed when held at 40 cm, simply extend the viewing distance and monitor if and when the target disappears.
- Set up an Autoplot tangent screen with the smallest light target and the red filter. Have the patient wear red/green filter glasses, oriented so that only the eye suspected of having the central suppression area is able to see the small red light on the Autoplot screen. The patient fixates the central fixation target with both eyes as the red stimulus light is brought toward that target. If the patient has a small facultative scotoma, the red light will disappear as it enters the suppression zone.
- Test for suppression with the AO vectographic distance slide. If it manifests, have the patient continue to fixate that line of letters as he walks toward the screen. When he reaches the point where the suppressed letters on the screen subtends an angle larger than his facultative scotoma, they will become apparent.
- Clearly, there are many ways to document the presence of a small, unilateral, central facultative scotoma. For all practical purposes, however, what has already been described should be sufficient.

□ If Small-Angle Strabismus? = Yes

The detection process is completed. Move on to the strabismus diagnosis process (see Figure 6.14 and below).

□ If Small-Angle Strabismus? = No

Look at the flow diagram (Figure 6.1). What does it reveal about the patient? He displays substandard stereoacuity and/or substandard visual acuity that is not attributable to either strabismus or ametropia. What possible explanations remain? Either an impediment to sight caused by a lesion within the sensory system or a nonobservable, nonpathological deficiency in the resolution capabilities of the sensory system. In simpler terms: an organic deficit or a functional deficit. The next step, then, is to differentiate between the two (see H in Figure 6.1 flow diagram and below).

H. EVIDENCE OF PATHOLOGY?

In most cases of reduced monocular visual acuity it is not difficult to distinguish between a functional and organic deficit. Organic deficits are usually apparent (i.e., accompanied by one or more abnormal fundus signs such as disc pallor, macular lesion, etc.), or they may be inferred on the basis of an abnormal response to a unilateral color test, swinging flashlight test, glare recovery test, electrodiagnostic testing, and so on. Functional deficits are usually accompanied by detectable strabismus and/or associated refractive conditions, such as significant anisometropia.

There are some cases, however, where it is exceptionally difficult to differentiate between the two, the dilemma being resolved only through exercising a deductive process: by ruling out what can be ruled out, and assuming that what remains is likely to be the cause.

Obviously, then, the first step should be to reassess the ocular health status (53). It is always possible, for example, to overlook a very small macular lesion, particularly when there was no reason, initially, to suspect its existence. Only after the reassessment is completed and no organic deficits noted should the optometrist assume a functional basis for the reduced visual acuity.

□ If Evidence of Pathology? = Yes

Diagnose and make appropriate recommendations.

□ If Evidence of Pathology = No

Assume amblyopia and initiate amblyopia diagnosis process (see Figure 6.15).

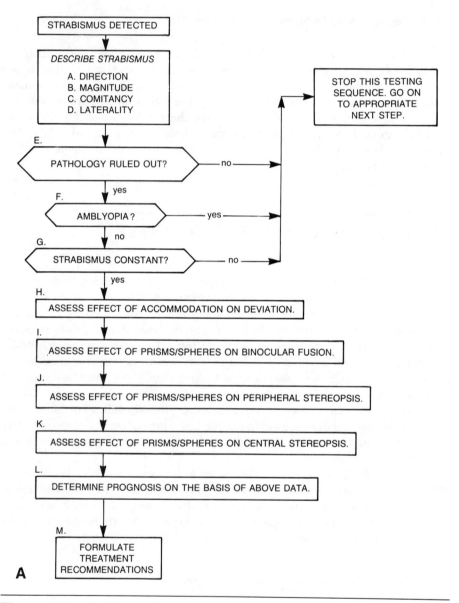

Figure 6.14 Strabismus diagnostic sequence.

Figure 6.14

(Continued)

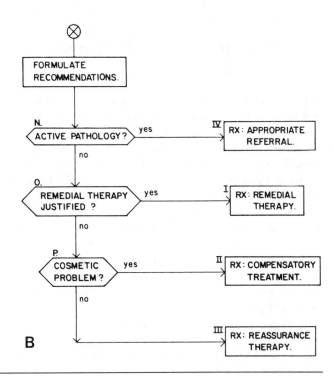

DIAGNOSIS OF A BINOCULAR ANOMALY

The preceding section was mainly concerned with the *detection* of two binocular anomalies: strabismus (overt and small-angle) and amblyopia. If either anomaly is detected, the optometrist is obliged to *diagnose* the condition: to define it well enough to make appropriate recommendations regarding its management. To do this, she must consider such factors as the potential reversibility of the condition and the probable relative effectiveness of various treatments, and weigh these against the short-term and long-term impact of the condition on the patient and the physical (time/money) and pyschological costs of the treatment.

This section focuses on those concerns and on nystagmus. It does not provide an exhaustive review of the topics of strabismus, amblyopia, and nystagmus. They are complex topics that warrant separate texts (15,24,25,51,52,54). The goals here are (a) to define efficient diagnostic steps that should be taken once the anomaly has been detected, and (b) to propose guidelines for making decisions about how the condition, once diagnosed, should be managed. An overview of what those treatments are likely to entail is presented in Chapters 9, 10, 11, 12, 13, and 14.

■

DIAGNOSIS OF STRABISMUS

Figure 6.14 maps out the diagnostic process that is useful once strabismus is detected, *if* the patient is old enough to engage in the tests. (See pp. 230–235 for the diagnostic process to be employed with younger children.) (Note: We recognize that the process shown in Figure 6.14 is not exhaustive; many traditionally popular tests are omitted. It is designed to obtain clinical data in an heuristic manner, so that the information needed to make valid treatment decisions is acquired efficiently, and other information, albeit interesting and conceivably pertinent at some future time, is ignored, at least for the present. In essence, it reflects a position that we believe to be reasonable; namely, that:

1. Some strabismus cases are very uncomplicated and can be successfully treated in a primary care practice, employing an office-managed, home-based lens/vision therapy regimen; *all* primary care optometrists should be able to identify such cases and proceed accordingly.

2. Some strabismus cases are relatively complex but, in the right hands, are amenable to treatment with lenses and vision therapy; *all* primary care opmetrists should be able to identify such cases and make appropriate referral to their more specialized colleagues.

3. Some strabismus cases will not respond favorably to lenses and/or vision therapy—they simply lack the neurophysiological potential for simultaneous binocular function; *all* primary care optometrists should be able to identify them and translate their findings into appropriate recommendations for the patient: i.e., the patient should be reassured, or referred for surgical consultation if cosmesis is a concern. We also acknowledge that some will object to our making a distinction between what all primary care optometrists should know and able to do, and what just a few more highly trained and experienced ones should be able to do. We would disagree with them and believe the present-day practices support our position.)

Notice that unless the process is truncated by evidence of significant amblyopia, all branches lead to one of the following recommendations:

1. Remedial therapy.*
2. Compensatory therapy.*
3. Reassurance therapy.
4. Refer for consultation.

*Remedial therapy refers to the instituting of training and/or surgical regimens that are designed to improve the functional level of the patient's binocular status. Compensatory therapy refers to the instituting of surgical and/or optical device regimens that are intended to improve cosmetic appearance by reducing the apparent magnitude of the binocular misalignment.

The first of these, remedial therapy, is recommended when the evidence suggests that the patient is physiologically capable of normal binocular vision if binocular alignment is achieved, albeit through the use of prisms and/or spheres; the second, when the evidence suggests the contrary; the third, when circumstances indicate that "no treatment" is the wisest and/or most practical course; and the fourth, an appropriate referral, when there is reason to suspect active pathology.

The flow diagram does not call for a detailed assessment of every aspect of the strabismus. It focuses on what is permitted to determining the probable benefit of a remedial approach. (Implicit in this remark is the assumption that remediation is always preferable to a compensatory treatment, if a choice exists.) It ignores what does not contribute directly to that goal, even though such information may ultimately be needed, if and when a remedial program is designed.

The process commences with a description of the basic characteristics of the deviation (see A in Figure 6.14 flow diagram and below). If the patient is ametropic, all testing is to be done with the correct compensatory prescription.

□ A. Direction

The direction of a strabismus is defined in terms of the relative positions of the visual axes. When one visual axis converges in excess of the other, the condition is called *esotropia, convergent strabismus*, or, simply, an *esodeviation*. The opposite condition is called *exotropia, divergent strabismus*, or an *exodeviation*. When the visual axis of one eye is higher than it should be, the condition is called *hypertropia;* the opposite, *hypotropia*. When there is a rotation of the eye, a tipping of the vertical meridian of the cornea, the condition is called *cyclotropia; incyclotropia* describes a tipping toward the nose; *excyclotropia*, a tipping away from the nose.

When the condition is exclusive to one eye, it is customary to indicate this as part of the directional label. Hence, a patient might display *right esotropia, left hypertropia*, and so on. And finally, an eye may deviate in more than one direction; for example, as a *right esohypertropia, a right exohypertropia*, and so on.

We recognize that is is a departure from convention to include surgery as a component of an optometric remedial therapy approach to the management of strabismus. Our reason: It is important to recognize that (a) reorienting an eye surgically may, if successful, hasten the rehabilitation effort dramatically; and (b) the less time the eyes function in a deviant posture, the better, particularly when strabismus manifests in the very young child.

This topic will be discussed more fully in Chapter 11. It is sufficient at this time for the reader to comprehend that this position does not argue against nonsurgical remedial (vision) therapy, but neither does it argue against surgery. In fact, it argues against nothing except losing the opportunity to provide a child with normal binocular vision because of an unwavering commitment to one specific treatment regimen and an equally unwavering prejudice against another.

☐ B. Magnitude

The magnitude of a strabismus at far and near fixation is usually measured in prism diopters. Some measurement methods are objective, based on examiner's observations. Others are subjective, based upon the patient's observations and reports. In this instance, an objective method should be used; the subjective procedure may be affected by the sensory adaptions that often accompany strabismus (see discussion regarding anomalous retinal correspondence [ARC] below).

ALTERNATE COVER TEST AND PRISM

The unilateral cover test is effective in detecting strabismus and may also, at times, be useful in measuring its magnitude. (This is especially true with noncomitant strabismics who manifest different magnitudes of deviation as a function of which eye is fixating. This phenomenon, however, goes beyond the scope of this book. Suffice it to say that noncomitant strabismus will become evident to the optometrist in other ways [see below]; there should be no need for her to investigate primary versus secondary deviations.) But the alternate cover test is far more effective. The principle of the alternate cover test is to prevent binocular function by shifting the cover from one eye to the other rapidly enough to prevent binocular looking (55). This does not mean that the occluder is removed immediately from each eye. On the contrary, it is desirable to keep the occluder over one eye for a few seconds before shifting it, rapidly, to the other eye.

In the unilateral cover test, heterotropia is signaled by a realignment shift in one eye that is triggered by introducing an occluder over the partner eye while the patient is viewing a target binocularly. In the alternate cover test, a realignment shift does not necessarily signal heterotropia; it could also be caused by a heterophoria. Hence, the alternate cover test is used to measure the magnitude of a strabismus *after* strabismus has been detected.

The general goal of the procedure is to determine the amount of horizontal and vertical prism needed to eliminate refixation shifts as the cover is alternated between the right and left eyes.

1. Patient fixates a farpoint, detailed target (e.g., 20/30 letters, if they are discernible by both eyes).

2. Examiner holds the occluder in one hand and a prism bar (or loose prism) in the other. She estimates the magnitude of the deviation in prism diopters, and then places a prism of this power before one of the patient's eyes, making certain to orient it properly (i.e., esotropia = base out; exotropia = base in; hypertropia = base down; hypotropia = base up).

3. The examiner moves the occluder quickly from one eye to the other, pausing when the transfer is completed, watching for the effect of the prism on any fixation shifts.

4. Examiner changes the amount of prism until alternate cover test reveals no refixation shifts. This is recorded as the magnitude of the strabismus.

5. Repeat this procedure while the patient fixates an accommodation-stimulating target held at nearpoint. (Note: This procedure does not apply when the patient's heterophoria may be significantly greater than the magnitude of the heterotropia: e.g., small-angle strabismus.)

ALTERNATIVE METHODS

The procedures described above should meet clinical needs in virtually every case. Should an alternative method be desired, however, there are many procedures available. These include using the major amblyoscope or other devices of that type, and are described fully in all standard strabismus textbooks (see, for example, [15,24,25]). There is no need, therefore, to expand on this topic here, other than to mention a recently published description of a procedure for measuring the amount of shift provoked by the cover test with a millimeter rule in lieu of prism (56). On average, each millimeter of shift, is equivalent to 4.7 degrees.

□ C. Comitancy

If the magnitude of a deviation at a given distance remains the same in all directions of gaze, it is described as *comitant*. If it varies then it is *noncomitant*. Noncomitant deviations imply extraocular muscle involvement. This, in turn, has led to the suggestion that noncomitant deviations should be classified either as *paralytic* or *incomitant* (24, p. 146). The former, of course, refers to extraocular muscle paralysis or paresis; the latter to faulty neuromotor interactions that result in overaction or underaction of an extraocular muscle in certain positions of gaze.

TO ASSESS

Look for changes in the magnitude of the deviation as the eye is directed to the nine diagnostic positions of gaze. This is most readily accomplished by observing the relative position of the corneal reflexes (as in the Hirschberg test). This, in turn, can be done in two ways: Patient's head remains stationary while fixation target is moved; or fixation target remains fixed and patient's head is moved so that, in order to retain fixation, the eyes must move accordingly. The latter method is usually best with young children.

ALTERNATIVE METHODS

Measure the deviation with the alternate cover and prism test (see above) in all diagnostic positions of gaze; or compare the magnitude of the deviation measured by the unilateral cover test (see above) with the right eye fixating and with the left eye fixating. If difference is revealed, suspect noncomittance.

☐ D. Unilateral or Alternating?

Some strabismics show a very flexible fixation pattern; sometimes their right eye is the deviating one, sometimes the left. Other strabismics show a unilateral fixation pattern; the same eye deviates at all times under all conditions.

The link between fixation pattern and amblyopia is obvious. The patient with 20/20 visual acuity in each eye is not apt to be a unilateral strabismic, just as the patient with 20/20 in one eye and 20/70 in the other is not likely to display an active alternating pattern.

To test. Separate procedures are not needed. Draw inferences from the patient's visual acuity and observe the patient's eyes as he engages in the various diagnostic tests, described above.

☐ E. Signs of Pathology?

In diagnosing a strabismus, special care should be taken to rule out the possibility of an active pathology. The optometrist should make particular inquiry regarding:

1. *Age of patient at onset*. Most strabismus manifests during the first 4 years of life. Onset of strabismus past the age of four should be viewed with careful suspicion.

2. *Abruptness of onset*. This is directly related to the first concern: age at onset. Once again, an abrupt onset is more apt to be a sign of pathology than is one that has been noted, off and on, for a long period of time.

3. *Accompanying symptoms*. Concern regarding an active pathology increases if the patient manifests constant diplopia, ptosis, and or other signs and symptoms that appear to be related to a central nervous system involvement.

IF SIGNS OF PATHOLOGY? = YES

Treat or make appropriate referral.

IF SIGNS OF PATHOLOGY? = NO

Before continuing with the diagnostic process, consider amblyopia and its potential impact. There is little benefit in probing subordinate binocular abilities until amblyopia has been ruled out or dealt with successfully (see F in Figure 6.14 flow diagram and below).

☐ F. Evidence of Significant Amblyopia?

No additional testing should be necessary to answer this query. Assuming that the patient's ocular health and refractive status have been thoroughly assessed, and appropriate actions taken, any persistent reduction in (best corrected) visual acuity should now be viewed as evidence of amblyopia.

IF EVIDENCE OF SIGNIFICANT AMBLYOPIA? = YES

Initiate the amblyopic diagnostic process (see Figure 6.15). This is especially important if best corrected visual acuity is 20/60 or less. Good decisions regarding management of strabismus are not possible until an effort has been made to improve visual acuity to maximum level.

IF EVIDENCE OF SIGNIFICANT AMBLYOPIA? = NO

At this point, it would be useful to determine the constancy of the strabismus (see G in Figure 6.14 flow diagram and below).

□ G. Strabismus Constant?

Here the optometrist attempts to determine whether the strabismus is present at all times (*i.e.*, *constant*) or interrupted by occasions when the patient displays bifoveal alignment (*i.e.*, *intermittent*). Subsequent testing will be decided on the basis of this information.

A description of procedures for detecting intermittent strabismus was included in the previous section. Those procedures do not pertain here, however. Clinical concerns are not the same at this stage, as when the detection process was underway. Then the question was, "Does the patient maintain bifoveal alignment *at all times?*" Now the question is, "Does the patient *ever* display bifoveal alignment; are there *ever* instances when his stereoacuity is adequate"

This question, if taken literally, could be very difficult to answer. It would require the strabismic patient to be within view of a trained observer for as many hours/days as is necessary to satisfy the word "ever." This is avoided by assuming that the patient who shows no capacity for bifoveal alignment during the time he is within the optometrist's view has a constant strabismus. True, there is always the possibility of committing a sampling error—of overlooking a period of bifoveal alignment because insufficient time was spent observing—but this is not very likely unless the patient arrives for his visit exceptionally tired or ill. So many powerful fusion-stimulating conditions are provided during an optometric evaluation that it is reasonable to conclude that if bifoveal alignment is never obtained during the testing process, it is equivalent to documenting a constant strabismus.

If, on the other hand, the strabismus is intermittent, an attempt should be made to determine whether it is condition-specific. That is, does it occur when the patient fixates at a certain distance (e.g., far off, close up) or in a certain direction (e.g., to the right, upward)? Such strabismus is termed to be periodic and implies a specific cause. Nonperiodic strabismus applies when the deviation is intermittent but occurs unpredictably; when it does not appear to be triggered by specific visual-spatial condition but, rather, seems to be linked with the patient's fatigue state.

TO TEST

Measure stereoacuity at farpoint and nearpoint. Apparent alignment is insufficient documentation. (For all practical purposes, it is not difficult to identify intermittent strabismus. The condition is usually observed well in advance of this stage of the evaluation.)

IF STRABISMUS CONSTANT? = NO

As already stated, for the question to be answered "no,"the optometrist must be able to document occasions of adequate stereoacuity; i.e., better than 60 seconds of arc at nearpoint: better than 2 minutes of arc at farpoint. When this is the case, further testing should focus on prognosis and treatment recommendations (see G in Figure 6.14 flow diagram and below).

IF STRABISMUS CONSTANT? = YES

This establishes that the patient is never able to display high-grade central stereopsis. In other words, it documents what he cannot do, but it does not rule out other aspects of binocularity; i.e., the extent to which the deviation is affected by accommodation and the patient's potential to perform binocularly when prisms and/or spheres are used to stimulate both of his foveas simultaneously—*as though* his eyes were in alignment. These are important prognostic considerations.

□ H. Assess the Effect of Accommodation on the Deviation

In some cases of strabismus, the angle of deviation is significantly altered by accommodation; i.e., when fixating at far as compared with when fixating at near, or when fixating through plus or minus lenses that go beyond what is called for by the manifest ametropia; i.e., lenses that relax or stimulate accommodation. The first aspect of this has already been accomplished; it was done when the magnitude of the deviation was measured at far and near (see above). To investigate the latter aspect, empirically place minus (for exotropes) or plus (for esotropes) lenses before the patient's eyes and measure the angle of deviation at far (with exotropes) and at near (with exotropes and esotropes). For example, if the patient displays exotropia, assess the effect of -2.50 to -4.00 diopter spheres (O.U.) as the patient fixates on a near and then a distant target, making sure that the patient exercises full accommodation; that is, keeps the target clear. If the patient manifests esotropia, assess the effect of about $+2.50$ to $+4.00$ diopter spheres (O.U.) as she fixates on a near target, again making sure that she relaxes accommodation as much as possible—that is, again, keeps the target clear. We will discuss the interpretation of these observations shortly; for now, simply consider any evidence of a link between accommodation and the angle of deviation (as revealed by the magnitude of the deviation at far as compared with near, or by the effect of plus/minus lenses) to be a *favorable* sign.

Once these measures have been made, they are applied in determining the patient's potential for binocular fusion and stereopsis. Before this is discussed, however, the terms *fusion, peripheral stereopsis,* and *central stereopsis* should be defined.

FUSION AND PERIPHERAL STEREOPSIS

The distinction between central and peripheral single binocular vision is clinically important. Parks (15) defines *central single binocular vision* as "the cortical integration of the images projected onto each macula from the area of conscious regard," and *peripheral single binocular vision* as an "extramacular function that serves the visual space peripheral to the area of conscious regard" (p. 42). (The area of conscious regard is that part of the visual field—about 3 to 5 degrees in diameter—that one attends to under ordinary circumstances; that projects onto the maximal resolving area of the retina.) He goes on to observe that peripheral single binocular vision can, and frequently does, exist even when central single binocular vision is absent, but that the reverse does not occur. The rationale for this phenomenon is fairly apparent, although it borders on being a tautology: Panum's area is less constricted peripherally; therefore, fusion is more attainable.

Conceptualizing single binocular vision as two separate but interacting processes (i.e., central and peripheral) forces a reconsideration of the traditional hierarchy of fusion proposed by Worth (57). He defined fusion as comprising three levels of ascending ability. First degree: simultaneous awareness of dissimilar targets, one presented to the right eye, the other to the left, in a haploscopic device (e.g., fish and bowl; bird and cage). In short, simultaneous perception. Second degree: the binocular blending of two similar targets, each of which contains one (small) unique component that is not present in the other; i.e., flat fusion. Third degree: the binocular blending of similar targets that contain some moderately disparate components, thereby producing the percept of depth; i.e., stereopsis.

The Worth scaling is not compatible with the concept of two parallel, interacting processes of single binocular vision. Parks argues convincingly that simultaneous perception is solely a peripheral function, best illustrated by physiological or pathological diplopia: the awareness of similar retinal images too disparate to fuse, in the presence or absence of central fusion.

He also points out significant differences between fusion and stereopsis, each a separate process requiring different stimuli that produce different responses, and differing also in what they contribute to central and peripheral single binocular vision.

For example: (a) Fusion has a motor component while stereopsis does not. The optimal condition for fusion is zero image disparity and fusional vergence serves to achieve that condition. Stereopsis, on the other hand, requires horizontal image disparity but has no motor component to serve this need. (b) Although the sensory aspect of fusion is equally good for both central and peripheral single binocular vision, the motor aspect is very deficient in the central process and excellent in the peripheral. Extramacular stimulation produces normal motor fusional responses (15,58); the fusional vergence amplitudes of a person having only peripheral single binocular vision are usually just as good as those of one who also has central single binocular vision (59). (c) Central single binocular vision yields precise stereoacuity; the stereopsis obtained from peripheral single binocular vision is crude.

With these concepts in mind, what now? Central single binocular vision has been ruled out; that, in fact, is one of the reasons why the diagnostic process was initiated. Thus, the next question in a sequence of questions designed to determine what to recommend in terms of clinical management is: *Is there evidence of fusion and/or peripheral stereopsis?*

Clearly, a *yes* answer will have a different impact on treatment and prognosis considerations than will a *no*.

☐ I. Assess the Effect of Compensating Prism/ Spheres on Binocular Fusion

The central question at this point is the patient's ability to display a potential for normal fusion; i.e., would she be able to obtain fusion *if* her eyes were aligned? It has already been established that, in her present state, she lacks central stereopsis. It has not yet been established, however, whether she is capable of binocular fusion when appropriate targets have been positioned so that, despite the binocular misalignment, both maculae are stimulated simultaneously; i.e., by using compensating prisms/spheres. To do this:

Place sufficient prism in front of the patient's eyes to neutralize the strabismus at distance and administer the Worth Dot test at distance and near (and midway between, if this appears to be useful) in moderate illumination. Then remove the prism and repeat the test. (Note: If the patient's deviation was significantly reduced by the plus or minus lenses [as described above], repeat this testing through those same spherical lenses as well.)

If the patient reports seeing two, three, or five dots (i.e., suppression or diplopia) when the compensating (prism/sphere) lenses *are not* in place, and four dots (fusion) when the compensating (prism/sphere) lenses *are* in place, interpret it as a *favorable* sign. Go on to test the patient's potential for peripheral stereopsis. (See below.)

If the patient reports seeing four dots without the compensating lenses and something different than that when they are in place, it suggests ARC. This is *not* a favorable sign. (See below.)

If the patient reports seeing two, three, or five dots both when the compensating lenses are and are not in place, it raises very serious doubts about her potential for normal binocular fusion.

□ J. Assess the Effect of Compensating Prism/ Spheres on Peripheral Stereopsis

To test the patient's ability to perceive peripheral stereopsis: Start at near, then at distance (and midway between, if this appears to be useful), first without, then with the (prism/sphere) compensating lenses.

The Titmus stereotest "fly," and the TNO "butterfly" are appropriate for near-point testing, as is any other device that presents a relatively large stereo target. For distance, use the large red/green eccentric circles in the Bernell TV Stereotrainer, or something else of that type.

If the compensating lenses significantly improve peripheral stereopsis (at any or all fixation distances), consider it a *favorable* sign and go on to test the effect of those compensating lenses on his central stereopsis. (See below.)

If the patient reports peripheral stereopsis without the compensating lenses that is at least as good (if not better) than when they are in place, it suggests ARC. (See below.) This is *not* a favorable sign.

If the patient does not display peripheral stereopsis under either condition (i.e., with/without compensating lenses), it raises doubts about his potential for normal binocular fusion.

□ K. Assess the Effect of Compensating Prism/ Spheres on Central Stereopsis

To assess the patient's potential for central stereopsis at near, administer a standard stereoacuity test, such as the Wirt circles from the Titmus stereotest, etc., first without, then with the compensating (prism/sphere) lenses in place. To test this at distance, use the smaller red/green eccentric circles on the Bernell TV Stereotrainer.

If the compensating lenses provide central stereopsis that was not present without them (at any or all fixation distances), consider it a *favorable* sign.

If the patient displays central stereopsis without the compensating lenses that is at least as good (if not better) than when they are in place, it suggests anomalous retinal correspondence. (See below.) This is *not* a favorable sign.

□ Test for Anomalous Retinal Correspondence

ARC describes a condition where "either the two foveas have different visual directions, or where the fovea of the fixating eye has acquired an anomalous common visual direction with a peripheral element in the deviated eye" (24, p. 251).

In measurement terms, ARC exists when the objectively measured angle of deviation (known as angle H) does not coincide with the subjectively determined angle of deviation (known as angle S). The difference between angles H and S is called the angle of anomaly (angle A). Hence, in NRC, angle A equals zero. If angle A does not equal zero, ARC is revealed.

ARC, in turn, may be *harmonious* or *unharmonious*. In harmonious ARC, angle S equals zero; or, said differently, angle A equals angle H. In unharmonious ARC, angle S does not equal zero; angle H does not equal angle A. (We are ignoring the subclassifications of unharmonious ARC. They are not relevant to the process under discussion here.)

All of this confuses at first, becoming clear when it can be related to concrete situations. One is best served by keeping in mind that angle H refers to the actual position of the two eyes as measured objectively by a trained observer; the extent to which they deviate from alignment. Angle S represents the match between the stimulation of specific points on the patient's retinas and where she, in turn, perceives these stimuli to be located in space. In effect then, the term ARC describes a situation wherein the patient responds to a given set of conditions *as though* she had normal binocular vision, yet the examiner is able to observe a misalignment of the visual axes. For example, if the patient's eyes are in a strabismic posture as she looks at a light stimulus through (red/green) anaglyph filters, and she reports seeing a single, red/green light, then she is demonstrating that although noncorresponding retinal points are being stimulated, she perceives the situation as though corresponding points were being stimulated, i.e., ARC. Similarly, if a condition is constructed wherein both of her foveas are stimulated, the patient with ARC is likely to perceive two stimuli, separated the equivalent of angle A.

There are a number of retinal correspondence tests and, interestingly, they often appear to yield contradictory outcomes. (See Flom and Kerr [60] for some pertinent comments on this.) All of them are similar in that they are designed to compare angle H to angle S, in one way or another. They differ in how they elicit angle S, this ranging from determining the relative position of bifoveally stimulated afterimages to the mapping of the positions of a right-eye perceived image and a left-eye perceived image within the patient's binocular receptive field. Some investigators have scaled these tests in terms of how closely the test conditions approximate real-space conditions, thereby attempting to explain why they may yield different outcomes.

All of this is described in any good strabismus text. It need not be elaborated upon here. The purposes of this volume are served by pointing out that (a) ARC is a sensory adaptation to strabismus. It enables that strabismic patient to see "as though" his two eyes were in alignment. (b) As such, patients with ARC, because they have adapted, are usually less responsive to remedial treatment than are those with NRC.

TO TEST

The retinal correspondence tests described above meet the needs of the primary-care optometrist. There is a tendency to overtest retinal correspondence. The purpose of clinical testing is to obtain information that leads ultimately to correct decisions regarding appropriate treatment. Hence, there is no good reason to test retinal correspondence until *after* it has been established that the strabismic patient does have some binocular function. The reason it is tested then is to gain information relevant to the next step in designing a treatment program. If the strabismic patient shows NRC, then the conditions (test) in which this normal binocular function was observed may be used as foundation for teaching higher order abilities. If he shows ARC, then the existing binocular function provides a poor foundation; treatment will have to be designed to work around it or re-structure it.

That is the reason we recommended tests that employ stimuli and conditions that closely resemble the stimuli and conditions used in probing binocular function. There is no sense at this stage of the diagnostic process in selecting a test that presents totally different stimuli and conditions. Such a test will not provide the information that inspired the testing in the first place: namely, "Does the binocular ability observed in the patient derive from an adaptation that precludes the development of normal single binocular vision?"

□ Is More Testing Needed?

The procedures described above mark the end of the initial phase of testing. It is now time to make some decisions regarding the prospect of remediation through lenses and/or vision therapy. (Note: The following comments presume that the patient manifests reasonably good visual acuity in both eyes; i.e., at least 20/40. If she does not, then the diagnostic validity of these procedures is significantly reduced. In those cases, as Figure 6.14 indicates, the amblyopia should be ad-dressed first.)

□ M. Formulate Treatment Recommendations

The flow diagram (Figure 6.14) indicates four options. Obviously, appropriate treatment or referral (option IV) is chosen when there is reason to suspect an active pathology that warrants direct and immediate attention (see N in Figure 6.14 flow diagram, and discussion above).

When (and if) this concern is ruled out, then selection of the proper option from among the remaining three depends upon a prognosis. Or, stated more specifically, on the answer to: What is the probability of the patient achieving an adequate binocular status (normal binocular vision), assuming that appropriate therapeutic procedures are followed? (See O in Figure 6.14 flow diagram and below.)

□ O. Is Remedial Therapy Justified?

The guidelines defined below (and summarized in Tables 6.8 and 6.9) reflect the position we assumed earlier when we proposed that the primary-care optometrist

Prognosis	Indicator
Very good	Patient displays central stereopsis and normal retinal correspondence when tested at far and/or near through compensatory prisms/spheres
Good	Patient displays improved peripheral stereopsis and normal retinal correspondence when tested at far and/or near through compensatory prisms/spheres
Fair	Patient displays normal binocular fusion (Worth Dot test) but no stereopsis when tested at far and/or near through compensatory prisms/spheres
Guarded	Deviation is 10 pd more eso/less exo at near than at distance and/or deviation reduces 10 pd or more in response to additional plus/minus spheres. No evidence of fusion/stereopsis
Poor	None of the above

Table 6.8   Prognostic Indicators

should be expected to treat certain types of cases only, leaving the more complex ones to optometric colleagues (if nonsurgical treatment seemed reasonable), to surgeons (if nonsurgical treatment seemed futile and the patient was justifiably concerned about his appearance), or to simply reassure (if nonsurgical treatment seemed futile and the patient was not concerned about appearance).

Four types of test were described above (Figure 6.14) in which *favorable signs* may or may not be observed. In reverse order—but in correct order of relative importance—they were the following:

1. The effect of compensating lenses on central stereoacuity
2. The effect of compensating lenses on peripheral stereoacuity
3. The effect of compensating lenses on binocular fusion
4. The effect of accommodation on the magnitude of the deviation (i.e., fixation distance; plus or minus spheres beyond what is needed to compensate for ametropia)

If the first of these (i.e., the effect of compensating prisms/spheres on central stereopsis) yielded a favorable sign, then the patient should be viewed, at least thus far, as a *very good candidate* for vision therapy. All else being equal, the patient can probably be successfully managed in a primary-care practice. (See Chapter 9 for a discussion regarding the other factors that influence the efficacy of vision therapy, and Chapter 11 for specific suggestions regarding vision therapy for constant strabismus.)

If compensating prisms/spheres did not improve central stereopsis but did enable the patient to obtain significantly improved peripheral stereopsis, then consider him to be a *good candidate* for vision therapy, but not quite so good as if he had responded positively to the central stereoacuity stimuli. Once again, all else being equal, the patient can probably be successfully managed in a primary-care practice.

If Prognosis Is	Consider the Following
Very good	Recommend vision therapy in your office
Good	Recommend vision therapy in your office
Fair	Refer patient to specializing colleague
Guarded	Refer patient to specializing colleague
	or
	Reassure (if cosmetic appearance is good)
	or
	Refer (if cosmesis is unacceptable) for a surgical consultation
Poor	Reassure or refer for surgical consultation, as discussed above

Table 6.9   Treatment Guidelines

If the compensating lenses did not enable the patient to obtain central or peripheral stereopsis but did enable him to obtain binocular fusion, consider him to be a *fair candidate* for vision therapy, although not so favorable as if he had also demonstrated stereopsis. Such patients are probably best served by referral to an optometrist who is more highly skilled or experienced in the management of complex vision therapy cases.

If the patient did not respond favorably in any of the above circumstances but did display a significant reduction in the angle of deviation when accommodation was stimulated or inhibited—by changing fixation distance and/or by introducing minus or plus lenses—then prognosis, although certainly significantly more guarded, is not completely negative. Once again, referral to someone specializing in the treatment of strabismus with vision therapy is probably justified. (This applies even to those patients who exhibited ARC in the fusion and/or stereopsis tests described above.)

If none of the above procedures yielded a favorable sign, then the prognosis for remediation through lenses/vision therapy is very poor. In practical terms, there is no good reason for further testing. The optometrist should consider other treatment options. (Others have developed different prognostic systems; see, for example, reference 61).

IF REMEDIAL THERAPY JUSTIFIED? = YES

The next step is to design and describe the treatment program to the patient/ parents: what it involves, what it will require of them, and so forth. This will probably necessitate a separate consultation where, along with discussion, additional testing may be carried out to obtain relevant information (see Chapters 9 and 11).

IF REMEDIAL THERAPY JUSTIFIED? = NO

Once it has been decided that a remedial program is not likely to produce the desired outcomes, still another decision has to be made: Is the strabismus apparent to the untrained observer? How does the patient/parent perceive the condition? On the basis of these will come subsequent recommendations (see P in Figure 6.14 flow diagram and below).

□ P. Does Strabismus Present a Cosmetic Problem?

This question confronts the optometrist after she has decided that remedial therapy is not justified. The following factors should influence her thinking:

1. The magnitude of the deviation in relation to the patient's physical appearance. Generally speaking, a deviation of 15 prism diopters is not apparent to the untrained observer. However, this is also influenced by the patient's interpupillary distance (I.P.D.), angle kappa, bridge-of-nose width, and other facial characteristics.
2. The patient's self-perception. Some patients are very concerned about the most trivial of blemishes; others are not so affected. Here, the optometrist's judgment will probably be intuitive, based on how she perceives the patient's attitude: distress and psychological trauma or, in contrast, apparent unawareness.
3. The family's attitude regarding the deviation. Some parents are extremely upset by their child's strabismus; others are inclined to ignore the deviation and be more concerned about the cosmetic impact of spectacles. Here again, individual judgments will prevail.

IF NO

Reassure the patient (and parents) and arrange for subsequent routine care (see discussion regarding reassurance therapy in Chapter 9).

IF YES

Recommend cosmetic lenses and/or a surgical consultation. The decision, in this instance, should be based on the extent to which the cosmetic problem can be alleviated by spectacles as compared with the prospects for significant cosmetic improvement from surgery, the patient's/parent's attitude about spectacles, and so on (see Chapter 11).

□ Guidelines for Evaluating the Very Young Strabismic Patient

The optometrist's concerns and goals with the young strabismic patient are the same as they are with the older ones. All that differs is how she goes about obtaining relevant information and how she uses that information in formulating recommendations.

As expressed above (see Figure 6.14), the optometrist's first task, once strabismus is detected, is to describe the condition in terms of direction, magnitude, comitancy, and laterality.

Direction
This does not differ from what has been stated above in regard to the older patient.

Magnitude
The difficulty one encounters in assessing the magnitude of a deviation in young children is their tendency to be noncompliant when it comes to sustaining fixation on a near or distant target. As a result, other methods usually have to be used. Of particular use under these circumstances is the reflection of a light source from the cornea.

HIRSCHBERG TEST (25)
This test was mentioned briefly in Chapter 4. It requires more discussion in this context. The Hirschberg test exploits the reflections (reflexes) of a light from the patient's two corneas, with the measurement being derived by comparing the relative location of one reflex to the other, and then translating any noted displacement into degrees or prism diopters of deviation. For example, if both reflexes appear to be centrally and symmetrically positioned when the patient fixates straight ahead, then there probably is no deviation; or more accurately, no overt deviation. If, in another instance, the examiner observes that one reflex is centrally located while the other is displaced toward the nose, then it signals an exodeviation. In the opposite condition, when one reflex is centrally located while the other is displaced away from the nose, it indicates an esodeviation. Thus, the magnitude of a deviation may be calculated by measuring the relative location of the two reflexes.

But, another factor has to be taken into account if the Hirschberg test is to provide accurate information: *angle kappa*. In most eyes, the optical axis and the visual axis do not coincide. A line projected from a fixation point in space through the optical centers of the cornea and the lens to the retina will not strike the macula. The separation between those two axes, as displayed by the position of the corneal reflex in relation to the apparent pupil of the eye is called angle kappa.

To measure angle kappa (62):

1. Patient fixates, with one eye, a penlight located centrally at about a 50-cm distance. (Other eye is occluded.)
2. Examiner sights with one eye from a point just above the penlight, taking note of the position of the corneal reflex in relation to the center of the patient's apparent pupil.
3. Angle kappa is represented by the distance, in mm, between the center of the light reflex and the center of the apparent pupil.

4. When the reflex is located precisely in the center of the apparent pupil, angle kappa equals zero. When the reflex is displaced nasalward from the center of the apparent pupil, angle kappa is described as being *positive*. The opposite, a displacement away from the nose, is known as a *negative* angle kappa.

In all instances, the measurement is in units of 0.5 mm. Thus, a patient with a +1.5 angle kappa shows a corneal reflex displaced 1.5 mm nasalward from the center of the apparent pupil.

Most persons display a positive angle kappa (up to about +1.5 mm), some display an angle kappa of zero, and even fewer, a negative angle kappa. Vertical angles kappa other than zero are not uncommon. These are recorded in similar fashion with vertical descriptors (hyper/hypo) used in lieu of the positive and negative designations.

5. Measure angle kappa in the other eye. The two should be equal. A detectable difference between the two eyes (e.g., more than 0.5 mm) signals the possibility of eccentric fixation.

Once angle kappa has been measured, the *Hirschberg* test may be carried out rapidly, as follows:

1. Patient fixates, with both eyes, a penlight bulb held centrally at a 50-cm distance.

2. Examiner sights monocularly over the bulb and notes the relative location of the two corneal reflexes. The position of the reflex in each eye should be approximately the same as when angle kappa was measured. If the eyes are not aligned accurately, the location of the reflex in one eye (the deviating one) will be different than where it was during the angle kappa measurement.

3. The difference is equivalent to the magnitude of the deviation. This may be calculated by measuring the relative location of the two reflexes. The standard rule of thumb for making the conversion into prism diopters is that 1 mm of displacement is equivalent to 22 prism diopters or 12 degrees (63).

KRIMSKY TEST

This is an extension of the Hirschberg tests wherein the examiner measures the separation of the corneal reflexes by determining the amount of prism power required to reposition the reflex of the deviating eye so that it is symmetrical with the reflex of the preferred eye (64). The deviation, then, is the amount of prism required to accomplish this.

Comitancy

Once again, the young child's tendency not to look where you want her to look gets in the way of an exact measure. Hence, the examiner may have to exercise some ingenuity to obtain this information. The most effective is to introduce something that will attract the child's attention (a toy, etc.) and either move it about into the various positions of gaze, or move the child's head about as she continues to fixate the target—which remains stationary. In either case, the examiner pays attention to the corneal reflex for evidence of comitance or noncomitance.

Laterality

There are usually two ways in which laterality is established in patients beyond the infant stage (see above). One, the examiner's observations; the other, the patient's visual acuity. This applies to the very young patient as well, although the evidence may be less precise than desired. In respect to the first: an alternating fixation pattern may be very evident. If this is the case, then obviously the strabismus is characterized as "alternating." On the other hand, even if an alternating pattern is not observed, that does not rule out the condition. More data is needed. This is usually obtained in one of two ways:

One, present the child an interesting visual target in one of her temporal fields; then in the other. The very young alternating strabismus—particularly, the esotrope—will "cross fixate." That is, she will look at objects to her right with her left eye, and those to her left with her right eye. This is clear evidence of an alternating fixation pattern.

Second, in lieu of more precise visual acuity measures, take note of the child's behavior when you occlude each of her eyes. The very young unilateral strabismic is likely to have significantly reduced visual acuity in the deviating eye. If that is the case, then occluding the eye that sees relatively well will elicit a behavior that is clearly different than the behavior elicited when the other eye is occluded. If such a difference is observed—if the child resists occlusion of one eye but not the other, then infer a unilateral strabismus accompanied by reduced visual acuity in the deviating eye.

IS MORE TESTING NEEDED WITH THE VERY YOUNG PATIENT?

One more concern remains. The optometrist should attempt to search for evidence of an innervational component contributing to the binocular deviation; i.e., determine the effect of accommodation on the magnitude of the strabismus. Information relevant to this derives from (a) the date of onset; (b) the effect of fixation distance on the magnitude of the strabismus; (c) the effect of (plus/minus) spherical lenses on the magnitude of the deviation. The first of these is important in that, in most cases, a strabismus that manifests during the first 6 months of life does not usually derive from an innervational dysfunction. Rather, it most often falls under the classification of a "congenital" or "infantile" strabismus, which implies an anatomical (neurological/muscle) anomaly of some sort. (See Chapter 4; also see p. 251 for a description of yet another congenital problem that is related to strabismus—the nystagmus blockage syndrome.) The latter are addressed just as they are with the older patient, so long as the examiner recognizes the need for rapid judgments because of the young child's tendency to avoid prolonged fixation on any given target.

Why not assess the effect of compensating prism/spheres on fusion and stereopsis? For the simple reason that the child lacks the communication skills needed to conduct these tests; if that is not the case then, by all means, take those measures.

FORMULATE RECOMMENDATIONS

The flow diagram shown in Figure 6.14 pertains to the very young patient as well. Once again, if pathology is suspected, the only acceptable option is to treat the pathology or make an appropriate referral. Once that concern is ruled out, then the decision about treatment depends upon prognosis. If remedial (nonsurgical) therapy is justified, then it should be instituted. If it does not appear to be justified, then the parents should be reassured (if cosmesis is not a concern) or (if cosmesis is a concern) the child should be referred for surgical consultation.

IS REMEDIAL THERAPY JUSTIFIED?

Remedial vision therapy that anticipates the patient "learning" binocular function from controlled experiences is not appropriate for the very young patient. The only types of nonsurgical treatment that might benefit the very young patient are those that (a) enhance the child's ability to see clearly with both eyes (i.e., amblyopia treatment); (b) enable the child to use both maculae simultaneously (i.e., compensating prisms); (c) take advantage of the fact that the child's binocular deviation derives, at least in part, from an innervational dysfunction and might therefore be aided by spherical lenses that foster more accurate eye alignment.

If amblyopia is suspected, then it becomes the initial treatment concern. (For treatment guidelines, see Chapter 12.) It is not likely that normal binocular vision will be established if the patient's visual acuity is very poor in one eye. In respect to the second type of treatment, the pivotal question is: "Does the patient adapt to a compensating prism?" (i.e., does the angle of deviation increase once the compensating prisms are placed before the patient's eyes?). If this occurs, then there is little justification for compensating prism. If it does not occur—if the angle of deviation does not alter after the prisms have been in place for a reasonable period of time ("reasonable" in this case, may vary from 15 minutes to a day)—then prisms should be viewed as desirable in that, at the least, they increase the possibility for both maculae to be stimulated simultaneously. This, in turn, improves the child's chances to obtain peripheral fusion and stereopsis.

With regard to the third type of situation—the patient whose strabismus appears, at least in part, to derive from innervational dysfunction—the key indicator is similar to what was described above, in the section devoted to older strabismus patients: Namely, the difference in the angle of deviation when measured at distance and near, and the effect of plus or minus spheres on that angle. If the angle of deviation differs significantly at distance as compared to near—if, at near, the eso increases, or the exo decreases—then an innervational component should be suspected. Similarly, if plus lenses at near reduces the esotropia, or if minus lenses has the same effect on exotropia then, again, it is evidence of an innervational component. Remedial therapy is justified in those cases, although, at this stage of the child's life, the therapy must be limited to application of appropriate lenses.

■ DIAGNOSIS OF AMBLYOPIA

Amblyopia has been defined as "the unilateral or bilateral decrease in vision for which no obvious cause can be detected by the physical examination of the eye" (65). Schapero and colleagues (66) define it as "the condition of reduced visual acuity not correctable by refractive means and not attributable to obvious structural or pathological ocular anomalies" (p. 35).

Present-day conventional wisdom identifies two major classes of amblyopia: *functional* and *organic,* although there are some investigators who contend that the designation of amblyopia is limited to functional etiologies. If an organic factor exists, they argue, the condition should not be termed amblyopia.

Griffin (25) lists three types of functional amblyopia: *hysterical, refractive,* and *strabismic,* and three that pertain to organic amblyopia: *nutritional, toxic,* and *congenital,* the last of these applying when the amblyopia does not respond to treatment yet no organic cause factors are identified.

Von Noorden (24) tends to accept this classification, but with some modifications. Under functional amblyopia, he lists *strabismic amblyopia, anisometropic amblyopia,* and *visual deprivation amblyopia* (amblyopia ex anopsia) derived from occlusion (67), ptosis, cataract, corneal opacity, and other visual impediments.

Parks (4) takes a more focused view, stating that amblyopia is a deprivation phenomenon, the "result of the child not using the foveal-cortical system adequately during its labile period, the first nine years of life." This, in turn, Parks goes on "impairs the cortical function of foveal discrimination" (p. 85).

Amblyopia is a prevalent condition. Von Noorden (24, p. 220), combining the data from many investigators, estimates that between 2 to 2 1/2 percent of the general population manifests some degree of functional amblyopia.

The diagnosis of amblyopia differs from the diagnosis of strabismus in two key ways: First, amblyopia is a sensory visual disorder that cannot be observed directly; it is inferred on the strength of what can and cannot be documented about the patient's visual acuity in relation to his ocular health and structural states, binocular status, and refractive status. As such, diagnostic testing subserves a deductive process, with the conclusion being based, ultimately, on what cannot be ruled out.

Second, there is no surgical treatment for amblyopia. All treatments are non-surgical, involving various, but not numerous, methods designed to sensitize, or resensitize, the fovea(s) of the amblyopic eye(s). Hence, unlike the diagnosis of strabismus, where an effort is made to determine how closely the patient can approximate a normal performance level, the diagnostic process in amblyopia—once its existence is established—attempts to answer two questions: (a) What method of foveal stimulation is most likely to be effective? and (b) How effective is it likely to be? The first of these requires a conclusion about the inferred cause of the condition. The second requires some "educated guessing." In most cases, prognosis is risky until after some treatment has been instituted and short-term effects assessed.

Before discussing the diagnostic sequence to be employed once amblyopia has been detected, it would be helpful to recall what steps of the examination sequence brought the patient to this stage. Was the amblyopia detected during the first process (Figure 6.1: the testing sequence designed for general assessment of binocular status) or the second one (Figure 6.14: strabismus diagnosis)? Although both of these sequences have an amblyopia detection component, they differ in what they reveal to the examiner. If amblyopia was detected in the first process, it means that the amblyopia is connected with inadequate stereoacuity and/or a (best corrected) visual acuity of less than 20/20 in each eye, but *is not connected with overt or small-angle strabismus*. If strabismus was noted in that sequence, the detection process would have halted and the diagnostic process begun before the detection of amblyopia juncture was reached. On the other hand, if amblyopia was detected during the *strabismus diagnostic process*, it means that the patient manifests strabismus.

There is, of course, a third possible amblyopia condition that would not have been identified in either of the two sequences already defined: the strabismic patient who has amblyopia but is able to display occasional central binocular vision or, at the least, peripheral single binocular vision. There is no need to define yet another diagnostic sequence for such a patient. He is best served by being treated primarily for the bifoveal misalignment problem, with only secondary concern devoted to his amblyopia. This will be discussed more extensively in Chapter 11. For now, it is enough to state that remediating bifoveal misalignment is apt to remediate amblyopia; the reverse is not so predictable.

Now to the process defined in the flow diagram in Figure 6.15.

□ A. Is the Condition Bilateral?

This question requires very little discussion. If the best corrected visual acuity of both eyes is inexplicably substandard (i.e., 20/30 or worse) and relatively equal, then the condition is, indeed, bilateral.

If only one eye is so affected, then the obvious answer is no, the condition is not bilateral.

IF IS CONDITION BILATERAL? = YES

Examine all available data to determine whether they support the diagnosis of bilateral amblyopia. If they do, then treatment recommendations may be formulated (see B in Figure 6.15 flow diagram and below).

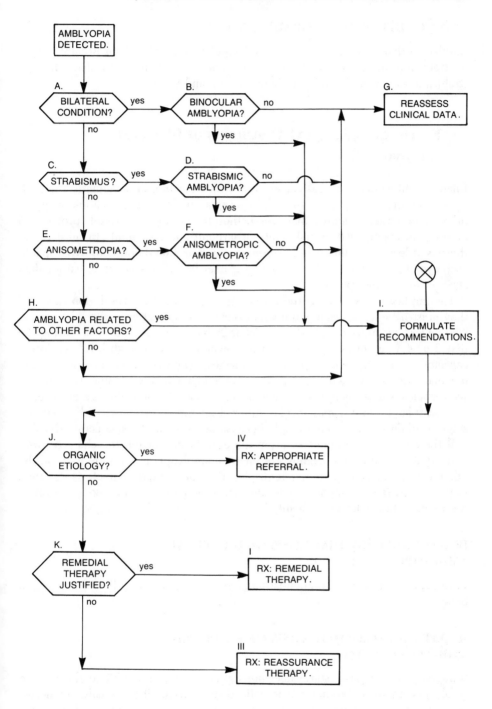

Figure 6.15 Amblyopia diagnosis.

IF IS CONDITION BILATERAL? = NO

Amblyopia that is limited to one eye (i.e., unilateral amblyopia) is usually related to strabismus and/or anisometropia. It probably is most efficient to focus first on strabismus (see C in Figure 6.15 flow diagram and below).

☐ B. Do Data Support Diagnosis of Bilateral Amblyopia?

Bilateral amblyopia is typically associated with (a) significant astigmatism in both eyes, often in combination with high hyperopia, (b) delayed application of appropriate compensatory lenses that, when they finally are prescribed, provide no better than about 20/40 visual acuity at farpoint and nearpoint. In most cases, there is at least 1.75 diopters of astigmatism and/or 4.00 diopters of hyperopia in each eye along with a history of the first glasses being prescribed no earlier than age four or five (68, p. 85).

The implication is clear. If the foveas are to develop high resolution capacity, they must have appropriate stimulation during the formative years. The patient who never sees more clearly than 20/50 or 20/60 at distance and near during the first 3 or 4 years of her life is not likely ever to develop high-level resolution capacities, even after she starts to wear glasses. (The reason that myopic eyes do not manifest such difficulties is evident: although a highly myopic eye will not see very clearly at farpoint, high resolution of nearpoint stimuli is always accessible.)

Most bilateral amblyopes display bifoveal alignment. However, their stereoacuity is often not adequate, simply because of the central visual acuity deficit.

If the clinical data obtained during the examination match the characteristics defined above, then the diagnosis of bilateral amblyopia is supported. If, on the other hand, the patient does not display the above-cited characteristics, then the diagnosis is not supported and alternative actions must be taken to explain the reduced binocular visual acuity.

IF DATA SUPPORT DIAGNOSIS OF BILATERAL AMBLYOPIA? = YES

Formulate treatment recommendations (see I in Figure 6.15 flow diagram and below).

IF DATA SUPPORT DIAGNOSIS OF BILATERAL AMBLYOPIA? = NO

If the patient's refractive status does not support a diagnosis of bilateral refractive amblyopia, then the optometrist is obliged to do what all responsible clinicians are expected to do when clinical evidence contradicts earlier-formed opinions: reconsider the evidence and collect whatever additional data are needed to provide appropriate care (see G in Figure 6.15 flow diagram and below).

□ C. Does Patient Manifest Unilateral Strabismus?

If the proposed testing sequence has been followed, then the answer to this question is already in the record.

IF DOES PATIENT MANIFEST UNILATERAL STRABISMUS? = YES

Examine all available data to determine whether they support the diagnosis of strabismic amblyopia. (See D in Figure 6.15 flow diagram and below.)

IF DOES PATIENT MANIFEST UNILATERAL STRABISMUS? = NO

The condition has now been established as (a) unilateral and (b) not accompanied by strabismus. The next logical step, therefore, is to consider anisometropia (see E in Figure 6.15 flow diagram and below).

□ D. Do Data Support Diagnosis of Strabismic Amblyopia?

Strabismic amblyopia is a unilateral condition caused by the "active inhibition within the retinocortical pathways of visual input originating in the fovea of the deviating eye" (24, p. 221).

The reduced visual acuity of the deviating eye reflects the age at which the strabismus manifested, the duration of the strabismus, and the extent to which the fovea of the deviating eye has been deprived of precisely focused, detailed stimuli (69,70,71). This latter, in turn, is directly related to the fixation pattern of the eyes (unilateral/alternating), the magnitude of the deviation, and in unilateral strabismus, the fixation accuracy of the deviating eye when the nondeviating eye is occluded. As such, the data that are relevant in supporting the diagnosis of strabismic amblyopia and formulating appropriate treatment recommendations include (a) the accuracy of fixation, and (b) the size and depth of the suppression area.

Accuracy of fixation refers to the patient's ability to align the fovea with a designated stimulus. Various methods for assessing this were defined earlier (see Chapter 4). These included (a) monocular visual acuity, (b) stereoacuity, (c) visuscopy, (d) position of corneal reflexes (Angle Kappa test), (e) unilateral cover test, (f) the position of entoptic phenomenon (Haidinger's brushes; Maxwell's spot) within the patient's central field of vision.

The first two in the list are ruled out, obviously. It is because they are abnormal that the need for more testing arises. One or more of the other methods may be useful and should be administered at this time, if feasible and if they have not already been performed.

Size and depth of suppression area were also discussed earlier, in the section devoted to the detection of small-angle strabismus. Although there are additional tests, the ones mentioned there—Worth 4-dot test, 4 base out prism test—will usually supply the information the clinician needs (see pp. 210–211).

In addition to the above, the amblyopic eye often responds idiosyncratically to different visual acuity test conditions.

CROWDING PHENOMENON

A nonamblyopic eye ordinarily demonstrates the same visual acuity threshold regardless of whether the letters are presented singly (single-letter acuity), in lines (line acuity), or full chart (chart acuity).

An amblyopic eye will often respond in a different manner, with the visual acuity threshold varying as a function of display format. Single-letter acuity is apt to be better than line acuity which, in turn, is better than full chart acuity. Flom and associates (72) showed this to be attributable to the amblyopic eye's sensitivity to contour interactions. In other words, in addition to letter size, the spaces between the letters, the "crowding," influences the patient's visual resolution abilities. Burian and Cortigmiglia (73) reported differences as great as 6/30 line acuity improving to 6/6 letter acuity, with the greatest differences noted among patients with relatively poor acuity.

There has been a fair amount of speculation regarding the clinical interpretation of the crowding phenomenon (e.g., [73,74,75,76,77]). Some propose that good single-letter visual acuity is a favorable prognostic sign, regardless of how poor line acuity may be. Other disagree. But, as Von Noorden points out, "Single E acuity represents the true potential functional ability of the eye which is masked by the amblyopic process" (24, p. 229). As such, it does provide useful information, regardless of how vulnerable the eye is to the crowding effect.

EFFECT OF NEUTRAL-DENSITY FILTER

The visual acuity of an amblyopic eye is purported to correspond roughly to the acuity of the normal eye when both are tested at scotopic luminance levels, somewhat poorer than a normal eye when tested at mesopic levels, and markedly worse than a normal eye at photopic levels (78). This characteristic is not shared by eyes where acuity loss is due to macular involvements (4, p. 86). Thus, the neutral-density filter should be a useful device for distinguishing organic from functional defects. However, personal clinical experience does not support the proposition with sufficient consistency to recommend it as a useful diagnostic test.

IF DO DATA SUPPORT DIAGNOSIS OF STRABISMIC AMBLYOPIS? = YES

Formulate treatment recommendations (see I in Figure 6.15 flow diagram and below).

IF DO DATA SUPPORT DIAGNOSIS OF STRABISMIC AMBLYOPIA? = NO

Search for alternative explanations for clinical signs and symptoms (see G in Figure 6.15 flow diagram and below).

☐ **E. Does Patient Manifest Significant Anisometropia?**

Undoubtedly, the answer to this question is already in the record. It now is simply a matter of establishing the criterion that defines "significant anisometropia" in this context.

A difference between the two eyes of 1.00 or more diopters (sphere or cylinder) has been shown to be significantly associated with subsequent strabismus and/or amblyopia (79,80). This conclusion, based on longitudinal data derived from 215 preschool children, appears to identify a reasonably sensitive criterion for sorting anisometropia into significant and nonsignificant categories, as long as one allows for the ambiguities and exceptions that are sure to be found on both sides of this cutting edge (81).

IF DOES PATIENT MANIFEST SIGNIFICANT ANISOMETROPIA? = YES

Examine all available data to determine whether they support the diagnosis of anisometropic amblyopia (see F in Figure 6.15 flow diagram and below).

IF DOES PATIENT MANIFEST SIGNIFICANT ANISOMETROPIA? = NO

It appears that the patient's reduced visual acuity cannot be explained by either strabismus or anisometropia. A limited list of alternative explanations remain (see H in Figure 6.15 flow diagram and below).

☐ **F. Do Data Support Diagnosis of Anisometropic Amblyopia?**

The underlying connection between anisometropia and amblyopia is somewhat different than the link between strabismus and amblyopia. In constant unilateral strabismus, by definition, the fovea of the deviating eye is out of alignment. Therefore, sensations stimulating that fovea are usually out of focus because the internal optical adjustments of the deviating eye are determined by the aligned eye.

In nonstrabismic anisometropia, the sensations stimulating the fovea of the more ametropic eye are out of focus *as long as a compensatory lens is not applied*. (This, of course, explains why anisomyopia is rarely connected with amblyopia. The fovea of a highly myopic eye may very well receive focused stimulation, if the stimulus is located sufficiently close to the eye. The same does not hold for anisohyperopia.) As such, a critical factor in anisometropic amblyopia is the age at which a compensatory lens was first applied and the extent to which the patient functioned binocularly once the lens was worn. In other words, the critical concerns are (a) the length of time during which the patient received poorly defined images on that fovea under both monocular and binocular viewing conditions, and (b) the quality of binocularity obtained once the lens was provided (82,83).

The first of these is answered from the case history. The second, from a determination of the aniseikonia-producing effects created by the unequal lens prescription.

IF DO DATA SUPPORT DIAGNOSIS OF ANISOMETROPIC AMBLYOPIA? = YES

Formulate treatment recommendations (see I in Figure 6.15 flow diagram and below).

IF DO DATA SUPPORT DIAGNOSIS OF ANISOMETROPIC AMBLYOPIA? = NO

Search for alternative explanations for clinical signs and symptoms (see G on Figure 6.15 flow diagram and below).

□ G. Reassess the Clinical Picture

A clinician always reserves the right, and indeed bears the obligation, to reconsider a previously formed opinion when she is confronted with contradictory evidence. The patient with reduced monocular or binocular visual acuity that cannot be linked with significant ametropia, anisometropia, strabismus, or some ocular anatomical anomaly, must be viewed with concern. In such cases, two lines of investigation are reasonable: one, a reassessment of the health and structural integrity of the visual components. This would include central and peripheral visual fields, monocular color vision, confirming the patient's ability to appreciate an entoptic phenomenon, and various other tests of retinal and central nervous system integrity, such as ERG and VEP. The second possibility: psychogenic factors. This can range from blatant malingering to true hysteria.

□ H. Other Possible Causes of Amblyopia

Some children are born with (or acquire in their early years) ptosis or opacities within the ocular media. They may become amblyopic even though the obstruction itself is eliminated (67). The key question in these instances is when was the

obstruction acquired and/or removed. In addition, some children undergo monocular occlusion very early in life because of an eye injury or, for that matter, a
binocular deviation. Sometimes the occlusion schedule is poorly designed and/or
managed, resulting in occlusion amblyopia.

All of these are possible explanations for amblyopia independent of high ametropia, anisometropia, or strabismus. If any are identified, then once again, consideration should be given to the formulation of treatment recommendations.

□ I. Formulate Recommendations

The flow diagram indicates three options. The first is exercised when there is
reason to suspect an organic etiology (see J on Figure 6.15 flow diagram).

If this is ruled out, then the decision comes down to treat or not; or, said
differently: Is remedial therapy justified? (See K on Figure 6.15 flow diagram and
below.)

□ K. Remedial Therapy Justified?

The basic assumption one should hold in the management of amblyopia is that
the situation is not hopeless. But, in fact, it may be.

There is no reliable method for predicting the potential effects of amblyopia
therapy. Certain indicators are worth looking at, however, if only to help the
optometrist determine the level of enthusiasm she should display when making
recommendations to the patient. These are:

1. *Age of patient*. The younger, the better. Most authorities are pessimistic
about the effectiveness of first-attempt amblyopia therapy with children who have
passed their ninth birthday (4). On the other hand, there is evidence of beneficial
effects from therapy among persons appreciably older than 9 (66).

2. *Age of onset*. Some amblyopic patients never experienced age-normal visual
acuity in the affected eye(s). Others did, then encountered an event that halted
further acuity development and may even have caused it to deteriorate somewhat.
The latter group is much more likely to benefit from amblyopia therapy. The
prospects of the former group are less bright (67).

3. *Fixation status*. If one considers eccentric fixation to be a maladaptation,
then central fixation has to viewed as the more favorable condition. In the event
that eccentric fixation does exist, the key indicators of its embeddedness are the
variability and magnitude of the eccentricity. Relatively small and/or variable
angles of eccentric fixation are more favorable than are large and steady deviations
(25).

There are other factors, of course (e.g., visual acuity, cause of amblyopia), but
the three listed above are the most critical. The order of their listing is of no

importance. The three are completely interrelated; each implies the other in some way. For example, eccentric fixation is more likely to be steady in the older patient.

In essence, then, there is no fixed formula. The optometrist has to consider the circumstances and make honest recommendations; but most often the best attitude is, "It's worth a try." The alternative—the future of the amblyopic eye that is left untreated—is too predictable to defend. If there is any possibility of improving the status of an amblyopic eye, the effort should be made.

IF REMEDIAL THERAPY JUSTIFIED? = NO

Give final reassurance and recommendations, and arrange for next visit (see Chapter 9).

IF REMEDIAL THERAPY JUSTIFIED? = YES

Recommend remedial therapy (see Chapter 12).

☐ The Very Young Amblyopic Patient

In most cases, amblyopia in the very young patient is diagnosed through inference rather than documentation of reduced visual acuity. As a rule of thumb, amblyopia—or a potential for amblyopia—should be suspected in the presence of significant bilateral ametropia (more so with hyperopia and astigmatism than with myopia), anisometropia (in excess of 1.00 diopter), and/or strabismus. Therefore, retinoscopy and a careful assessment of the child's binocular status are important.

Obviously, if an accurate measure of visual acuity can be obtained, that is of great value in detecting or ruling out amblyopia. However, if such measures are not possible, as is more often the case with very young children—if the methods described in Chapter 3 do not provide adequate data—then the optometrist will have to rely on such probes as taking note of the child's reaction to unilateral occlusion or any other informal procedure that might reflect a visual acuity difference between the two eyes.

In any event, when signs of possible amblyopia are seen, they should be taken seriously. The patient should be treated as though he manifested amblyopia, and, as always, the effects of that treatment should be monitored very closely. To do otherwise on the basis of wishful thinking is not acceptable.

DIAGNOSIS OF NYSTAGMUS

Nystagmus, although not necessarily a binocular anomaly, is included in this section because it often manifests in children with strabismus.

Figure 6.16 portrays a diagnostic process that will serve effectively when nystagmus is detected.

The process begins with a description of the pertinent clinical characteristics of the condition (see A through H in Figure 6.16 flow diagram and below).

The following observations should be made with the patient maintaining his habitual head position. If he ordinarily turns his head in one direction, or tilts it, then he should continue to do so during this part of the work-up.

□ A. Age of Onset

Nystagmus may be either congenital or acquired. Indeed, it may be inherited (84). Obviously, the case history is the best single source of information, but not the only source (see below); and, in fact, it may not be helpful in certain cases (e.g., when the patient was adopted several months or more following birth, or when the nystagmus is not very prominent and simply "may have been present but not noticed" by his parents during the child's early months). A very reliable (but not quite infallible) indicator of congenital nystagmus is the direction of the oscillations on upgaze. A persistence of horizontal nystagmus on upgaze is the "hallmark of congenital nystagmus" (85, p. 27).

□ B. Rhythmic Pattern

Nystagmus is characterized as either *pendular* or *jerk*, depending upon the rhythm of the oscillations.

In pendular nystagmus, the eyes tend to move at the same rate and amplitude in both directions, whereas in jerk nystagmus there is a slow phase in one direction followed by a fast restorative phase in the opposite direction. When naming a jerk nystagmus, the direction of the fast phase is cited (e.g., slow movement to patient's left, fast movement to patient's right = *right jerk nystagmus*).

The usual cause of pendular (ocular) nystagmus is sensory deprivation resulting from an afferent visual defect; e.g., albinism, achromotopsia, bilateral macular scars, bilateral congenital cataracts, or some other similarly devastating condition (86). If the sensory deficit exists at birth, the nystagmus will usually appear before the child is 4 months old. If the sensory deficit is not present at birth, then the patient's age when it does occur will strongly influence the subsequent emergence of nystagmus. The so-called "2-4-6 Rule" states that if the child loses vision before the age of 2, he will develop nystagmus; if he maintained good vision until at least the age of 6 years, he will not develop nystagmus; and for the years in between, the fourth birthday probably marks the point when the likelihood of nystagmus following a severe binocular vision loss falls below the 50-percent level (85,86).

The usual cause of jerk nystagmus is a motor (efferent mechanism) defect that may be drug-induced, linked with a central nervous system lesion, or simply inherited. It may appear at birth (congenital) or any other time of life (87).

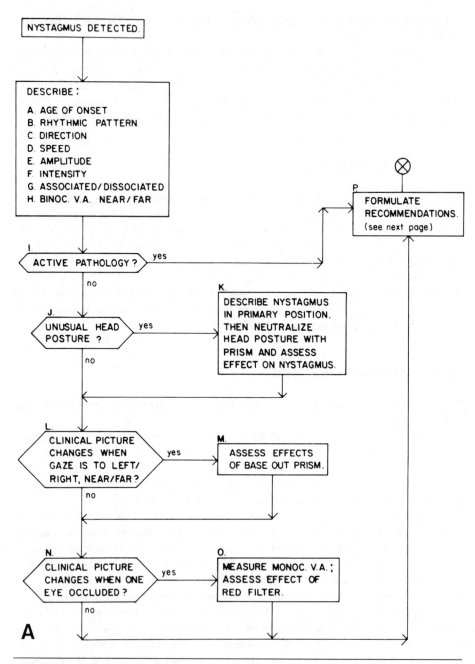

Figure 6.16 Nystagmus diagnosis.

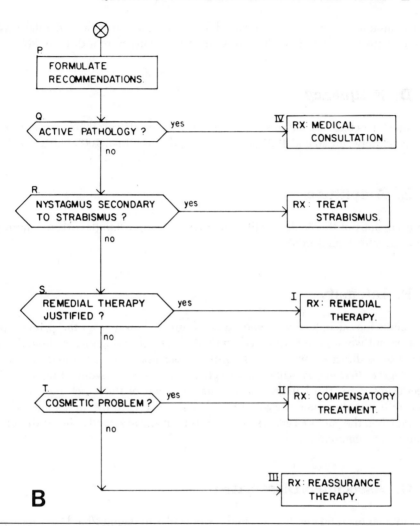

Figure 6.16 (Continued)

It is also not unusual to observe a mixture of the two patterns in a single patient; i.e., where a pendular rhythm prevails in the primary position, changing to a jerk pattern on gaze to either side (24). In these instances, however, it is not too difficult to identify the prevailing (pendular or jerk) rhythm.

□ C. Direction

Sensory defect (pendular) nystagmus is always horizontal. Jerk nystagmus may be horizontal, vertical, rotary, or mixed. Among these, the horizontal type is the most common, stemming from many different origins. Vertical and rotary nystagmus, with few exceptions, indicates central nervous system disease (86).

□ D. Frequency

The rate of ocular oscillations may vary from *slow* (fewer than 40/minute) to *moderate* (between 40 and 100/minute), to rapid (more than 100/minute) (86,88).

□ E. Amplitude

The excursions of the ocular oscillations may vary from *fine* (less than 1 mm) to *coarse* (greater than 3 mm).

□ F. Intensity

Nystagmus may manifest only when gaze is directed away from the primary position or/and when gaze is directed straight ahead. If nystagmus is elicited only when gaze is directed away from the primary position, it is called first degree or third degree: *first degree* when the direction of the quick movement matches the direction of gaze, third degree when the direction of the quick movement is opposite to the direction of gaze. *Second degree* refers to the nystagmus that is present when the patient's gaze is directed straight ahead as well as in the direction of the quick component (88).

□ G. Associated/Dissociated?

Most nystagmus is bilateral (associated). Monocular nystagmus has been observed in cases of congenital syphillis, meningitis, strabismus, unilateral amblyopia combined with high refractive error and multiple sclerosis. It may also appear in very young children, as a sign of myesthenia gravis or a brain-stem neoplasm (88).

Two dissociated yet bilateral types of nystagmus also warrant mention, if only because of their unusual nature. One, seesaw nystagmus, as its name suggests, is characterized by one eye moving up (and intorting) as the other eye moves down (and extorting); then the pattern reverses. It may be congenital, but most often it is associated with a lesion of the chiasm (87,88). The other type, usually associated with posterior fossa lesions, is characterized by each eye oscillating more or less independently from the other; i.e., one eye may be oscillating vertically, the other horizontally. (Technically, latent nystagmus might also be included in this category, but it is discussed separately; see N below.)

□ H. Binocular Visual Acuity

If nearpoint visual acuity is significantly better than farpoint, it suggests that convergence produces a positive change in the clinical picture. This will influence diagnosis and subsequent recommendations (see L in Figure 6.16 flow diagram and below).

Infants pose a special problem in this regard. Measuring visual acuity in any infant is not a simple task; measuring the visual acuity of an infant with nystagmus is even more of a challenge. As an adjunct to the methods proposed earlier, Smith (85) offers a very helpful suggestion. If a vertical response can be superimposed upon a child's basic nystagmus pattern by use of an optokinetic tape or drum, then, the likelihood is that the fundus is normal and that the child will probably have reasonably good visual acuity. This type of response is known as type I. If a vertical response cannot be superimposed on the child's nystagmus (type II), then prognosis is much more guarded. Typically, an ocular examination of this child will reveal a condition that impairs sight (e.g., macular dysplasia, pervasive opacities in the media, achromotopsia).

A significant difference in monocular visual acuity when measured under monocular and binocular viewing conditions also is pertinent. This will be discussed shortly (see N in Figure 6.16 flow diagram and below).

□ I. Reason to Suspect Active Pathology?

As a general rule, any one of the following should be viewed as a sign of potential pathology, and even more so when they occur in combination.

1. Acquired.
2. Dissociated.
3. Vertical or rotary.
4. Third degree.

IF REASON TO SUSPECT ACTIVE PATHOLOGY? = YES

Recommend a neurological consultation (see Q in Figure 6.16 flow diagram).

IF REASON TO SUSPECT ACTIVE PATHOLOGY? = NO

Assume a congenital nystagmus that may or may not be amenable to some treatment approach. This will now have to be determined, commencing with a probe for signs of gaze asymmetry, such as an unusual head posture (see J in Figure 6.16 flow diagram and below).

□ J. Unusual Head Posture?

An anomalous head position indicates that the amplitude and frequency of the nystagmus probably decrease significantly when conjugate gaze is in a particular, off-center direction; this, in turn, causing an improvement in visual acuity: concordant nystagmus (89). For example, if a neutral (null) zone is achieved with dextroversion, the patient will maintain a compensatory head turn to the left. If a null position is acquired through downward gaze, the patient will tend to elevate his chin and "look down his nose." (See, also, Nystagmus Blockage Syndrome; p. 251.)

IF UNUSUAL HEAD POSTURE? = YES

It is useful to document the extent of improvement the patient obtains from his asymmetric gaze head turn by reassessing the nystagmus while he fixates straight ahead. Once this is accomplished, the next step should be a determination of the potential benefit to be derived from lateral prisms that neutralize the head turn/tilt (see K in Figure 6.16 flow diagram and below).

IF UNUSUAL HEAD POSTURE? = NO

Look for changes in the clinical picture as a result of the patient directing his gaze (upon request) to the left, the right, near, far (see L in Figure 6.16 flow diagram and below).

□ K. Describe the Nystagmus When Gaze Is in Primary Position and Determine the Effect of Lateral Prism on Head Turn/Tilt

The first step does not require further discussion. Simply repeat the observations defined in steps B through H above as the patient's gaze is directed straight ahead.

Once this has been done, introduce sufficient prism to neutralize the patient's head turn/tilt and determine its effect on the nystagmus. For example, if the patient shows a neutral zone on dextroversion, then base-left prism before each eye should reduce the head turn. Reassess the nystagmus (B through H) with the prism in place. Then proceed to L in the Figure 6.16 flow diagram.

□ L. Does Clinical Picture Change When Gaze Is Shifted to Left/Right, Near/Far?

In addition to the above-mentioned concordant nystagmus, two other clinically pertinent, gaze-related phenomena are observed often enough in nystagmus patients to justify mention.

First: discordant nystagmus, where the frequency and amplitude of the oscillations are dampened by avoiding abduction. In such cases, only the right eye fixates in left gaze, only the left eye in right gaze, much like the crossed-fixation pattern of the esotrope. Indeed, most of these patients are strabismic, but apparently not for the same reason as the cross-fixating esotrope without nystagmus.

The second gaze-related phenomenon: a dampening of the nystagmus through convergence. This is usually determined both by direct inspection and by a comparison of farpoint and nearpoint visual acuities. A significant improvement of acuity at nearpoint (in a fully corrected ametrope) reveals clearly the beneficial effect of convergence.

IF DOES CLINICAL PICTURE CHANGE WHEN GAZE IS SHIFTED TO LEFT/RIGHT, NEAR/FAR? = YES

Determine the potential value of base out prism (see M in Figure 6.16 flow diagram and below).

IF DOES CLINICAL PICTURE CHANGE WHEN GAZE IS SHIFTED TO LEFT/RIGHT, NEAR/FAR? = NO

Investigate the effect of monocular occlusion on the nystagmus (see N in Figure 6.16 flow diagram and below).

NYSTAGMUS BLOCKAGE SYNDROME

A number of clinicians have reported a type of nystagmus that decreases in adduction. Cianci proposed that one third of infants with esotropia display nystagmus in abduction, a neutral point in adduction, and a head turn toward the side of the dominant eye. He also noted that there is often a shifting of the head from side to side with alternate fixation (90,91,92). Lafon (93) was the first to suggest that this form of nystagmus might be the cause of the esotropia, rather than vice versa. Von Noorden has also written about the condition, stating that he believes it to be a fairly common phenomenon, having encountered the syndrome in 12 percent of 789 consecutive patients with infantile esotropia (24).

□ M. Assess the Effect of Base-Out Prism on Nystagmus

Base-out prism before each eye reduces the abduction demands on each eye. This might benefit the discordant nystagmus patient.

Base-out prism may also benefit the patient whose nystagmus is reduced by convergence. In such cases, the next step is to determine the amount of prism that will improve farpoint visual acuity without disrupting farpoint binocular fusion.

□ **N. Does Clinical Picture Change When One Eye Is Occluded?**

Latent nystagmus is a congenital condition that manifests only when one eye is occluded. It is not apparent when both eyes are open. Characteristically, it is a horizontal jerk-type nystagmus with the slow component directed toward the covered eye. It is often seen in young strabismic patients.

Latent nystagmus is detected by direct observation of each eye as the partner eye is occluded.

IF DOES CLINICAL PICTURE CHANGE WHEN ONE EYE IS OCCLUDED? = YES

Measure monocular visual acuities. Then determine the effect of a red filter on any reduced monocular acuity (see O in Figure 6.16 flow diagram and below).

IF DOES CLINICAL PICTURE CHANGE WHEN ONE EYE IS OCCLUDED? = NO

Formulate recommendations (see P in Figure 6.16 flow diagram and below).

□ **O. Measure Monocular Acuities (Under Monocular and Binocular Viewing Conditions) and Assess Effect of Red Filter on Any Existing Amblyopia**

Measuring monocular visual acuity in latent nystagmus presents a special problem because of the very nature of latent nystagmus. Therefore, in those cases where the nystagmus manifests only when one eye is occluded, measure visual acuity under binocular viewing conditions as well as by the standard (i.e., one eye occluded) method. The former may be accomplished with a vectographic chart, or by blurring the nonfixating eye with a high plus (+ 8.00D) lens, or by using a very narrow occluder (e.g., a pencil that obstructs central vision only).

□ **P. Formulate Recommendations**

The flow diagram shows five options. Medical consultation (IV) is usually selected when the evidence shows that the nystagmus is acquired. If active pathology is not ruled out, the recommendation should be to obtain a medical (usually neurological) consultation (see Q in Figure 6.16 flow diagram).

The second (treat strabismus) is considered when certain characteristics are noted in the strabismus-cum-nystagmus patient (see R in Figure 6.16 flow diagram and below).

The third (initiate remedial therapy) is not exercised often, but should at least be considered if the patient is highly motivated and teachable (see S in Figure 6.16 flow diagram and below).

The fourth (compensatory) and fifth (reassurance) alternatives are the ones used most often; the fourth when the patient manifests an unsightly head position, and the fifth when all other options are ruled out (see T in Figure 6.16 flow diagram).

□ R. Is the Nystagmus Secondary to Strabismus?

Cases have been reported in which nystagmus was eliminated following the re-mediation of strabismus (94). Conceivably, these are honest misinterpretations of actual events; congenital nystagmus has been known to disappear in some patients as they mature (84). On the other hand, the notion of a cause-effect link between strabismus and nystagmus should not be rejected. Healy (94), in her report on such cases, states that the patient whose nystagmus will disappear when binocular function is restored displays certain identifying characteristics. Among the most important of these: even before treatment commences, the nystagmus ceases when the patient fuses second degree targets set at the objective angle in a major amblyoscope. (All of her patients were hyperopic esotropes with normal retinal correspondence.)

□ S. Remedial Therapy Justified?

The remediation of nystagmus is a relatively new notion. Until recently, very little has been reported; even now, the procedures are not well validated and, in some instances, depend heavily on the patient's ability to learn how to control his nystagmus by combining external signals with introspection (see Chapter 13).

As a general rule, nystagmus therapy should be proposed only with reservation, as an "experiment" that might be helpful.

□ T. Cosmetic Problem?

Nystagmus is almost always a cosmetic problem—to the patient. This is so even when the oscillations are almost invisible to the casual observer. But, when the nystagmus produces an unsightly head turn or tilt, then the problem increases, and compensatory treatment should be considered. Steps K and M in the diag-nostic process are designed to probe the potential value of compensatory treat-ment. The treatments, themselves, are described in Chapter 13.

When compensatory treatment is not feasible, reassurance therapy should be provided (see Chapter 9,).

■

PRACTICAL SUGGESTIONS

6-1. If a stereoacuity test stimulus is too complex for a child, attempt to simplify it. For example, it is not necessary to present all four lines, or even the five circles of one line, in the AO farpoint vectographic stereotest. You can eliminate one, two, or even three of the circles, and show the others—oriented vertically or horizontally—by effective use of the mask built into the projector.

For the very young child, simplify the task even further by using a (two-alternative or more) forced-choice condition and simplifying the language requirements imposed on the patient. Several examples follow.

AO farpoint vectographic test. Use the built-in projector masks to show only two rings at a time—a disparate (stereo) one alongside a nondisparate one—and ask the child, "Which ring (or circle) looks as though it is closer to us, the one on this side (touch the proper hand, or point), or the one on this side (touch the other hand)?" The two rings need not be situated side by side. If it works better to have them oriented one above the other, present them that way. (If the child is able to deal with more than two circles at a time, but not with all five, then adjust the projector mask accordingly. But remember that the value of additional circles is to reduce the possibility of lucky [undetected] guesses—to increase its reliability—nothing more. Hence, if when using only two circles, you are convinced, by observing the child's behavior, that he perceives the stereo effect, then trust your judgment; there is no need to confound the situation by introducing more stimuli than the child can accommodate. See Practical Suggestion 1-37.)

Frisby stereotest. Cut the 6-mm and/or the 3-mm test plate into four squares, each containing one of the stimuli. Attach a gray plastic backing to two of these: one that contains the disparate stimulus and one that does not. (The purpose of the gray backing is to provide a background that is nondistracting and to eliminate telltale shadows; the latter will be apparent if a white background is held in contact with the stimulus.) The two squares may then be displayed to the child from a reasonable (nearpoint) distance along with the request to "Show me (or point to) the ball." Threshold is measured by the thickness of the plate and/or the test distance. However, threshold measurements may not be practical with the very young; you may have to settle for documentation of fairly low stereoacuity—but stereoacuity nonetheless; something worth noting. (For example, the youngster may respond to the 6-mm plate, but only when it is held no further away than 33 cm. This does not necessarily indicate stereoacuity threshold; rather, it may indicate "interest" threshold.) This procedure has been shown to be effective with children as young as 13 months of age. (See reference 27, Chapter 6.)

Titmus stereotest. Show the child the "fly" and ask: "Which looks closer to you: the fly or the picture frame?" (Run your finger around the frame of the picture as you do this.) When using the animal stimuli (rows A, B, C), use a cardboard mask that allows the child to see only two (or three) of the animals at a time.

Randot stereotest. Follow the suggestions offered for the Titmus stereotest above.

Random-dot E stereotest. Always present the E in the upright (crossed disparity) position and avoid discussing the stereo illusion. Introduce the test as described on p. 191, and, as additional explanation, identify the 'E' as "3 lines that go this way," showing three horizontal fingers as you do. Then ask the child to "Point to the picture with the three lines."

TNO. Refer to the disc from which a 60-degree wedge has been eliminated as 'Pac Man,' after the video game. Have available a cardboard replica of this figure and teach the child to "Point where Pac Man is going now." Also remember that when using any of these tests, they must be properly positioned and illuminated. In regard to position, they should be held at the standardized distance (or the examiner should take the nonstandardized distance into account when determining stereoacuity) and positioned perpendicular to the visual axes. With those tests that are covered by a plastic protector, it is advisable to have adequate ambient illumination above the test and to hold the test plate so that it is somewhat below the patient's eye level, thereby reflecting some of that ambient light.

6-2. Some patients are too young for a stereoacuity test. The Bruckner test has been proposed as a useful alternative. This test, originally called the "transillumination" test (95) is now identified by the name of its author. It is purported to facilitate the detection of strabismus and amblyopia in young children, whose subjective responses are often unreliable.

The test calls for a bright light source (a direct ophthalmoscope will do) that is used to illuminate both pupils from a distance of 1 meter. The examiner evaluates the brightness differences of the (right and left eye) fundus reflexes. If both eyes are in alignment, there should be no difference in brightness; if strabismus is present, the fixing eye will display a darker reflex than the deviating eye, due to the difference in fundus pigmentation in the macular and peripheral portions of the retina. (Other explanations for the difference have been proposed [96], but all agree that when a between-eye difference is observed, the duller reflex is in the fixing eye.)

As described by Tongue and Cibis (97), the Bruckner test also includes comparing the positions of the corneal light reflexes (Hirschberg test), as well as comparing pupillary action and fixation movement of each eye separately under the same illumination. They suggest that,

as illumination is switched from both eyes to the eye with the brighter fundus reflex, slight pupillary dilation will be observed. Subsequently, two things may occur. If the patient's fixation switches to foveal fixation with this eye, the pupil will constrict and the fundus reflex will become darker. In this case, amblyopia is unlikely. If amblyopia is present, fixation usually does not change, the pupil will not constrict, and the fundus reflex remains unchanged or brighter than that of the opposite eye while it was fixing.

The patient may also exhibit a wavering unsteadiness of fixation with that eye. The monocular illumination step is thus a fixation pattern assessment with the added advantage of monitoring pupillary behavior and fundus reflex brightness changes. (p 1042.)

For some reason or other, this aspect of the test has not gained much attention by U.S. optometrists.

The Bruckner test has been cited as a useful tool for nonprofessionals to use in mass vision screenings where the goal is identification of bincular anomalies in preschool children. Griffin and Cotter (98) take a contrary position, offering evidence that—because uncorrected ametropia can also produce unequal reflexes— the test, in the hands of lay persons who are unable to assess other visual functions, is likely to generate an unacceptable number of false-positives.

6-3. When conducting a cover test, it may be helpful to

1. use a translucent occluder that enables you to observe the movements of the patient's eye behind the cover. (The patient should not be able to see anything but light through the occluder.)

2. have the patient alter fixation periodically so as to avoid your confusing a (desired) fixation behavior with a (nonhelpful) "staring" behavior. For distance fixation, have the patient look at different stimuli (e.g., different letters within a full array of letters), or at you, then back to the distant stimulus. For near fixation, periodically move the target from side to side before you shift the occluder, watching the patient's eyes to make sure that she is fixating the target.

3. have the patient hold the near fixation target.

4. take note of a different response produced when the occluder is place before one eye as compared with the other. If the patient is strabismic, it indicates an incomitant deviation. If the patient is heterophoric, it probably indicates anisometropia, in which one eye is required to accommodate significantly more than the other; i.e., one eye will be significantly more hyperopic or myopic than the other.

5. keep the occluder in place before an eye for more than a fraction of a second. If it is moved back and forth too rapidly, some patients will not take up fixation as the test requires.

6-4. Stay on the lookout for an increase in the magnitude of esotropia as a cycloplegic drug is taking effect. This is evidence of an accommodative (innervational) component as a potential contributor to the esotropia. As such, it may be interpreted as a favorable prognostic indicator for remedial (lens/vision therapy) treatment. (See p. 222.)

6-5. There are at least two ways to assess the effect of lens-evoked changes in accommodation (i.e., as produced by extra plus or minus lens power; see p. 222) on the magnitude of a strabismic deviation. You may find one easier to interpret than the other: (a) Place the pair of (plus/minus) lenses before both eyes as the patient fixates on a near/distance target, and attempt to observe any change in the angle of deviation. (b) Position an occluder in front of one of the patient's eyes in such a way that the eye remains visible to you, yet the patient is unable to see the fixation target with it. Place the (plus/minus) lens in front of the nonoccluded eye as the patient fixates the (near/distance target). If the lens induces a change in the patient's accommodative state, and if that change in accommodation has any effect on the patient's binocular status, it should be evident in the occluded eye; i.e., if he is esotropic, the occluded eye will be observed moving temporally with the introduction of a plus lens before the partner eye; if he is exotropic, the eye will move nasally when a minus lens is placed before the partner (nonoccluded) eye.

6-6. Notice that prognosis for the treatment of strabismus is not so much dependent upon the direction, magnitude, etc., of the condition as it is upon the extent to which the patient is able to demonstrate potential for binocular function.

■

REFERENCES

1. Parks MM. Stereoacuity as an indicator of bifixation. In: Arrugo A, ed. International strabismus symposium (University of Giessen, 1966). Basel and New York: S. Karger, A.G., 1966.
2. Simons K, Reinecke RD. Amblyopia screening and stereopsis. In: Symposium on strabismus: transactions of the New Orleans Academy of Ophthalmology. St. Louis: Mosby, 1978.
3. Morgan MW. Anomalies of binocular vision. In: Hirsch M, Wick R, eds. Vision of children. Philadelphia: Chilton Books, 1963.
4. Harwerth RS. Behavioral studies of amblyopia in monkeys. AJOPO 1982; 59(7):535–55.
5. Archer SM, Helveston EM, Miller KK, Ellis FD. Stereopsis in normal infants and infants with congenital esotropia.
6. Crawford MLJ, Smith EL III, Harwerth RS, von Noorden GK. Stereoblind monkeys have few binocular neurons. Inv Ophthal Vis Sci 1984; 25:779–81.
7. Crawford MLJ, von Noorden GK, Meharg LS, Rhodes JW, Harwerth RS. Binocular neurons and binocular function in monkeys and children. Inv Ophthal Vis Sci 1983; 24:491–95.
8. Harwerth RS, Smith EL III, Duncan GC, Crawford MLJ, von Noorden GK. Effects of enucleation of the fixating eye on strabismic amblyopia in monkeys. Inv Ophthal Vis Sci 1986; 27:246–54.
9. Mitchell DE, Murphy KM, Kaye MG. The permanence of the visual recovery that follows reverse occlusion of monocularly deprived kittens. Inv Ophthal Vis Sci 1984; 25:908–17.
10. Bechtoldt HP, Hutz CS. Stereopsis in young infants and stereopsis in an infant with congenital esotropia. J Ped Ophthal Strab 1979; 16(1):49.
11. Fox R, Aslin RN, Shea SL, Dumais ST. Stereopsis in human infants. Science 1980; 207(18):323.
12. Banks MS, Aslin RN, Detson RD. Sensitive period for the development of human binocular vision. Science 1975; 190:675–77.

13. Birch EE, Held R. The development of binocular summation in human infants. Inv Ophthal Vis Sci 1983; 24:1103–1107.
14. Schor CM. Development of stereopsis depends upon contrast sensitivity and spatial tuning. JAOA 1985; 56(8):628.
15. Parks MM. Ocular motility and strabismus. New York: Harper & Row, 1975.
16. Romano RE, Romano JA, Puklin JE. Stereoacuity development in children with normal single binocular vision. Am J Ophthal 1975; 79(6):966.
17. Ogle KN. Binocular vision. Philadelphia: Saunders, 1950.
18. Walk RD, Gibson EJ. A comparative and analytical study of visual depth perception. Psych Monog 1961; 75(15).
19. Bower TGR, Broughton JM, Moore MK. Infant responses to approaching objects. Perc & Psychophys 1970; 9:193.
20. Gordon RF, Yonas A. Sensitivity to binocular depth information in infants. J Exp Ch Psych 1976; 22:413.
21. Cooper J. Feldman J. Operant conditioning and assessment of stereopsis in young children. AJOPO 1978; 55(8):532.
22. Feldman J, Cooper J. Rapid assessment of stereopsis in pre-verbal children using operant techniques: a preliminary study. JAOA 1980; 51(8):767.
23. Howard HJ. A test for the judgment of distance. Am J Ophthal 1919; 21:1656.
24. Noorden GK von. Binocular vision and ocular motility. St. Louis:Mosby, 1980.
25. Griffin JR. Binocular anomalies. Chicago: Professional Press, 1976.
26. Frisby P, Mein J, Saye A, Stanworth A. Use of random-dot stereograms in the clinical assessment of strabismic patients. Br J Ophthal 1975; 59:545.
27. Gruber J, Dickey P, Rosner J. Comparison of a modified (two-item) Frisby with the standard Frisby and Random-dot E stereotests when used with preschool children. AJOPO 1985; 62(5):349–51.
28. Hering R. Zur lehre vom ortssinn der netzhaut. Beitrage zur Physiologie. Leipsig: W. Englemann, Vol. 3, 1861.
29. Lang J. A new stereotest. J Ped Ophthal & Strab 1983; 20(2):72.
30. Julesz B. Foundations of cyclopean perception. Chicago: University of Chicago Press, 1971.
31. Rutstein RP, Eskridge JB. Stereopsis in small angle strabismus. AJOPO 1984; 61(8):491–98.
32. Garzia RP, Richman JE. Stereopsis in an amblyopic small angle esotrope. JAOA 1985; 56(5):400
33. Rosner J. The effectiveness of the random-dot E stereotest as a preschool vision screening instrument. JAOA 1978; 49(10):1121
34. Hammond RS, Schmidt PP. A Random-dot E stereogram for the vision screening of children. Arch Ophthal 1986; 104:54–60.
35. Walraven J. Amblyopia screening with random-dot stereograms. Am J Ophthal 1975; 80(5):893.
36. Hine N. Survey of the clinical uses and reliability of random-dot stereograms. Aust J Optom 1980; 63(3):123.
37. Cooper J. Clinical stereopsis testing: contour and random-dot stereograms. JAOA 1979; 50(1):41.
38. Carmon A, Bechtoldt HP. Dominance of the right cerebral hemisphere for stereopsis. Neurophsychologica 1969; 7:29
39. Benton AL, Hecaen H. Stereoscopic vision in patients with unilateral cerebral disease. Neuropsychology 1970; 20:1084.

Question 6: What Is the Patient's Binocular Status? □ 259

40. Hamsher K deS. Stereopsis and unilateral brain disease. Inv Ophthal 1978; 17(4):336.
41. Reinecke RD, Morton G, Simons K. Stereopsis and orthoptics: Past, present and future. In: Moore S, ed. Orthoptics: past, present and future. New York: Stratton Intercontinental Med Book Corp., 1976.
42. Hinchliffe HA. Clinical evaluation of stereopsis. Br J Orthop 1978; 35:46
43. Simons J. A comparison of the Frisby, Random-dot E, TNO and Randot circles stereotests in screening and office use. Arch Ophthal 1981; 99:446.
44. Cooper J, Feldman J, Medlin D. Comparing stereoscopic performance of children using the Titmus, TNO, and Randot stereotests. JAOA 1979; 50(7):821.
45. Reinecke RD. Stereoacuity assessment in amblyopia. Trans Ophthal Soc UK 1979; 99:398–400.
46. Amigo G, Fiorentini A, Pirchio M, Spinelli D. Binocular vision tested with visual evoked potentials in children and infants. Inv Ophthal 1978; 17(9):910.
47. Shea SL, Fox R, Aslin RN, Dumais ST. Assessment of stereopsis in human infants. Inv Ophthal 1980; 19(11):1400–1404.
48. Setayesh AR, Khodadoust AA, Daryani SM. Microtropia. Arch Ophthal 1978; 96:1842.
49. Swan KC. Colored filters and screens for studying monocular perception in binocular vision. Doc Ophthal 1973; 34:371–80.
50. Jampolsy A. The prism test for strabismus screening. J Ped Ophthal 1964; 1:30.
51. Hugonnier R, Hugonnier S. Strabismus, heterophoria, ocular motor paralysis. St. Louis: Mosby, 1969.
52. Gibson HW. Textbook of orthoptics. London: Hatton Press, 1955.
53. Sherman J, Richter SJ, Epstein A. The differential diagnosis of visual disorders in patients presenting with marked symptoms but no observable ocular abnormality. AJOPO 1980; 57(8):516.
54. Greenwald I. Effective strabismus therapy. Duncan, Okla.: OEP Foundation, 1979.
55. Eskridge JB. The complete cover test. AAAO 1973; 44(6):602.
56. Paliaga GP, Ghisolfi A. Giumta G, Decarli A. Millimetric cover test—a linear strabismometric technique. J Pediatr Ophthal 1980; 17(5):331.
57. Worth C. In: Chavasse FB. Worth's squint or the binocular reflexes and the treatment of strabismus. Ed. 7. London: Bailliere, Tindall and Cox, 1939.
58. Luria SM. Duction, stereoacuity and field of view. AAAO 1971; 48(9):228.
59. Pratt-Johnson MB, Barlow JM. Stereoacuity and fusional amplitude in foveal suppression. Cd J Ophthal 1975; 10:56–60.
60. Flom MC, Kerr KE. Determination of retinal correspondence. Arch Ophthal 1967; 77:200–13.
61. Flom MC. In: Hirsch M, Wick R, eds. Vision of children: an optometric symposium. Philadelphia: Chilton Books, 1963.
62. Flom MC. A minimum strabismus examination. AAAO 1956; 27(11):642.
63. Jones R, Eskridge JB. The Hirschberg test— a re-evaluation. AAAO 1970; 47(2):105.
64. Krimsky E. The corneal light reflex. Springfield, Ill.: Thomas, 1972.
65. Burian HM. Thoughts on the nature of amblyopia exanopsia. Am Orhtop J 1956; 6:5.
66. Schapero M, Amblyopia. Philadelphia: Chilton Books, 1971.
67. Levi DM. Occlusion amblyopia. AJOPO 1976; 55(1):16.
68. Burian HM. Pathophysiologic basis of amblyopia and its treatment. Am J Ophthal 1969; 67:1.
69. Thomas J, Mohindra I, Held R. Strabismic amblyopia in infants. AJOPO 1979; 56(3):197.
70. Mohindra I, Jacobson SG, Thomas J, Held R. Development of amblyopia in infants. Trans Ophthal Soc UK 1979; 99:344.

71. Awaya S, Sugawara M, Miyake S, Isomura Y. Form vision deprivation amblyopia and the results of its treatment—with special reference to the critical period. Jpn J Ophthal 1980; 24:241–50.

72. Flom MC, Weymouth FW, Kahneman D. Visual resolution and contour interaction. J Opt Soc Am 1963; 53:1026.

73. Burian HM, Cortimiglia RM. Visual acuity and fixation pattern in patients with strabismic amblyopia. Am Orthop J 1962; 12:169.

74. Schlossman A. Prognosis, management and results of pleoptic treatment. Int Ophthal Clinics 1961; 1(4):8.

75. Stuart JA, Burian HM. A study of separation difficulty: its relationship to visual acuity in normal and amblyopic eyes. Am J Ophthal 1962; 53:471.

76. Tabolara L. Potere di separazione e possibilita di ricupero visivo nell amblyopia degl strabici. Boll Ocul 1958; 37:508.

77. Cibis L, Hurtt J, Rasicovici A. A clinical study of separation difficulty in organic and functional amblyopia. Am Orthop J 1968; 18:66.

78. Burian HM. The behavior of the amblyopic eye under reduced illumination and the theory of functional amblyopia. Doc Ophthal 1967; 23:189.

79. Ingram RM, Walker C. Refraction as a means of predicting squint or amblyopia in preschool siblings of children known to have these defects. Br J Ophthal 1979; 63:238.

80. Ingram RM. Amblyopia: the need for a new approach? Br J Ophthal 1979; 63:236–37.

81. Oliver M, Nawratzki I. Screening of preschool children for ocular anomalies: amblyopia. Br J Ophthal 1971; 55:467–71.

82. Amos JF. Refractive amblyopia: its classification, etiology and epidemiology. JAOA 1977; 48(4):489.

83. Martin G. Astigmatic amblyopia. Translated by Ciuffreda KJ. AJOPO 1978; 55(2):133.

84. Harcourt B. Hereditary nystagmus in early childhood. J Med Genetics 1970; 7:253.

85. Smith JL. Nystagmus. Am Orthop J 1973; 23:27.

86. Bedrossian EH. The surgical and non-surgical management of strabismus. Springfield, Ill.: Thomas, 1968.

87. Hepler RS. Central nervous system aspects of nystagmus. Am Orthop J 1973; 23:23.

88. Gay AJ. Eye movement disorders. St. Louis: Mosby, 1974.

89. Franceschetti A, Monnier M, Dieterele P. Analyse du nystagmus congenital par la methode electro-nystagmographique (ENG). Bull Schweiz Akad Med Wiss 1952; 8:403.

90. Cianci AO. La esotropia en el lactante, diagnostico y tratamiento. Arch Chil Oftalmol 1962; 19:117.

91. Cianci AO. La esotropia con limitacion bilateral de la abduccion en el lactante. Arch Oftalmol B Aires 1962; 37:207.

92. Cianci AO. Management of esodeviations under the age of two. Int Ophthalmol Clin 1966; 6:503.

93. Lafon C. La vision des nystagmiques. Ann Ocul 1914; 151:4.

94. Healy E. Nystagmus treated by orthoptics. Am Orthop J 1962; 12:89.

95. Bruckner R. Exacte strabismusdiagnostik bei 1/2-3 jahrigen kindern mit einem einlached verlahren, dem "Durchleuchtungslest." Ophthalmologica 1962; 144:184–98.

96. Roe LD, Guyton DL. The light that leaks: Bruckner and the red reflex. Surv Ophthalmol 1984; 28:665–70

97. Tongue AC, Cibis GW. Bruckner test. Ophthalmology 1981; 88:1041–44.

98. Griffin J, Cotter S. AJOPO 1986; 63:957–61.

7

Question 7
Does the (Binocular) Patient Display Adequate Sensory-Motor Adaptability (i.e., the Capacity to Adapt Efficiently to Reasonably Stressful Conditions)?

☐

Coordination of accommodation and convergence—the precise, synchronous interactions of a number of remarkably sensitive anatomical components and sensory-motor processes—begins to develop very early in most children (1, 2). The fundamental assumptions of this chapter are that (a) normal (comfortable, clear, single, simultaneous) binocular vision requires *efficient* coordination of those two systems: the ability to achieve, sustain, and/or shift bifoveal alignment and optical focus under a great variety of task conditions, rapidly, accurately, and effortlessly, virtually automatically; (b) *inefficient* performance will have detrimental effects on comfort, and/or clarity, and/or binocularity, especially when sustained attention at nearpoint is required.

Undoubtedly, the most valid method for assessing the efficiency of sustained visual performance is to observe that performance over prolonged periods of time. It is one thing to extrapolate from a single set of measures, and another to obtain a series of related measures, taken as the patient engages in a variety of representative tasks at different occasions, under different circumstances. The latter will yield more valid data, but it is impractical. The less valid, single-measure approach must suffice.

The flow diagram shown in Figure 7.1 depicts a sequence of steps designed to assess a patient's binocular performance efficiency, all based on the extrapolate-from-a-single-set-of-measures approach. It reflects conventional wisdom, based in

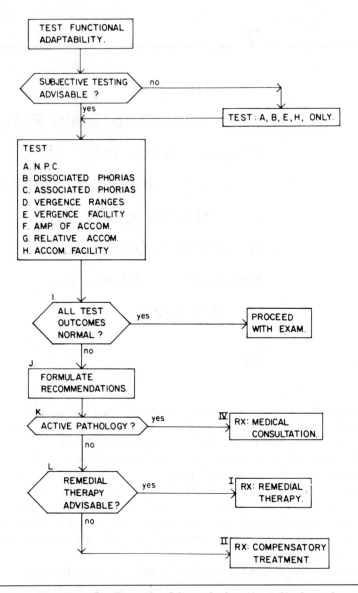

Figure 7.1   Question #7: Does the (binocular) patient display adequate sensory-motor adaptability?

part on knowledge that has been validated under controlled laboratory conditions, in part on knowledge acquired by clinical observations, and in part on reasonable assumptions (3,4,5,6,7,8).

It also reflects the central nature of the question that heads this chapter. The testing sequence—or the core of it, at least—is to be implemented with *all* binocular patients, even those who occasionally lapse into a nonbinocular status;

i.e., intermittent strabismics. There is no good reason to skip over this portion of the evaluation, and many good reasons why it should be performed, even when the patient is symptom free. The best reason: It may serve to prevent a future binocular deficiency and all that this implies in regard to the patient's ability to meet the visual requirements of his daily life.

An inspection of the flow diagram reveals clearly its focus on accommodation and convergence, both as separate as well as synkinetic processes. The depth to which these are probed depends on the patient's age. As the flow diagram indicates, all tests should be administered when feasible. With the young, immature child, administer the objective tests only.

A. NEARPOINT OF CONVERGENCE (NPC)

Measures of the patient's convergence, break, and recovery thresholds should be made under three stimulus conditions. (NPC is also discussed under Question #4. In that context, the discussion was limited to the process investigated by condition #2 below):

1. The patient fixates on a detailed accommodation-stimulating target, such as vertical line of small letters or a line drawing about which attention-provoking questions may be posed.
2. The patient fixates on a small, nondetailed light source; e.g., a penlight.
3. The patient fixates on a small, nondetailed light source (e.g., a penlight) while a red filter is held in front of one eye (9).

Threshold is recorded in terms of distance from the patient. Two thresholds are measured in each condition: an *objective NPC* and a *subjective NPC*. The former refers to the distance between the fixation target and the patient *when the examiner observes* a loss of binocular fixation. The latter refers to the distance between the fixation target and the patient *when the patient reports* diplopia. The reader should be advised that some authorities use the terms objective NPC and subjective NPC when referring to the outcomes of procedures #2 and #3 above (10, p. 210). That differs from how the terms are used here. In this context, *objective* means examiner-observed; *subjective* means patient-observed.

Test outcomes are evaluated in three ways:

1. The adequacy of the objective amplitude of convergence. Normally, this falls somewhere between 2 and 8 cm (11).
2. The intertest relationships among the three objective NPC measures; that is, the similarity of these findings and the clinical implications of any observed differences. In particular:

a. A comparison of the objective NPC when measured under stimulus conditions #2 and #3: a penlight with and without the red filter over one eye. The red filter is purported to inhibit voluntary convergence and therefore provide a more accurate assessment of fusional convergence (9; 12, p. 396). Based on this, its proponents argue that it is a more valid measure of what the optometrist wants to learn when she investigates the NPC. Assumptions aside, patients whose NPCs are significantly affected by the monocular red filter do appear to be unusually prone to the symptoms of convergence insufficiency.

b. A comparison of the objective NPC when measured under stimulus conditions #1 and #2: letters versus a penlight. The implication: an NPC that is closer with a target that requires full accommodation may be attributed to a high AC/A ratio. If the reverse occurs, if the NPC is more remote when an accommodation-stimulating target is used, then the difference between the two measures may be attributed to the inhibition of convergence once the patient reaches the limits of her amplitude of accommodation; i.e., when the letters blur.

3. The intratest relationships.

a. The extent to which the objective and subjective NPC's of a single condition coincide. When there is a lack of concurrence, the objective NPC is likely to be the more remote of the two; that is, the examiner will see the loss of bifoveal alignment before the patient reports it.

There are different ways of explaining this, ranging from the patient simply being a slow responder, to the delayed awareness of diplopia being caused by a central suppression area.

b. The relationship between break and recovery points. The two should not be significantly different (i.e., no greater than 6 cm). When they are, when the patient displays difficulty in regaining binocular alignment even as the target is being moved farther away, it suggests an explanation similar to the one put forth by advocates of measuring NPC with a monocular red filter: that the break point reflects voluntary convergence; the recovery point, fusional convergence. Hence, the latter may well be more clinically relevant of the two.

B. DISSOCIATED PHORIAS

Phorias may be measured in a number of ways. Most optometrists prefer the Von Graefe method, wherein a measure is made of the relative positions of the visual axes while fusion is disrupted by a dissociating prism.

There is no need to describe this method. It is amply covered in basic optometry texts (13,14). Nor is there any reason to argue against its use, if the child is able to respond reliably to the procedure.

However, a significant number of children, especially children under the age of 6, are apt to be confused by some aspects of the Von Graefe phoria test. They need something different.

A reasonable substitute is the *Alternating Cover Test* (see Chapter 6). This procedure is very useful for measuring vertical and horizontal phorias, once it has been established that the patient does have single binocular vision and that what is being measured is not a heterotropia.

The test depends upon objective assessment rather than subjective responses. (If a subjective measure is wanted, the Maddox rod is far less confusing than the Von Graefe method.) The child need not speak. All she has to do is fixate on an appropriately positioned target. In this regard, it is important to remember that the optimal target is one that requires discriminating observation (e.g., small but legible letters) at both farpoint and nearpoint testing distances. In the young emmetrope (or appropriately corrected ametrope), orthophoria (more or less) is expected at farpoint, with orthophoria to 6 prism diopters exophoria considered to be normal for nearpoint.

On the basis of these measures, the AC/A ratio may be calculated, or simply estimated. The latter is usually adequate, with a difference between the two phorias (distance and near) in excess of 10 prism diopters indicating an abnormally high or low AC/A ratio. For example, if the patient shows at least 10 prism diopters more esophoria (or less exophoria) at near than at distance, it signals a high AC/A ratio; if the patient shows at least 10 prism diopters more exophoria (or less esophoria) at near than at distance, low AC/A ratio (15, p. 61).

■
C. ASSOCIATED PHORIAS (FIXATION DISPARITY)

Some years ago, it was observed that fusion could be maintained without precise bifoveal alignment; that within Panum's area, small amounts of horizontal and/or vertical bifoveal misalignment will not disrupt the central processes (16). Typically, as much as 10 minutes of arc is tolerable in the horizontal dimension, less than that in the vertical. Ames and Gliddon (17) termed this *retinal slip*. Later, the phrases fixation disparity and associated phoria were introduced (18). The two terms are used interchangeably here, despite certain technical differences (see below).

Clinical measurement of fixation disparity can be accomplished in the following three ways:

1. Patient views a pair of vertically or horizontally oriented targets. Usually, these are vernier lines that are constructed so that when appropriate filters are in place, each target is visible to one eye only, yet everything else in the patient's visual field is visible to both eyes simultaneously. Hence, the binocular patient sees both targets within a fused binocular context. If he has no fixation disparity, the relative position of the two targets is not affected by the filters. If, in fact, they are in precise alignment, he will see them that way. The patient who reports a deviation from alignment therefore reveals a fixation disparity that is measured by determining the amount and direction of prism needed to align the targets. For example, if 3 prism diopters, base out, are needed to align the targets, it would be described as 3 prism diopters eso fixation disparity.

There are a number of commercially produced devices available that have been designed according to these principles (e.g., *for farpoint testing:* A.O. Co. Vectographic Slide; Bernell fixation disparity test; Mallet fixation disparity test; *for nearpoint testing:* A.O. Co. Vectographic fixation disparity test; Mallet test; Bernell test).

2. Patient is shown a series of pairs of polarized targets that vary in the degree to which they are in alignment. The patient's task is to select the pair that appears to be aligned when viewed through compatible polarized filters. If he selects the pair that are, in fact, aligned, he has no fixation disparity. If he has a fixation disparity, he will select a pair that are out of alignment. The magnitude and direction of his fixation disparity are then determined by the misalignment of the pair he selected, as measured in minutes of arc (the Disparometer is designed on this principle, and is available from Vision Analysis, P.O. Box 14390, Columbus, Ohio) (19).

3. Here, again, filters are used as the patient views a pair of targets; in this instance, however, at least one of the targets is moveable. His task is to place the targets in precise alignment. Fixation disparity is determined on the basis of where he positions the targets. If he aligns them precisely—if what he sees through the filters matches the true positions of the targets—then he has zero fixation disparity. If he misaligns the targets, he reveals a fixation disparity, with the magnitude and direction calculated by the degree of that misalignment.

Although at present there is no apparatus produced specifically for this method, one can easily be devised.

☐ Farpoint Measures

Use two flashlights that are capable of projecting focused spots; one equipped with a red filter; the other, a green filter. The patient's task: while wearing red/green filters, superimpose the spot from one flashlight, held by him, over the spot from the other, held by the examiner. Make certain that this is carried out in a setting where there is sufficient illumination for the patient to be able to see nonfiltered ("fusion-lock") stimuli—stimuli visible to both eyes simultaneously—in addition to the anaglyph targets. (If this is done in total darkness, it may be interpreted as a measure of the dissociated phoria.)

☐ Nearpoint Measures

Construct a Brock Posture Board (20), an instrument now out of production (see p. 212). It too employs anaglyphic materials. Draw a small red pencil spot in the center of a white sheet of paper. Place the paper on a sheet of red plastic. Thus, if a white penlight is held under and against the sheet of red plastic, it will be seen as a red spot by the patient equipped with red/green filters—visible only to the eye behind the red filter. The red pencil spot will appear as a black spot, visible only to the other eye. The patient's task: superimpose the red light spot on the black pencil spot. (Again, provide some fusion locks, this time on the sheet of white paper; e.g., letters or geometric designs drawn with a black pencil so that they are seen simultaneously by both eyes.)

In both of these conditions, fixation disparity is measured by calculating any separation between the two supposedly superimposed stimuli.

The three methods for measuring the associated phoria differ in three significant ways:

1. Method #1 measures the prism needed to neutralize the optical effects of the fixation disparity. Methods #2 and #3 measure the optical effects of the patient's fixation disparity. The results may differ (21).

2. All three methods are vulnerable to environmental influences (22,23,24). For example, if the targets are displayed in the center of a fairly uncluttered visual field, there is no compelling need for the patient to exercise full accommodation. If, in contrast, the targets are displayed in the center of a page of print, or if printed letters are part of the central target and if the patient is stimulated to keep the print clear, then accommodation will be stimulated. This factor very often influences test outcomes. Hence, it is important to take it into account when doing test-retest comparisons.

3. Methods #1 and #2 require fairly sophisticated language skills. The patient must communicate orally regarding the relative position of the targets. Method #3 does not require spoken responses. As a result, it is the method of choice with young children; certainly with children not yet 6 years old.

☐ Fixation Disparity Curves (FDC)

A fixation disparity curve is generated by first measuring the patient's fixation disparity in the standard manner, then remeasuring it as she looks through a series of prisms of increasing powers. The recommended procedure for determining a horizontal FDC calls for prism power to be increased in 3-diopter increments, starting with base in and proceeding to base out (19). Vertical FDCs may also be generated, but, thus far, these have not been shown to provide any useful clinical information.

Ogle (25) showed that FDCs vary among individuals. Four types of response patterns have been identified. These are purported to be related to patient's symptoms (or lack of them) and to have implications in respect to treatment recommendations (26).

A type I FDC, reported to be representative of the majority (60 percent) of the population, tends to be relatively unaffected by moderate amounts of prism, responding only when higher amounts of prism are used. For example, a type I curve for a patient with a zero horizontal fixation disparity is one that continues to show approximately zero fixation disparity even when the patient looks through 3 prism diopters base in and base out, but then responds strongly and equally as larger amounts of base in and base out prism are used.

A type II curve is one that shows very little response to base out prism but marked response to base in prism.

A type III curve mirrors the type II in that it shows very little response to base in prism, but marked reaction to base out.

A type IV curve tends to be flat, with very little, if any, measurable reaction to base in or base out prism.

Of the four, type I has been identified as representative of the patient who will be most responsive to therapy, with type IIIs running a reasonably close second.

D. FUSIONAL VERGENCE AMPLITUDES

It was noted earlier that practical constraints require the optometrist to assess visual performance efficiency on the basis of limited observations and reasonable extrapolations. One key factor in the extrapolation process is the patient's fusional vergence amplitudes; i.e., the extent to which positive and negative vergence is stimulated by disparate retinal images projected from a single object, rather than by accommodation. These, in combination with related phoria measures, make up a substantial portion of the date base for judging a binocular patient's general ability to adapt efficiently to reasonably stressful conditions.

What justifies such sweeping extrapolations from such minimal data? One reason, of course, is that the empirical clinical evidence appears to validate that interpretation. In addition, it seems reasonable. Consider an analogous situation:

Suppose we wish to assess an individual's ability to stand at a work bench for prolonged periods of time. How could this be accomplished? One straightforward method would be to have him stand at a work bench until fatigue forced him to give up that posture. A second method: introduce controlled, quantifiable stress into the situation and assess its relative effects; that is, determine what kind and how much stress is needed to cause a change in his posture, and how that compares to the "normal." For example, weights could be placed on his shoulders while he stands at the work bench, and an assessment made of the relative effects of the different weights. Or, he could be placed on an unstable base, thereby requiring him to devote extra attention and energy to maintaining balance as he stands at his works bench. The point is evident: in these instances, the goal is to evaluate, and compare to some established norm, the individual's ability to continue to perform a task despite the introduction of counterproductive forces. That is what fusional vergence testing attempts to accomplish, and it appears to do so with reasonable reliability.

Unfortunately, the standard test procedures for measuring positive and negative fusional vergence amplitudes are not always applicable with young patients. The phenomena of blur, break, and recovery are illusions that frequently confuse, yielding either no data from the child or, worse yet, unreliable data.

In situations where the standard test methods are applicable, they should be used. Where they are not appropriate, alternative tests will have to be used or decisions will have to be made without the information they supply. Vergence facility testing is an appropriate alternative in many instances.

E. VERGENCE FACILITY

One key aspect of performance efficiency is overlooked in the standard measurements of fusional vergence amplitudes: speed of response. Standard methods do, indeed, measure the extent to which the patient can make fusional vergence adjustments in order to maintain the two retinal images within Panum's area, but they do not assess how easily and rapidly these can be performed. Data that revealed this would be useful (27).

Therefore, even when fusional vergence amplitudes are reliably measured in the standard manner, there is reason to assess the facility with which the patient can adapt to controlled, quantifiable stress when it is introduced abruptly, in relatively large increments. Vergence facility is measured as follows (see Figure 7.2):

□ At Farpoint

1. Present the patient with a vertical row of small but legible letters (e.g., 20/30) and confirm that these appear to be both *single and clear*.

2. Place a 6-diopter prism, base in, in front of one eye, while asking the patient, "How many rows of letters do you see now?" If she reports seeing two, then request that she tell you "as soon as they come together into a single row and become clear." (Note: Watch the patient's eyes so as to confirm objectively what she is reporting. The fusional vergence movements should be apparent.)

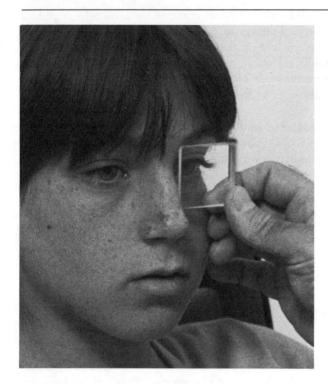

Figure 7.2
Assessing vergence
facility.

3. If (and as soon as) clear fusion is regained, remove the prism, again requesting the patient to report as soon as the row of letters is single and clear. (Continue to watch her eyes.)

4. As soon as she reports fusion and clarity without prism, reintroduce the prism, repeating step #2, above. Continue in this manner until the patient has successfully accomplished three cycles (a cycle = fusion and clarity with prism, then without) or until 30 seconds have elapsed, whichever, occurs first. Consider three cycles within 30 seconds to be "passing" performance.

5. *If the patient satisfies criterion* (i.e., three cycles accomplished within 30 seconds), increase prism power in 2-diopter increments until threshold is reached. Record the highest prism power that she could adapt to successfully within those same time constraints.

6. *If the patient does not satisfy criterion* (i.e., if she cannot successfully adapt to the 6-diopter prism, base in), reduce prism power in 2-diopter steps and repeat the procedure until she does satisfy the three cycles within 30 seconds criterion. Then, in order to take into account the possibility that she may have "caught on" slowly, increase prism power in 2-diopter increments until threshold is determined. For example, if initially the patient could not satisfy criterion through the 6-diopter prism nor the 4-diopter prism, but could deal successfully with the 2-diopter prism, then retest with the 4-diopter prism. If she passes, go up to

6-prism diopters, and so on until the task again becomes too difficult. Record the highest prism power to which she could adapt.

7. Repeat the process with base out prism, starting with 12 prism diopters.

□ At Nearpoint

1. Repeat the procedures described above, this time using small letters held at 40 cm. Measure base in facility first, starting with 12 prism diopters; then measure base out, starting with 14 prism diopters.

2. Record the highest prism power (both base in and base out) to which the patient can adapt at the rate of three cycles within 30 seconds.

□ Performance Criteria

These have been established arbitrarily but appear to be clinically valid. In effect, they are comparable to the "recovery" measures of positive and negative relative convergence when determined in the standard way. (See 28,29,30 for other opinions regarding criteria.) Consider the following to be satisfactory: **At farpoint,** base in: 6 prism diopters/plano. At farpoint, base out: 12 prism diopters/plano. **At nearpoint,** base in: 12 prism diopters/plano. At nearpoint, base out: 14 prism diopters/plano.

□ Vergence Facility Testing with Younger Children

The procedures just described depend, in part, on patient's responses, with confirmation obtained from examiner's observations. Unfortunately, it is sometimes difficult to see the patient's eyes make fusional vergence shifts under these test conditions. Hence, to assess vergence facility in very young children, certain procedural modifications should be made.

One method that tends to work adequately is to use stereopsis targets instead of letters (31). All else remains the same. At farpoint, use two or three rings from the 2 minute of arc line in the A.O. Vectographic slide. At nearpoint, use the Random-dot E stereotest, or whatever other stereotest that was used for investigating the patient's binocular status. "Passing" criteria for the 3-year-old and above are the same as those shown for the older patient.

F. AMPLITUDE OF ACCOMMODATION

If NPC was measured with a detailed target, this will have already been accomplished. Unless there is reason to measure monocular amplitudes, no other testing is necessary.

■

G. RELATIVE ACCOMMODATION RANGES

An adaptable binocular system will also display an efficient capacity to exercise and inhibit accommodation in some reasonable amount while vergence remains fixed (14,32).

This is typically measured with the familiar tests of positive and negative relative accommodation. These tests ignore two basic factors, however. One, farpoint function; the other, the time required to accomplish the action (33). For these reasons, and also because the standard method tends to elicit unreliable responses from young children, accommodation facility should be assessed in addition to, or in place of, the standard measures.

■

H. ACCOMMODATION FACILITY

☐ At Farpoint

1. Present the patient with a vertical row of small but legible letters (e.g, 20/30) and comfirm that they appear to be single and clear.

2. Place a pair of −2.00D spheres before the patient's eyes, while asking, "Tell me as soon as these letters appear to be single and clear." (Note: Lenses may be from trial case and held in the examiner's hand, or they may be mounted in so-called "flipper" frames. See Figure 7.3.)

3. When (and if) the print clears (remaining single), remove the −2.00D spheres, again requesting that the patient report as soon as the print clears and appears single.

4. When she reports clarity without the lenses, reintroduce them, repeating step #2 above. Continue in this manner until the patient has successfully accomplished three cycles (a cycle = letters clear and single through lenses, then again clear and single when lenses are removed), or until 30 seconds have elapsed, whichever occurs first. Judge the accomplishment of three cycles within 30 seconds to be "passing" performance.

5. If the patient satisfies criterion (i.e., accomplishes three cycles within 30 seconds), increase lens power in 1.00D increments until threshold is reached. Record the highest lens power that she could adapt to successfully within these same time constraints.

6. If the patient does not satisfy criterion (i.e., if she cannot successfully adapt to the −2.00D spheres), reduce lens power to a −1.00D sphere and repeat the

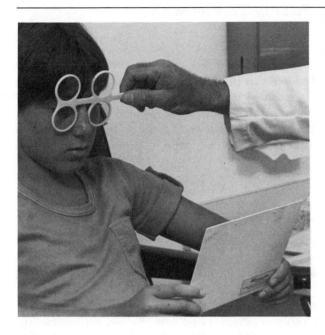

Figure 7.3
Assessing
accommodation facility.

procedure. If she then is successful, repeat the test with −2.00D spheres and continue, as described above. If, however, even the −1.00D sphere is insurmountable, stop testing and record this threshold as zero.

□ At Nearpoint

1. Repeat the procedures described above, this time using small letters held at 40 cm. Also, because it is nearpoint, probe both positive and negative relative accommodation; the former with a −2.00/plano combination, the latter with +2.00/plano. In other words, start off by testing the patient with the +2.00/plano combination, working up or down in 1.00-diopter increments in accord with the patient's ability to meet the demands of the task. Then repeat with the −2.00/plano combination.

2. Record the highest plus/plano and minus/plano pairs to which the patient could adapt at the rate of three cycles within 30 seconds.

□ Performance Criteria

Consider the following to be satisfactory: **At farpoint,** −2.00/plano; **at nearpoint,** +2.00/plano and −2.00/plano.

□ Accommodation Facility Testing with Young Children

Once again, the optometrist must settle for less information in her attempt to collect valid data. The procedures described for vergence facility testing apply here as well. That is, use a stereoscopic target for fixation, making sure that the one you select is one that the patient has already responded to appropriately, perhaps during the assessment of her binocular status. In addition, keep watch on the child's pupils. They should constrict and dilate in accord with the related changes in accommodation.

□ Additional Tests

A number of innovative studies recently have been reported that seem to signal impending major breakthroughs in our understanding, diagnosis, and treatment of the binocular problems discussed in this chapter (34,35,36). Foremost among these is an intriguing series of reports by Schor and various collaborators, explicating the intimate interconnections and clinical relevance of six key phenomena: *tonic accommodation, tonic vergence, vergence accommodation, accommodative vergence, adaptation of tonic accommodation, and adaptation of tonic vergence* (37,38,39,40,41). Noting that we currently have clinical methods for measuring only two of these (tonic vergence—the horizontal phoria; accommodative vergence—the AC/A ratio), Schor describes methods for measuring the other two. His method for determining tonic accommodation is described in Chapter 5 (see p. 158). The method for determining the convergence-accommodation (CA/C) ratio is described below.

The CA/C RATIO

The CA/C ratio is analogous to the gradient AC/A; it refers to the mean change in open-loop accommodative (diopter) response produced by the change in vergence. Hence, to assess the CA/C ratio, one measures the change in resting focus of accommodation before and during convergence or divergence. First, the examiner determines the patient's (baseline) tonic accommodation using Nott retinoscopy, as described in Chapter 5 (see p. 158). Then a prism (usually 10 prism diopters base in) is introduced and Nott retinoscopy is repeated. (Retinoscopy should be performed as soon as the patient has fused the DOG target—within 5 to 10 seconds—so as to prevent any additional prism adaptation from influencing the accommodative response.) Any change measured by retinoscopy reflects a change in accommodation that is attributable to the change in vergence. Hence, to calculate the CA/C ratio, the measured change in accommodation is divided by the added prism. According to Schor, CA/C ratios above 1 diopter per meter angle (D/MA) are to be considered *high*, whereas ratios below 0.5 D/MA are *low* for patients age 22 and younger. Another interesting observation: the CA/C ratio is not immutable. It, and the AC/A ratio, can be changed through appropriately designed and effective vision therapy (42).

ADAPTATION* OF TONIC ACCOMMODATION

Schor also stresses the value of assessing the extent to which a patient's tonic accommodation is altered by adapting to (plus or minus) lenses that either inhibit (plus spheres) or stimulate (minus spheres) accommodation. To accomplish the latter, he suggests again using the 0.2 cycles per degree (cpd) DOG target. The target is positioned 40 cm from the patient and a transparent visual acuity target (or thin line) is superimposed over it. The patient views the visual acuity target (monocularly) for 30 seconds, through lenses (in a trial frame or phoropter) that stimulate an additional 3.00D of accommodation. (Monocular stimulation prevents convergence from contributing to the accommodative response.) According to Schor, this situation will typically result in a large enough accommodative after-effect (1 to 2D) to be measured by Nott retinoscopy. Once the adaptation is complete (after 30 seconds), the transparent visual acuity target is removed, and the subject passively views the 0.2 cpd DOG target while Nott retinoscopy is employed to measure the duration of the tonic aftereffects of accommodation, i.e., until accommodation returns to the baseline resting position. According to Schor, if tonic aftereffects last less than 10 seconds, the patient has *low adaptation;* if the aftereffects last between 10 and 45 seconds, it indicates *moderate adaptation;* and aftereffects that persist for 1 minute or longer may be classified as *high* or *robust adaptation*.

ADAPTATION* OF TONIC CONVERGENCE

Much has been written about this phenomenon, most of it under the rubric of prism adaptation (42,43,44). In essence, it is the extent to which a patient's het-erophoria (tonic vergence state) is altered by stimulating fusional vergence with prisms and the persistence of that aftereffect. Standard methods for assessing this have not been defined; obviously, the degree of adaptation depends upon the amount of prism, its orientation, and how long it is worn.

As noted above, this line of research appears to have great promise. Clearly, more work is needed: standard testing protocols have to be defined; norms have to be determined. In the interim, the optometrist is urged to keep informed, to try what appears to be reasonable, and to evaluate the outcomes of those trials. When considered in conjunction with advances being made in our understanding

---

*The reader should be advised that the word adapt is used differently by different authors. In the context of this chapter, we intend the word adapt to mean "to overcome" the obstacle to fusion and/or clarity produced by prisms and/or spheres. Many vision scientists use the work adapt to mean "change," such as the extent and duration of the change in tonic accommodation that results from looking through plus or minus spheres, or the extent and duration of the change in tonic vergence that results from maintaining binocular fusion while looking through base in or base out prisms. We presume that both usages are correct, but we also recognize the potential confusion such ambiguity can generate.

of how dual innervation of the ciliary muscle affects accommodation, it has the flavor of importance.

I. ALL TEST OUTCOMES NORMAL?

Although each of the tests described in this section has its own expecteds/norms, they are best interpreted in terms of how they interrelate. Over the years, a number of methods for doing this have been developed (e.g., [2,3,4]), and, although each has its unique characteristics, they are not all that different from each other.

All of them, however, require fairly precise measures of phorias, relative vergence amplitudes, and relative accommodation amplitudes—something that is not generally obtainable from the young patient. With this age group, the optometrist is well advised to make decisions solely on the basis of vergence and accommodation facility test outcomes in combination with farpoint and nearpoint dissociated phorias. They are objective tests. They yield fairly reliable data. And, for clinical purposes, they provide much the same information obtained from the standard relative vergence and relative accommodation tests, although not in quite so precise a form.

When the outcomes from this short battery all fall within normal limits, assume that the patient has sufficient binocular adaptability—unless, of course, something else has been observed that contradicts that assumption.

☐ If Yes

Proceed to question #8, (Chapter 8), but continue to keep in mind any signs/symptoms that might have been explained by a deficit in binocular efficiency, had one been found. These signs/symptoms continue to require explanation.

☐ If No

Formulate recommendations (see J in Figure 7.1 flow diagram and below).

J. FORMULATE RECOMMENDATIONS

The prognosis in cases of binocular inefficiency is usually very favorable. There are three treatment options.

1. When the evidence points to a systemic etiology, refer the patient for appropriate medical consultation.

2. If the patient appears to be sufficiently motivated and teachable, recommend remedial therapy: A regimen of structured activities that is designed to improve—reeducate—the substandard visual functions.

3. When remedial therapy is contraindicated, recommend compensatory treatment. This usually takes the form of spherical and/or prismatic lenses that enable the patient to cope with the deficit; i.e., perform satisfactorily despite the substandard function.

Rarely does the optometrist have to resort to reassurance therapy in cases of binocular inefficiency.

K. SIGNS OF ACTIVE PATHOLOGY?

The first decision to be made at this stage in the process centers on the possibility that the observed deficit may be a sign of some general health problem. Potential etiologies range from congenital defects, to infectious and toxic conditions, to central nervous system involvements, to hysteria (12,45).

Typically, in cases where the problem does derive from a systemic pathology, the deficit is apt to be apparent in both positive and negative relative accommodation and convergence. In other words, it tends to be general rather than localized. In addition, there usually are other indications that point toward something more complex than a visual function disorder.

☐ If Yes

Recommend a medical consultation.

☐ If No

Assume a functional deficit. Consider the advisability of remedial therapy (see L in Figure 7.1 flow diagram and below).

L. REMEDIAL THERAPY ADVISABLE?

Three major, interrelated factors have to be considered when attempting to determine the advisability of remedial therapy for binocular inefficiency. First, the specifics of the therapy; i.e., what it will require of the patient in terms of time, energy, and money. Second, the patient's motivation and ability to profit from instruction. Third, the consequences of bypassing remediation; i.e., either ignoring the condition or recommending a compensatory treatment.

Binocular inefficiency characteristically manifests as (mild to severe) ocular discomfort, and/or occasional episodes of blurred vision, and/or occasional disruptions of binocular fusion (i.e., intermittent strabismus with or without an awareness of diplopia), and/or simply a tendency to avoid the kinds of tasks that produce the symptoms.

Such signs and symptoms have strong influence over the patient's motivation. The college student who cannot keep up with his assignments because of substandard fusional convergence will probably be much more motivated (and teachable) than the 6-year-old with an intermittent exotropia that is noticed only by her parents and only when she is "daydreaming." On the other hand, the parents of a first grader are likely to be more successful than the parents of a tenth grader in insisting that a remedial program be followed.

Thus, when it comes to evaluating the patient's motivation, there are no set rules other than that the optometrist should be aware that very few patients/ parents understate their motivation, many overstate it.

In regard to what a remedial program will require of the patient in terms of time, effort, and money, the specifics are discussed in Chapter 14. In general, effective remedial programs ordinarily consist of two segments. The first is likely to extend over a 4- to 8-week period and require daily out-of-office sessions of about 30 to 45 minutes, periodic office visits (perhaps once every 2 weeks), and a small investment in equipment. The second segment will require much less time per day, far fewer office visits, but a long-term commitment to the kind of drill and practice needed to convert an established inefficient pattern of behavior to a different and efficient performance pattern that is carried out automatically; in other words, to replace one habit with another.

Certain conditions are relatively easy to remediate; others are not. In essence, they all stem from an inefficient linkage between convergence and accommodation. They vary in the nature of those linkages. To treat them is to attempt to alter that linkage in one way or another.

The treatment goal is the same in all cases. The critical determinant of how easily that goal will be achieved is the nature of the condition when the treatment is begun.

Some years ago, Duane (46) proposed a classification system that employed such terms as convergence insufficiency, convergence excess, divergence insufficiency, and divergence excess.

More recently, Schapero (47), elaborating on this, described ten different types of conditions made up of the various combinations of three variables; tonic convergence (actually, the dissociated phoria at farpoint), fusional convergence, and the AC/A ratio. He then went on to propose various treatment strategies for the ten conditions. It was a useful contribution; it warrants study.

Most recent is the highly interesting work of Schor and others, cited above, which explicates the exquisite interrerlationships between tonic accommodation, tonic convergence, accommodative-convergence, convergence-accommodation, and the extent and duration of the changes that are produced in those tonic states when stimulating and inhibiting spheres and prisms are introduced.

In the final analysis there is not yet a hard and fast rule that specifies what type of treatment is appropriate for what type of case. It reduces to this: all else being equal (i.e., patient motivation, teachability, etc.), the cases most susceptible to remediation, are those where (in order of increasing difficulty): (a) the deficit is present only at one fixation distance; i.e., farpoint *or* nearpoint; (b) the deficit is exophoria combined with reduced positive fusional convergence—with nearpoint deficits being easier to remediate than farpoint deficits (48); (c) the deficit is esophoria combined with reduced negative fusional convergence—with nearpoint deficits being easier to remediate than farpoint deficits; (d) the deficit is present at both farpoint and nearpoint—with exophoria-based deficits being easier to remediate than esophoria—based deficits.

It is important to keep in mind that the scaling assumes a set of discrete clinical problems. In reality, of course, these are only points along a continuum. As such, the scale is not infallible, but it will help in making some predictions about the relative difficulty (i.e., time, effort, etc.) of a remedial program.

In summary, the best way to deal with the question regarding the advisability of recommending remedial therapy is to be reasonably optimistic but not to lose sight of the critical role that the patient/parent plays. Weigh the relative tractability of the condition against the patient's parent's motivation and teachability. Remediation is a worthwhile goal when it is desired and attainable. When it is not desired and when it is unobtainable, compensatory treatment should be recommended without hesitation. Spectacles are not an anathema.

□ If Yes

Design and initiate the program (see Chapters 9 and 14).

□ If No

Recommend appropriate compensatory treatment (see Chapters 9 and 14).

■ PRACTICAL SUGGESTIONS

7-1. When administering vergence and accommodation screening tests, urge the patient to "try." The patient who can catch on quickly to what she has to do to pass one or both of these batteries is not an appropriate candidate for vision therapy.

For example, if the patient fails the vergence facility screening test, ask if (a) she sees two images; (b) if so, can she "try harder" to fuse them into one if you alter the fixation distance. If she then performs satifactorily, retest at the standard distance. Similarly, if the patient fails the accommodation facility screening test, retest at a different distance; then, if she can perform appropriately, retest at the standard distance.

7-2. A very satisfactory near point fixation disparity test can be constructed using a polarized lens from one of the commercially produced vectographic tests vision therapy kits:

   1. Type on white paper a horizontal row of three letters: "x o x."
   2. Type a short vertical line just above and just below the "o" in the above array.
   3. Cut a polarizing filter lens in half—horizontally—and scotch tape half over the upper short vertical line; scotch tape the other half over the lower short vertical line, but turn the filter over before you do—so that it is polarized orthoganally to the upper one. Thus, when the two vertical lines are observed through polarizing filters, only one eye will see the upper line; and the other eye, only the lower line.
   4. Both eyes will see the center line of letters, the "x o x." It is not affected by the polarizing filters.
   5. Thus, if the patient reports that the center line of letters is single and clear but the two vertical lines (the upper and the lower) are out of alignment, he is manifesting an associated phoria that may be measured with neutralizing prism.

7-3. Another way to construct a device for measuring nearpoint- (or, for that matter, farpoint-) associated phorias is to make a device similar to the one described above, but in this case using black ink for the center line of letters (the stimulus that both eyes see), a red vertical line (above the black letters), and a green vertical line (below the black letters). If the correct red and green colored pencils are used, the patient will be able to see one line with one eye only and the other with the partner eye, when she is wearing standard red/green filters.

7-4. Developmental studies have shown that young children often lack the capacity to project a straight line between two separate points. In other words, they have difficulty deciding when two stimuli are in vertical or horizontal alignment. The implications of this in regard to the Von Graefe method for measuring phorias is obvious. It therefore is wise (a) to use vertical lines of letters when measuring horizontal phorias (thereby reducing the gap between the right eye and left eye stimuli) or (b) to use an alternative method, such as the Maddox rod.

■

REFERENCES

1. Brookman KE. Ocular accommodation in human infants. AJOPO 1983; 60(2):91–99.
2. Banks MS. The development of visual accommodation during early infancy. Child Dev 1980; 51:646–66.
3. Donders FC. On the anomalies of accommodation and refraction of the eye. Translated by Moore WD. London: The New Sydenham Society, 1864.
4. Sheard C. On accommodative exophoria and the accommodation association with the act of convergence. Am J Phys Opt 1920; 1:34.
5. Percival A. The prescribing of spectacles. Bristol: J. Wright, 1928.
6. Neumueller J. Proximal convergence and accommodation. AAAO 1942; 19:16.
7. Health GG. The use of graphic analysis in visual training. AAAO 1959; 36:37.
8. Hofstetter HW. The zone of clear single binocular vision. AAAO 1945; 23:301.
9. Capobianco NM. The subjective measurement of the near point of convergence and its significance in the diagnosis of convergence insufficiency. Am Orth J 1952; 2:40–42.
10. Noorden GK von. Binocular vision and ocular motility. 2nd ed. St. Louis: Mosby, 1980.
11. Morgan MW. Anomalies of binocular vision. In: Hirsch M, Wick R, eds. Vision of children. Philadelphia: Chilton Books, 1963.
12. Noorden GK von, Brown D, Parks M. Associated convergence and accommodative insufficiency. Doc Ophthal 1973; 34:393–403.
13. Grosvenor T. Primary care optometry. New York: Professional Press, 1982.
14. Borish I. Clinical refraction. Chicago: Professional Press, 1970.
15. Parks MM. Ocular motility and strabismus. New York: Harper & Row, 1975.
16. Panum PL. Untersuchunger uber das sehen mit zwei augen, Kiel, 1958. Cited in: Ogle KN. Researches in binocular vision. New York: Hafner, 1964.
17. Ames A Jr, Glidden GH. Ocular measurements. Trans sect Ophthal AMA 1928; 102.
18. Ogle KN, Mussey F, Prangen A deH. Fixation disparity and the fusional processes in binocular single vision. Am J Ophthal 1949; 32:1069–87.
19. Sheedy JE. Actual measurement of fixation disparity and its use in diagnosis and treatment. JAOA 1980; 51(12):1079–84.
20. Brock F, Folsom, WC. A clinical measure of fixation disparities. JAOA 1962; 33(7)497–502.
21. Sheedy JE, Saladin JJ. Phoria, vergence and fixation disparity in oculomotor problems. AJOPO 1975; 54(7):474–81.
22. Herzau M. Fixationsdisparitat bei verschiedenen darbietungsbedingungen. Graefes Arch klin exp Ophthal 1975; 197:193–202.
23. Mallett RJ. Effect of fixation disparity. Ophthal Optician. Letters to the editor 1979; October 27:815–16.
24. Semmlow JL, Hung G. Accommodative and fusional components of fixation disparity. Inv Ophthal 1979; 18(10):1082–86.
25. Ogle KN. Binocular vision. New York: Hafner Pub., 1950.
26. Sheedy JE, Saladin JJ. Association of symptoms with measures of oculomotor deficiencies. AJOPO 1978:55(10):670–76.

27. Vaegan Pye D. Independence of convergence and divergence: norms, age trends and potentiation in mechanized prism vergence tests. AJOPO 1979; 56(3):143–52.
28. Buzzelli AR. Vergence facility: developmental trends in a school age population. AJOPO 1986; 63(5):351–55.
29. Suchoff IB, Petito GT. The efficacy of visual therapy: accommodative disorders and non-strabismic anomalies of binocular vision. JAOA 1986; 57(2):119–25.
30. Grisham JD. Treatment of binocular dysfunctions, in Schor CM, Ciuffreda KJ. Vergence eye movements: basic and clinical aspects. Boston: Butterworths, 1983.
31. Rosner J. A procedure for measuring the nearpoint fusional vergence reserves of young children. JAOA 1979; 50(4):473–74.
32. Hebbard FW. Case analysis. O-Eye-O 1961; 4:111–15.
33. Haynes HM. The distance rock test—a preliminary report. JAOA 1979:50(6):707–13.
34. Carroll JP. Control theory approach to accommodation and vergence. AJOPO 1982; 59(8): 658–69.
35. Semmlow JL, Hung GK. Experimental evidence of separate mechanisms mediating accommodative vergence and vergence accommodation. Doc Ophthal 1981; 51:209–24.
36. McCormack GL. Vergence adaptation maintains heterophoria in normal binocular vision. AJOPO 1985; 62(8):555–61.
37. Schor CM. Adaptive regulation of accommodation vergence and vergence accommodation. AJOPO 1986; 63(8):587–609.
38. Schor CM, Narayan V. Graphical analysis of prism adaptation, convergence accommodation, and accommodative convergence. AJOPO 1982; 59(10):774–84.
39. Schor CM, Robertson KM, Wesson M. Disparity vergence dynamics and fixation disparity. AJOPO 1986; 63(8):611–18.
40. Schor CM. Models of mutual interactions between accommodation and convergence. AJOPO 1985; 62(6):369–74.
41. Tsuetaki TK, Schor CM. Clinical method for measuring adaptation of tonic accommodation and vergence accommodation. AJOPO 1987; 64(6):437–49.
42. North R, Hensen DB. Adaptation to lens-induced heterophorias. AJOPO 1985; 62(11):774–80.
43. Sethi B, Henson DB. Vergence-adaptive change with a prism-induced noncomitant disparity. AJOPO 1985; 62(3):203–206.
44. Birnbaum MH. An esophoric shift associated with sustained fixation. AJOPO 1985; 62(11):732–35.
45. Duke-Elder S. Systems of ophthalmology. Vol. V. St. Louis: Mosby, 1970.
46. Duane A. A new classification of the anomalies of the eye, based upon physiological principles. Ann Ophthal Otolaryngol 1896; 6:84.
47. Schapero M. The characteristics of ten basic visual training problems. AAAO 1955; 32(7):333–42.
48. Cooper J, Duckman R. Convergence insufficiency: incidence, diagnosis and treatment. JAOA 1978; 49(6):673–80.

8

Question 8
Is the Patient's
Developmental Status
Appropriate for
His or Her Age?

□

The inclusion of this question represents another milestone for the optometric profession. The present-day optometrist has evolved from the traveling spectacle salesman of the last century into a highly trained primary-care practitioner who, in addition to the extended scope of her prescribed professional role, assumes the obligation of administering screening tests for a variety of general health problems that her patients might display.

Today's optometrist, for example, uses a sphygmomanometer fairly routinely. Her purpose: to screen for elevated blood pressure, a critical clinical sign of hypertension. This does not imply that she will diagnose hypertension, only that she will advise those patients who display a higher-than-normal blood pressure to contact their physicians.

Why blood pressure? Three reasons: first, hypertension is an insidious, devastating disease. Its long-term effects are very damaging. Second hypertension is usually a manageable disease if treated properly. Early detection, therefore, is very desirable. Third, screening for elevated blood pressure is inexpensive in terms of time, space, equipment, and personnel. These three facts, in combination, designate blood pressure as a concern of the primary-care practitioner.

A central assumption of this chapter is that screening young patients for developmental deviations represents a similar set of circumstances: The long-term effects of a developmental deviation can be devastating; early detection can lead to early intervention, which often has ameliorating effects; screening for a developmental deviation is inexpensive in terms of time, space, equipment, and personnel (1).

The flow diagram shown in Figure 8.1 depicts two screening protocols: one for children age 4 years and below, the other for children age 5 years and above (see A in Figure 8.1 flow diagram and below).

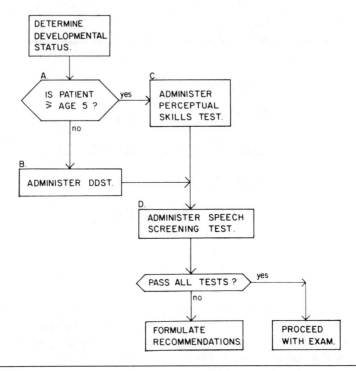

Figure 8.1   Question #8: Is the patient's developmental status appropriate for his age?

A. IS THE PATIENT YOUNGER THAN AGE FIVE?

The question appears to be completely unambiguous. A glance at the child's birthdate should be all that is needed to procure the answer. It is not always so, however. In those cases where a developmental deviation is suspected, it probably is best to commence testing the child as though he were younger than his birthdate indicates. A simple rule of thumb: when in doubt, screen first with a less demanding instrument. If this is too easy for the child, it will soon become apparent and a more appropriate test can then be administered with no harm done.

☐ If No

Assess his general development on the basis of case history and informal observations. Implement screening tests for visual perceptual skills and auditory perceptual skills (see C in Figure 8.1 flow diagram and below).

□ If Yes

Administer the Denver Developmental Screening Test (see B in Figure 8.1 flow diagram and below).

___■_____

B. THE DENVER DEVELOPMENTAL SCREENING TEST (DDST)

The original version of the DDST (available from Denver Developmental Materials, Inc., P.O. Box 6919, Denver, Colorado 80206) was published in 1967 (2). It was designed to be administered by nonprofessional personnel after minimal training, thereby serving as an economical method for detecting atypical development in young children.

In 1971, the scoring criteria were revised in order to make the test both more valid and more reliable (3). This was accomplished.

The DDST appears to be an excellent instrument for the primary-care practitioner who serves young children. (For alternative tests, see below.)

The test is made up of four sections, called sectors. These are the *Personal-social, Fine motor-Adaptive, Language,* and *Gross Motor.*

Each sector comprises a number of items that describe various easily observed changes in a child's behavior that normally occur during the first 6 years of life. In general terms, the items of each sector show that, as the child matures, he acquires the ability to perform more elaborate behaviors under less structured and supportive conditions. For example:

Personal-social. As he matures, the child tends to be less anxious and dependent, socially and physically, and more adept at serving his own needs.

Fine-motor adaptive. As he matures, the child tends to be able to sustain at tasks of increased complexity and engage in those tasks in effective, meaningful, reasoning ways.

Language. As he matures, the child tends to be able to produce and respond appropriately to verbal (and nonverbal) language of increasing complexity.

Gross motor. As he matures, the child tends to be able to engage in motor activities that require increasingly complex body coordinations.

Figure 8.2 shows the DDST record form.

A key feature of the DDST is its format. Notice the age scale located at both the upper and lower margins of the test form. Notice also that each test item is contained within a rectangle that spans a period of time, rather than being located at a single point along the age continuum. The position of the rectangle on the

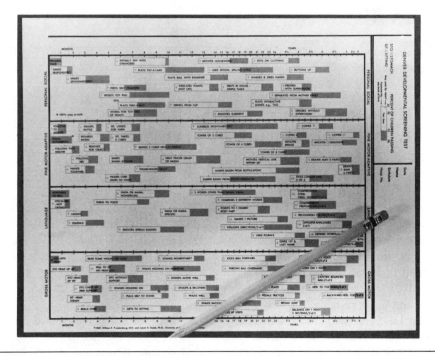

Figure 8.2 DDST recording form.

record form, along with two of its features, portrays the span of time that separates the age when only a small percentage of children are able to perform a behavior to the age when most children have mastered that behavior.

The test item shown in Figure 8.3 will serve as an example:

The left edge of the rectangle indicates the age at which 25 percent of normal children are able to pass the item; i.e., walk up steps in a way that satisfies the criteria of the DDST. The age scale places this at 14 months.

The short vertical line extending upward from the rectangle signifies the age at which 50 percent of the children are characteristically able to perform the task represented by the item; in this instance, age 17 months.

The line that separates the shaded portion of the rectangle from the white serves as the 75-percent marker; age 21 months in regard to walking up steps.

And finally, the right edge of the rectangle indicates the age at which 90 percent of a normal group of children are expected to show mastery of the item. For walking up steps, this is age 22 months.

The advantages of such a display format in comparison to the typical list of milestone ages is obvious. Clearly, it is much more useful to know that most children acquire the ability to walk up steps between the ages of 14 months and 22 months than to be informed the age at which the "average" child is able to perform the behavior, with no mention made regarding the normal variance around that average.

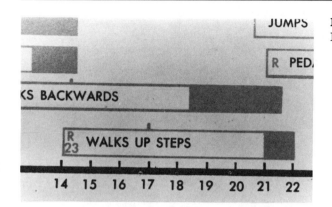

Figure 8.3
DDST test item.

Two other item characteristics should be noted. One, some items contain an "R" (see Figure 8.3). This signifies that the examiner need not personally observe the child perform that behavior; a parent report of this ability will satisfy the test. Second, some items contain a numeral (again, see Figure 8.3). This refers to additional data relevant to the item that will be found on the reverse side of the test sheet. Figure 8.4 shows that side.

This is all the explanation needed to commence using the DDST.

☐ To Administer the DDST

The steps listed here are basic guidelines. The reader is urged to purchase the test manual for complete information.

1. Calculate the child's age and locate this on both (upper and lower) age scales. Then connect these two points with a vertical line, called the "age line."

2. Test all items that are intersected by the age line.

3. Record directly on the test items themselves: P for pass, F for fail, R for those items the child "refuses" to do, and N.O. for the few items that the child cannot do simply because she has never had an opportunity to try (e.g., "pedals a bicycle").

4. Continue testing until all items intersected by the age line have been administered and/or until three P's and three F's have been recorded in each sector.

5. If an item that is situated completely to the left of the age line is failed, it is classified as a "delay"; i.e., an inability to perform a behavior that 90 percent of the children her age are able to do. Failing an item that is not so situated on the age line is simply a "fail," not a delay.

6. Test outcomes are judged to be either *abnormal, questionable, or normal*. (The test authors suggest that children who score abnormal or questionable on one occasion should be rechecked about 2 or 3 weeks later in order to confirm the outcomes of the first screening. Clearly, that will vary with the case. In many instances, a single assessment is obviously sufficient.)

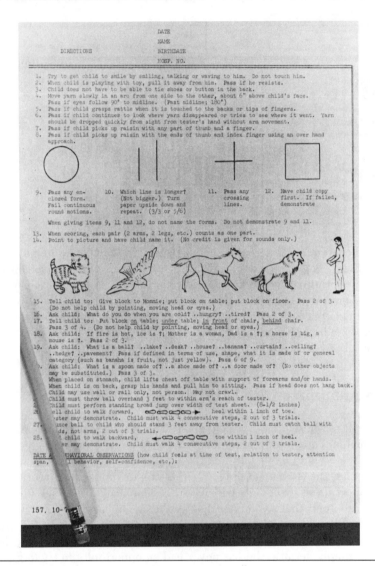

Figure 8.4   Reverse side of DDST record form.

Abnormal
1. If two or more sectors have two or more delays; or
2. If one sector has two or more delays and one other sector has one delay and, in the same sector, all items intersected by the age line are failed.

Questionable
1. If any one sector has two or more delays; or
2. If one or more sectors has one delay and, in the same sector, all items intersected by the age line are failed.

Normal
1. If the performance is neither abnormal nor questionable.

□ The Abbreviated DDST

In 1981, the guidelines for administering that DDST were revised in order to shorten testing time. On the basis of extensive re-analysis of the original normative data, it was determined that 100% of the children who failed the full DDST could have been identified by their performance on as few as twelve selected items (4). These twelve items comprised the three items in each of the four sectors that are immediately to the left of—but not touching—the child's age line. Hence, the new guidelines suggest that if any of these items is failed (constituting a delay) or refused (constituting a potential delay), a full DDST should be completed. If, on the other hand, all twelve of those items are passed, there is no need for further testing. In effect, then, the Abbreviated DDST serves as a prescreening test for identifying those children who should, or should not, be given the full test battery.

□ Advising the Parent

The DDST is a screening test. It is not foolproof. It will produce both false-positives and false-negatives. Hence, test outcomes should be interpreted for the parents in a considered fashion.

Nonetheless, children who do not perform normally on the DDST should be viewed as "at risk," until shown otherwise. There is no justification for a pat on the back and the false reassurance that "she'll grow out of it." On the contrary, actions should be taken. What kind of actions and by whom depend upon where the main area(s) of deficit appeared. This topic will be discussed in Chapter 15.

All that remains now is a short screening for speech disorders (see D in Figure 8.1 flow diagram and below). Then, unless there are some "loose ends," some observations that have yet to be adequately explained, the next step is to report all this information to the parents in conjunction with appropriate recommendations (see Chapter 15).

OTHER TESTS APPROPRIATE FOR SCREENING CHILDREN WHO ARE YOUNGER THAN AGE FIVE YEARS

Many other tests have been designed to identify young children who are not developing at an expected rate. Most of these are very similar to each other; most resemble the DDST in respect to the kinds of behaviors they examine, although they may differ in the format of that assessment (i.e., how they are administered, the age range they were designed for, and the interpretation given to test outcomes). Among those that the optometrist should have some familiarity with are the following:

☐ Bayley Scales of Infant Development*

This test is for infants from birth to 30 months of age. It consists of a *Mental Scale* and a *Motor Scale*. The former attempts to measure sensory-perceptual acuities and discriminations; early acquisition of object constancy and memory, learning, and problem-solving ability; vocalizations and the beginning of verbal communication; and early evidence of the ability to form generalizations and classifications. The Motor Scale looks at the child's capacity to control his own body, coordinate large muscles, and the fine manipulatory skills of the hands and fingers. The full test requires about 45 minutes and is designed to yield an Intelligence Quotient (IQ) score that has been shown to be reasonably well correlated with Stanford-Binet IQs of children ages 24 through 30 months.

☐ Goodenough Harris Drawing Test**

This test consists of evaluating the child's response to a request that he draw a man, a woman, and himself (5,6). Drawings are scored on the basis of the presence or absence of certain anatomical features; e.g., fingers, nostrils, eyebrows. The score is then compared with norms that have been developed for children as young as age three. In general terms, this test provides an overview of the child's attentiveness to details rather than his ability to draw the human form.

☐ Vallett Developmental Survey†

This test is designed for use with children between the ages of two and seven. It consists of 233 tasks in the areas of motor integration and physical development, tactile discrimination, auditory discrimination, visual-motor coordination, visual discrimination, language development, verbal fluency, and conceptual development. Age norms are provided for each of the tasks.

*N. Bayley, 1969; available from The Psychological Corp, Atlanta, GA.
**F. Goodenough, D. Harris, Atlanta: The Psychological Corp., 1963.
†R. Vallett, Palo Alto: Consulting Psychologists Press, 1966.

□ Assessment of Reflexes and Other Behaviors

This does not refer to a formal test, rather it acknowledges that the most valid predictor of a newborn's early development is her health status at birth, and the best predictor of the child's subsequent acquisition of basic learning aptitudes is the extent to which she displays normal early development. The APGAR test (see Chapter 2) is an example of a predictor that is based on the child's status at birth. Among the behaviors assessed by the APGAR test is the normalcy of the baby's reflexes. The normal, healthy neonate is expected to display a number of reflexes at birth (i.e., innate, automatic responses to specific stimulation), most of which are then expected to disappear as volitional behaviors develop, usually during the first year of life (7,8). As such, both the presence of a reflex and the age of its expected disappearance are important observable indices. If an expected reflex does not manifest, or if a reflex persists significantly beyond the age at which it ordinarily disappears, it should be noted. Similarly, if a volitional behavior is not developed at more or less the expected age, it too should be noted. Either circumstance is likely to signal something gone wrong.

It therefore behooves the optometrist to be familiar with this information. A representative listing of reflexes is shown in Table 8.1, organized in accord with the age when they are expected to disappear. A listing of developed, volitional behaviors follows in Table 8.2.

■

C. SCREENING FOR PERCEPTUAL SKILLS DYSFUNCTION

Optometrists are not yet agreed as to whether or not the diagnosis and treatment of perceptual skills disorders fall within their professional scope. But that is irrelevant to this discussion.

In this context, screening elementary school children (up to about the age of 12) for perceptual skills dysfunction is a primary-care obligation, for reasons already defined: perceptual skills dysfunction has been linked directly with unsatisfactory school performance; hence, it is not a trivial concern. Perceptual skills dysfunction can often be remedied; hence, early detection is desirable. Perceptual skills screening procedures are economically administered; hence, they should be done routinely rather than only in those cases where there is reason to suspect a problem (1).

Therefore, it does not matter how the optometrist perceives her role in the diagnosis and treatment of perceptual skills dysfunction (this will be addressed more thoroughly in Chapter 15). So long as she considers herself to be a primary-

Expected to disappear by age 4 months

Rooting reflex

Stimulus: Touch corner of infant's mouth with finger and draw the finger toward the infant's cheek. Insert finger into infant's mouth.

Response: Infant turns head toward the stimulated side and begins sucking motions. Infant sucks strongly on examiner's finger.

Significance: Absence indicates a general suppression of central nervous system.

Stepping reflex

Stimulus: Support baby in upright position; then move him forward and tilt him slightly to one side.

Response: Baby performs rhythmic stepping movements.

Significance: Absence indicates a general depressed infant.

Palmar reflex

Stimulus: Apply pressure on both of baby's palms while he is lying on his back.

Response: Eyes close, mouth opens, and head moves to midline.

Significance: Absence indicates a general depression of central nervous system.

Palmar (automatic hand) grasp

Stimulus: Examiner presses finger against infant's palm.

Response: Infant grasps examiner's finger.

Significance: Absence indicates a general depression.

Expected to disappear by age 6 months

Moro reflex

Stimulus: Sudden loud noise, head drop, or full body drop.

Response: Baby throws extends arms outwards, then brings them back, in a startled (convulsive) manner; fingers fan out, then fist is clenched lightly; spine and lower extremities are extended.

Significance: Absence or weakness indicates serious disturbance of central nervous system.

Expected to disappear by age 12 months

Plantar or toe grasp

Stimulus: Apply pressure with finger against balls of infant's feet.

Response: Plantar flexion of all toes.

Significance: Absences indicates defect of lower spinal cord.

Expected to persist throughout life

Blink reflex

Stimulus: Flash of light.

Response: Bilateral blink.

Significance: Absence indicates severe vision deficit.

Table 8.1   Neonatal Reflexes

care practitioner, the optometrist has an obligation to screen for perceptual skills dysfunction.

Two screening tests will be described in detail, along with an overview of what the two tests test. Then, alternative screening tests that accomplish the same goals will be listed. Finally, some discussion regarding how perceptual skills link with

Expected to appear by age
One month
　　Held upright, child's feet on hard surface, will not support her weight
　　Child regards mother's face, establishes eye-to-eye contact; is alert to surroundings
　　Child may move her eyes and head toward a sound source
　　Stops crying and turns toward sound of soothing voice
　　Child begins to coo responsively to mother's voice
　　When pulled into sitting posture, head lags until child is in vertical position; it is
　　　　then held erect for a moment or two; back is rounded
Three months
　　When held suspended from waist, face down, child elevates head above body
　　　　plane; arms and shoulders extended
　　When lying face down on bed, child flexes knees under body, elevates buttocks,
　　　　flexes arms, turns head to one side
　　When lying supine, child positions head in midline, hands open, together near
　　　　face. Kicks vigorously, alternating legs
　　When pulled into sitting position, there is little or no head lag for a few seconds;
　　　　then head falls forward
　　Sustained hand regard; holds rattle for a few minutes; engages in finger play
　　Recognizes mother on sight; follows an object, held 6 to 12 inches from face, with
　　　　eyes and head in 180-degree arc; watches hands and feet and recognizes bottle
　　Startle reaction at loud noises; quiets to mother's voice and shows excitement at
　　　　sound of running bath water
　　Vocalizes; coos when spoken to
　　Laughs aloud; enjoys being held
Four months
　　When held in sitting position, baby's head is erect and back is straight; head
　　　　wobbles when swayed
　　Turns head to side at which sound is heard; eyes look in same direction if sound is
　　　　at ear level
　　Babbles
　　Shows preference for mother; is sociable; vocalizes to initiate social interactions
Six months
　　When lying prone on bed, holds head high, supported by extended arms and flat
　　　　palms. Rolls over to back
　　When lying supine on bed, raises head to look at feet, then grasps foot; holds arms
　　　　out to be picked up
　　Pulls self up to sitting position when hands are grasped
　　Sits alone on floor, supported by hands forward
　　Bounces up and down when held in standing position
　　Transfers toy from one hand to the other; takes most things to mouth
　　Moves eyes in unison; no evidence of misalignment. Reaches for objects accurately;
　　　　inspects objects at length; distinguishes strangers; adjusts position to see objects
　　Turns head in search of sound; responds to mother's voice and own name
　　Vocalizes to certain sounds; e.g., "muh," "goo;" raises arms when mother says
　　　　"come;" looks toward family member when named

Table 8.2　Developed Behaviors (Continues on next page)

Cries easily; makes loud noises; plays contentedly with own hands and small toys; turns to own name

Twelve months

Crawls upstairs

Stands alone

Drinks from cup with assistance

Piles two or three blocks

Can throw objects forward

Drops toys and watches them fall

Watches small toy pulled across floor from a distance of 10 feet

Recognizes familiar persons from 20 feet or more

Sees and picks up very small objects, e.g., crumbs, threads

Knows and turns to own name

Understands up to 10 words (no, bye-bye, pat-a-cake, hot, [own name], give it to me, sit down). Jabbers expressively, i.e., produces vocal inflections, voices most vowels and many consonants

Protests loudly when separated from mother; demonstrates affection to familiar persons/objects; gives toys to adult on request; plays pat-a-cake and waves bye-bye on request

---

Table 8.2   (Continued)

classroom performance. Recommended treatment(s) will be discussed in Chapter 15.

□ The Test of Visual Analysis Skills (TVAS)*

This test is applicable with children as young as age four, although there is no practical reason to use it in addition to the DDST with prekindergarten children (9). There are sufficient items in the DDST that assess visual perceptual skills development. These will be identified later in this section. For the present, accept as a useful rule of thumb: use the TVAS with children age 5 years and above.

The test consists of 18 items, each involving a copying task. The items are shown, in reduced size, in Figure 8.5.

TO ADMINISTER

With children in the first grade and below, use Response Form A (see Figure 8.6). This 8 1/2 × 11-inch sheet of paper contains spaces for the first twelve items of the test. Typically, children of that age/grade will not proceed beyond item 12 (10).

---

*For a thorough description of the TVAS, see (9, pp 30/43). The 18 TVAS test items, each mounted on a laminated card, may be purchased from the Optometric Students Association, College of Optometry, University of Houston, Houston, TX 77004. A sample of Response Forms A (Figure 8.6) and B (Figure 8.7) be sent along with the test items.

T.V.A.S.

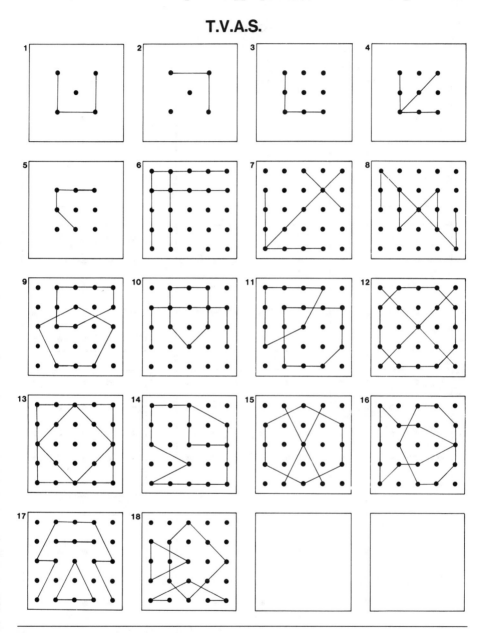

Figure 8.5 TVAS items.

With children in second grade and beyond, use Response Form B (see Figure 8.7). It contains spaces for the last twelve items of the test (items 7 through 18); this on the assumption that children beyond first grade rarely have difficulty with the first six items.

FORM A

NAME _____ DATE _____

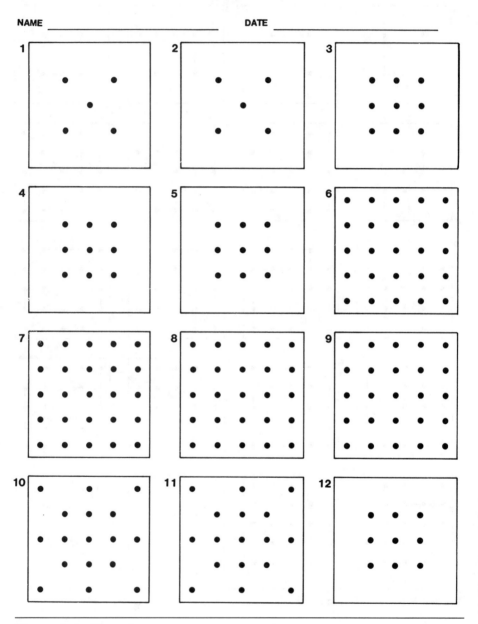

Figure 8.6 Form A.

FORM B

NAME _____   DATE _____

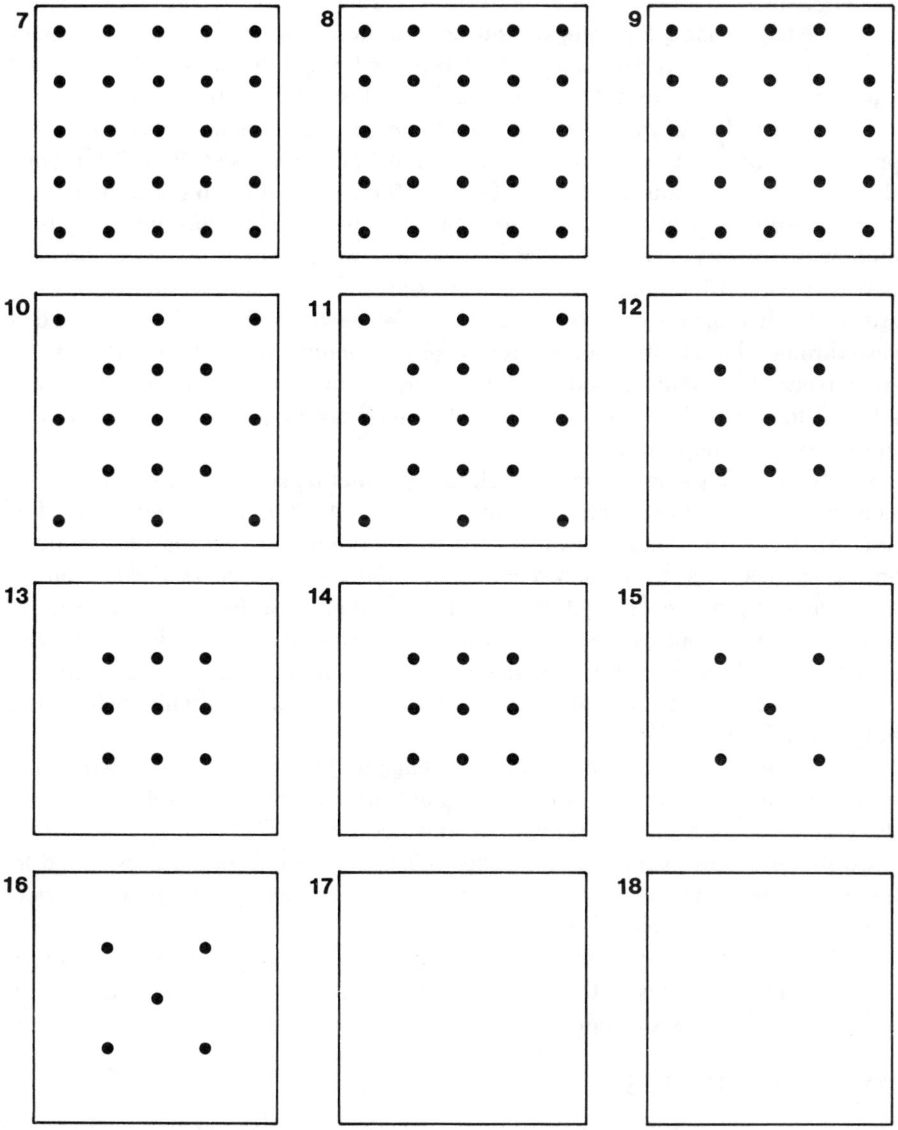

Figure 8.7   Form B.

Obviously, if these expectations are not upheld in a given instance, simply alter the guideline. In other words, if a first-grade successfully copies the first twelve items of the TVAS, and if testing is to continue (not essential as a screening process), then give her Form B, locate the response space for item 13 (halfway down the page), and administer the subsequent items. Similarly, if a second-grade child cannot accurately copy item 7, then remove Form B (without overt or implied criticism), give him Form A, and recommence testing with item 1.

Seat the child at an appropriately sized table, give him a pencil (with an eraser), present the first item he is to copy (item 1 if Form A is used; item 7 for Form B), and say, "Copy this here." (Point first to the model, then to the proper space on the response form.) "Make yours look like mine." (There are no restrictions on how the directions are stated as long as the examiner does not show the child how to accomplish the task; i.e., where to start, what to do next, etc. Also, there are no restrictions on erasures or on time. However, if the child is inclined to rush through the activity, thereby performing inadequately, ask him to slow down; conversely, if the child spends an inordinate amount of time on each item in an attempt to be precise, reassure him that it need not be perfect and urge him to move along a little faster.)

Continue in this manner until the child has either (a) failed two items in succession, or (b) successfully completed item 9. (Note: An item is "passed"if the child draws the correct number of lines and locates them, with reasonable accuracy, on the correct dots. An *incorrect number of lines*, or an *incorrect placement on the map*—i.e., on the *wrong* dots—constitutes an error, a "failed" item. Neatness is *not* a factor, so long as the child shows the abilities just described; i.e., drawing a line that fails to pass through the dot it was intended to traverse does not constitute an error if the examiner is convinced that the child knew what to do but simply failed to do it.)

When (and if) the child gets to item 10, change the instructions to: "Now some of the dots are missing from your map; don't draw in the dots; pretend they are there and draw the lines *as though* the dots were there."

Continue in this manner until (a) the child goes beyond the level expected for her grade, (b) all 18 items have been accurately completed, or (c) two successive items are failed—whichever occurs first.

Performance in items 10 through 18 continues to be judged on the basis of the correct number of lines in the correct locations; i.e., the examiner must be able to "pretend the dots are there."

TO SCORE THE TVAS

The score on the TVAS is *the number of the last item passed*. For example, if items 1, 2, and 3 were passed, 4 failed, 5 passed, 6 and 7 failed, then his score is 5.

EXPECTEDS

Table 8.3 shows the TVAS scores expected of children from prekindergarten and above. Notice that the ceiling is expected by the end of the third grade.

TVAS Score	Expected for Children in:
1	Preschool
2	Preschool
3	Kindergarten
4	Kindergarten
5	Kindergarten
6	Kindergarten
7	Kindergarten
8	Grade 1
9	Grade 1
10	Grade 1
11	Grade 2
12	Grade 2
13	Grade 2
14	Grade 2
15	Grade 2
16	Grade 2
17	Grade 3
18	Grade 3

From: Rosner J. Helping children overcome learning difficulties. New York: Walker Publishing Co., Inc. 1979, p. 42.

Table 8.3   TVAS Expecteds

If the child fails to score at the expected level, interpret it as indicative of a visual perceptual skills disorder.

WHAT THE TVAS TESTS

First, some definitions. The terms perception and perceptual skills are often used interchangeably. That is incorrect, and the ambiguity it generates is counter-productive to effective communication.

Perception
"The act of becoming aware through the senses; physical sensation interpreted in the light of experience" (Webster's New Collegiate Dictionary, 1974). The salient point here is that perception is a subjective, dynamic, interpretive act that reflects the perceiver's personal values and prejudices in interaction with existing environmental conditions. As such, perception is an exceptionally complex, highly individualized behavior.

Two examples: the *Rorschach test* is an assessment of personality as inferred from perception; i.e., from what the individual perceives when shown a series of "inkblots." The patient is asked to report what he "sees," meaning what comes to his mind, when he looks at the inkblots, *at that time, under those conditions*. This is then compared with what the prototype "normal" individual reports (11).

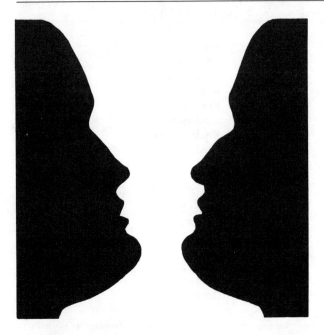

Figure 8.8
Ambiguous visual
illusion.

A second example: *optical illusions,* such as the one shown in Figure 8.8 also illustrate the act of perception. Obviously, there is far less of an emotional aspect to reporting what one perceives here. The test conditions are more concrete and unambiguous. One "sees" either a vase or the silhouette of two facial profiles, depending upon where in the drawing he fixates and how he identifies this. In other words, if a "nose" is perceived, then a face will be seen—at least until the percept is altered by some distracting element in the drawing or in the environment.

Both of the above examples highlight the same concept: perception is an individualized interpretive behavior that is strongly influenced by the physical and psychological states of the perceiver and the environment in which he is placed. It is not easily tested. Deviations in perception are usually difficult to define, let alone test. It is not what the optometrist assesses when he screens for perceptual skills dysfunction.

Perceptual Skills
"The ability to identify the task-pertinent concrete features of a sensory array" (9). It follows, therefore, that *visual perceptual skills* are employed in identifying the task-pertinent concrete features of a *visual* array. The phrase *task-pertinent concrete features* refers to those features (attributes) of an array that are (a) readily defined in absolute, unambiguous, concrete terms (e.g., the quantity, length, orientation of the lines that make up a geometric design) and (b) relevant to the accomplishment of a particular task. This suggests that one's perceptual skills may be inferred on the basis of how satisfactorily he accomplishes tasks that can be

performed satisfactorily only if certain concrete attributes of a given visual array are identified. That, in turn, suggests that defining "normal" perceptual skills is not exceptionally complex. And, in fact, that is the case.

An example: the TVAS was suggested as a screening test for visual perceptual skills.* It provides a series of copying tasks. In each of the first nine items, the correct response depends upon the child's ability to identify (a) all of the lines that make up the design and (b) the dots connected by those lines. In the final nine items, where the dots are gradually eliminated, a correct response depends still on the same two abilities plus (c) the ability to map out a spatial area (i.e., the space within the square) on the basis of fewer reference points (dots).

The pertinent concrete features of the visual array in these tasks are the lines, the dots, and the spatial interrelationships between these and the square that contains them. Such other features as the width and color of the lines are ignored by the child, and properly so. They are not pertinent to this task; they are concrete, but they are not task-pertinent.

A second example: the comment was made earlier that the DDST contained sufficient items to screen the visual perceptual skills of prekindergarten children. These are found in the fine-motor adaptive sector. Many test items in that sector assess the child's ability to copy a cube construction or a geometric design. True, these require fine-motor actions, but they also require visual analysis skills. The child must be able to identify the task-pertinent concrete features of the construc- tions she is to reproduce, something not guaranteed by fine motor abilities. What are the concrete features of the block tower that are pertinent to the task of reproducing it? The number of blocks and the spatial relationships among them. What are the features of the plus sign and the square, both items in the DDST, that are pertinent to the task of copying them? The finite number of lines that make up each design and the spatial interrelationships of those lines.

A common theme emerges from these examples. Tests of visual analysis skills are designed to examine a child's ability to analyze a spatially organized array into its separate structural components and map out the interrelationships among these components (12).

The TVAS and the DDST also illustrate another important characteristic of visual perceptual skills: they develop. They are species-specific. They evolve through the process of natural growth. So long as the child is fortunate enough to have a properly operating neuromotor system and is provided with a reasonably supportive environment, formal lessons are not required. Visual perceptual skills will be acquired, and, in fact, the rate of their acquisition is predictable. Also predictable is the age at which the development curve flattens: somewhere be- tween 10 and 12 (13). (This does not imply that one's visual analysis skills cannot go beyond what is shown by the typical 10- to-12-year-old. However, it does acknowledge that skills beyond that basic level are not derived from nature alone.

*The terms visual perceptual skills, visual analysis skills, and spatial analysis skills are used inter- changeably in this volume. The first, because it is well established; the latter two, because they are more precise (9).

They are the outcome of specific experiences over and above what nature tends to guarantee.)

The sequence defined in the DDST is revealing. According to the DDST, 50 percent of children in the 42-month age group are able to copy a plus sign. (Or, as defined in the DDST, "produce a pair of crossing lines," when asked to copy a plus sign.) More than 90 percent of this same age group can copy a circle, yet far fewer than 25 percent of them can copy a square. The average child is 54 months old before she can do that.

This progression was observed and documented long before the publication of the DDST. Indeed, Binet and Simon (14) recognized it when they set about designing the standardized IQ test during the first decade of this century. Since then, many investigators of child development have confirmed the phenomenon: as a child grows, she acquires the capacity to reproduce spatial arrays of increasing complexity, thereby demonstrating that she has become more competent at identifying a greater variety of task-pertinent concrete features, even when they are embedded in complex and distracting contexts.

The development phenomenon is also revealed by the changes that occur over time in a child's unsatisfactory performance. Take, for example, the characteristic differences in how the 4-, 5-, and 6-year-old respond to the task of copying a design that is appropriate only for the 6-year-old. The asterisk (see Figure 8.9) is such a design; it is often used in tests of visual perceptual skills. Normative data indicate that, on average, this design is not copied accurately by children younger than age 6. But, what is of interest here is that there are age-related differences in the unsatisfactory performance.

The 4-year-old is apt to produce something like what is shown in A, indicating no concern with either finite quantities or refined spatial relationships. The 4 1/2- to 5-year-old is likely to produce B, showing that a sense of specificity is developing, but has not yet reached a satisfactory level—satisfactory, that is, in terms of *this task*, this specific design, an array that contains *these* task-pertinent features. The child who produces C is usually between 5 and 5 1/2. She has developed further than A and B, obviously. She has reached the level where she can identify the *correct number* of lines that make up the design, but she is not so capable, yet, in mapping out all the spatial relationships.

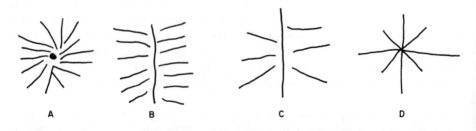

Figure 8.9   Four responses to copying an asterisk.

What do A, B, and C lack that D does not lack? The visual analysis skills necessary to accomplish the copying task in a satisfactory manner; restated in behavioral terms, they lack, in varying degrees, the ability to identify those features of the asterisk that are relevant in the task of copying it, and to ignore those features that do not count.

Observing age-related changes in how children copy the asterisk is interesting for yet another reason. We have noted that children much younger than age 6 are able to copy a plus sign (+). The same is true of the x. But, even though the average 5-year-old can copy both the + and the x, she cannot copy the asterisk, which is made up of an x and a +. Why? Same features; just too many of them in a single array. The context is too complex.

□ Alternative Visual Perceptual Skills Screening Tests

A number of visual perceptual skills screening tests have been published. They are all similar in that they attempt to assess the child's ability to analyze spatially organized patterns and then compare this with what is "normal" for her age. They all differ in one way or another; in the patterns they present, the format in which these are presented, and so on. These unique differences will produce unique outcomes. That is, a child will not necessarily perform at precisely the same level in one test as she does in another. But, that does not justify the use of more than one screening test. The small amount of extra information derived from a second test is hardly sufficient reason for using it, just as using two different visual acuity tests is not warranted simply because a patient may read a few more letters with one than the other (15).

The list of tests covered in this section is not exhaustive. The ones included here were selected because they are among the most popular. They are most likely to be cited in reports that accompany the patient to the optometrist's office. The descriptions that are provided here are insufficient for applications. The reader who wishes to administer any of these tests is advised to procure the test manuals from the respective publishers.

BENDER VISUAL-MOTOR GESTALT TEST*

The Bender (16) is the school psychologist's test of choice for evaluating a child's ability to analyze spatially organized sensory arrays. (They also apply it in other ways, but remarks here will be limited to its use as a test of visual perceptual skills.) It is a copying test, made up of nine designs that are applicable with children ranging from age 5 to 11 years. The patterns are shown in Figure 8.10.

*Lauretta Bender, A Visual Motor Gestalt Test and Its Clinical Use (New York: American Orthopsychiatric Assn., 1938).

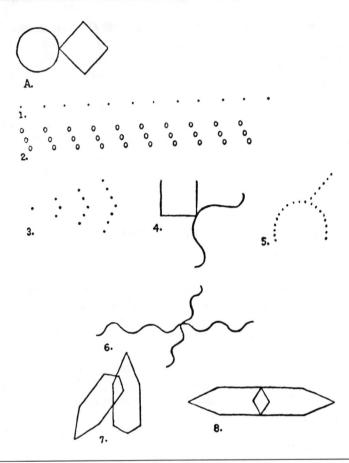

Figure 8.10   Patterns from the Bender Visual-motor Gestaldt Test (from Bender L. A visual-motor gestaldt test and its clinical use. New York: Am Orthopsych Assn, 1938).

A look at these reveals one of the test's advantages: The designs that are to be copied are not usually encountered elsewhere. As such, it is not likely that the child taking the test will have had previous instruction in how to reproduce these designs.

Although the original version of the test did not have a standardized method for scoring, two systems have since been developed: one by Watkins (17), the other by Koppitz (18). Both yield age-equivalent scores; that is, performance is reported as representative of a particular age level. Thus, the 7-year-old with normal skills will be reported as functioning on a 7-year-old level.

DEVELOPMENTAL TEST OF VISUAL PERCEPTION*

This test is usually identified as the "Frostig" (19). It may be group administered (i.e., classroom). It comprises five subtest areas and yields a "Perceptual Quotient" (PQ), an index (similar to IQ) that is derived by converting the child's raw score on the various tests into a scale score that takes his age into account. A PQ of 100 represents normal performance for his age; a PQ above 100 represents above-average performance for his age, and so on.

The main advantage of the Frostig is the aforementioned fact that it was standardized for group administration. The major disadvantage: it is a long test and, in fact, has been found to overtest in that each subtest category appears to be measuring the same fundamental ability (20). This latter fact probably explains why the test seems to have lost favor in recent years.

DEVELOPMENTAL TEST OF VISUAL-MOTOR INTEGRATION**

This test, usually identified as the VMI, is also very popular in schools. It is a copying test made up of 24 designs that range in difficulty from the 2-year-old level to the 15-year-old level. Scores are typically reported as age equivalents (21). The fact that this test is normed to age 15 seems to argue with the previously made statement that visual perceptual skills usually achieve full natural development by ages 10 to 12, and that any improvement in skills beyond that is attributable to experience and learning rather than normal development. The two statements do not conflict. In our opinion, the last few items of the VMI—those designed as appropriate for children older than age 12—do, indeed, test something beyond naturally developed visual perceptual skills. Precisely what that "something else" is has not yet been clearly established, but we believe that it is more closely related to personality factors—e.g., tenacity, compulsiveness—than to basic visual analysis skills.

GESELL COPY FORM TEST†

This test originated in the Gesell laboratory (22). Its purpose was to document one way in which children change as they grow and develop. It is made up of seven geometric designs of increasing complexity, representative of the copying abilities of children in the 4- to 7-year-old range: circle, plus sign, square, triangle, divided rectangle, vertical and horizontal diamonds. Gesell did not produce a formal, standardized scoring method. Like Bender, he left interpretation to the clinician. A scoring method was subsequently developed (23).

The Gesell Copy Form test has been very popular with optometrists for two reasons. First, it was available at the time optometrists began to take a clinical interest in visual perceptual skills. Second, Gesell's interest in vision had great

*Consulting Psychologists Press, Palo Alto, Calif.
**Follet Publishing Co., Chicago, Ill.
†New York, Harper & Row.

impact on the profession. (Some of this history is described in Chapter 15.) Its major drawback: the items are not difficult enough; the test may not produce useful information with children older than 7 years.

SLOSSON DRAWING COORDINATION TEST (SDCT)*

The SDCT is a copying test made up of designs that range from (purportedly) a 1-year-old level of difficulty to a 12-year-old level (24). Scores are usually reported as "percentage correct" and are related to age expecteds. A unique and clinically useful aspect of this test is that the child is required to copy each test design three times. Hence, a distinction may be revealed between the child who learns from her errors and the child whose performance does not change across trials. Obviously, the former type of performance offers a better prognosis than the latter. A disadvantage of the test: It provides only one test item for each year of development, thereby setting the stage for unreliable test outcomes.

RUTGERS DRAWING TEST (RDT)**

There are two forms of the RDT, A and B, each printed on an 8 1/2 × 14-inch sheet of paper. Form A (Figure 8.11) was designed for testing children between the ages of 4 and 7 years; Form B (Figure 8.12), for children between the ages of 6 and 10 years.

Form A consists of two "demonstration" items (the first, a vertical line; the second, a horizontal line) and 14 test items; Form B contains 16 test items—there are no demonstrators. The child's task: copy all of the designs in the spaces immediately below the printed items. Each of the child's copies is then scored on a three-point scale (0 to 2), and the total score is compared with norms, thereby yielding an "equivalent drawing age" for the child.

MOTOR-FREE VISUAL PERCEPTION TEST (MVPT)†

This test is unique because it is "motor free." The child is not asked to copy a design. Rather, she is confronted with a multiple choice format that requires nothing more complex in motor behavior than to point. The test yields a *perceptual age* that ranges from younger than age 4 to older than age 9 years.

Motor-free tests are often of particular interest because many young children lack refined motor skills. As such, when the child responds unsatisfactorily to a copying task, there is the question of possible cause: motor deficit or/and visual perceptual skills deficit? The concept of a motor-free test is therefore reasonable. Unfortunately, however, it has significant flaws; and, in fact, the question that

---

*Slosson Educational Publications, Inc., P.O. Box 280, East Aurora, NY 14052.
**The RDT was developed and distributed by Anna Starr, now deceased. A copy of Form A and Form B, and instructions for administration and scoring, may now be procured from the Optometric Students Association, College of Optometry, University of Houston, Houston, TX 77004. Insofar as we have been able to determine, the test was never copyrighted. Hence, the samples obtained from OSA may be reproduced for office use.
†P. Colarusso and D. Hammill, Academic Therapy Publication, San Rafael, California, 1972.

Figure 8.11
Rutgers Drawing Test
(Form A).

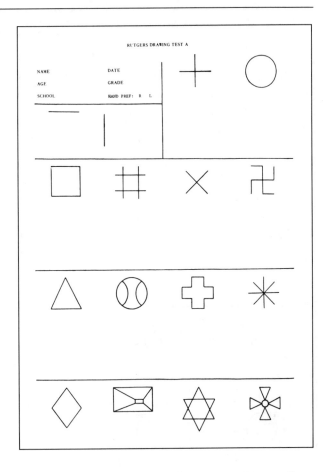

spawned the motor-free test can easily be answered without resorting to the test itself.

The flaw: motor-free tests usually require the child to identify a matching or a nonmatching figure, or some variation thereof. This usually does not require a thorough analysis of the designs. So long as a difference is observed, no further analysis is needed. For example, it is one thing to be able to identify a picture of yourself, and another to draw a self-portrait. Accomplishing the first does not indicate that you can also accomplish the other. Another example: recall the discussion regarding how children develop the ability to copy an asterisk. It is well documented that children who produce unsatisfactory copies, such as are shown in A, B, and C in Figure 8.13, will "point to" the correct asterisk when it is presented in a multiple-choice format. They simply cannot copy it. The point: copying a design necessitates a complete and accurate analysis. Discriminating similarities and differences does not (25).

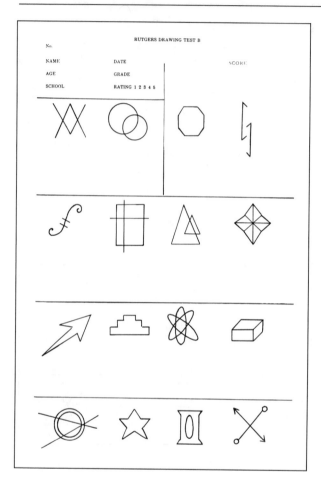

Figure 8.12
Rutgers Drawing Test (Form B).

How, then, can a potential motor problem be ruled out? Once more, the DDST offers a helpful clue. There are two items in the Fine motor-adaptive sector of the DDST that involve copying a square. One states simply, "Copies □." The other, "Imitates □ demonstration." The first, the more difficult of the two, refers to a situation where the child is shown a drawing of a square and is asked to copy it. In the second situation, the examiner shows the child how to draw a square and asks her to imitate the actions, step by step. The two require the same motor behaviors from the child, but not the same analytical skills. In the former, the child must perform the analysis, identify the task-pertinent features: the separate lines and their spatial interrelationships. In the second, the examiner carries out the analysis and models it for the child in sequential fashion. This is a remarkably effective yet simple way to make a distinction between a motor problem and an analysis problem. The child who can produce the design only when someone else does the analysis clearly has an analysis problem, not a fine motor problem.

A	Say **cowboy**	Now say it again, but don't say **boy**	**cow**
B	Say **steamboat**	Now say it again, but don't say **steam**	**boat**
1	Say **sunshine**	Now say it again, but don't say **shine**	**sun**
2	Say **picnic**	Now say it again, but don't say **pic**	**nic**
3	Say **cucumber**	Now say it again, but don't say **cu (q)**	**cumber**
4	Say **coat**	Now say it again, but don't say /**k**/ (the **k** sound)	**oat**
5	Say **meat**	Now say it again, but don't say /**m**/ (the **m** sound)	**eat**
6	Say **take**	Now say it again, but don't say /**t**/ (the **t** sound)	**ache**
7	Say **game**	Now say it again, but don't say /**m**/	**gay**
8	Say **wrote**	Now say it again, but don't say /**t**/	**row**
9	Say **please**	Now say it again, but don't say /**z**/	**plea**
10	Say **clap**	Now say it again, but don't say /**k**/	**lap**
11	Say **play**	Now say it again, but don't say /**p**/	**lay**
12	Say **stale**	Now say it again, but don't say /**t**/	**sale**
13	Say **smack**	Now say it again, but don't say /**m**/	**sack**

Figure 8.13 The Test of Auditory Analysis Skills (TAAS) (from Rosner J. Helping children overcome learning difficulties. New York: Walker Publishing Co., Inc., 1979).

□ The Test of Auditory Analysis Skills (TAAS)*

This test is applicable with children as young as age four and, because the DDST does not contain similar items, it should be used with that prekindergarten age group (26).

The test consists of 13 items, each involving the analysis of a spoken word into subcomponent parts. No other materials are needed.

TO ADMINISTER

1. Start with Item A (see Figure 8.13). This is a "demonstration item," intended to familiarize the child with the test. As such, it may be "taught" in the event that the child does not respond appropriately.

To teach Item A: Examiner says: "Say cowboy." Child states word. This demonstrates that she heard and remembers it. It also enables the examiner to take note of any speech problems that might affect how the child responds to the next step in this item: "Say it again, but this time do not say . . . [or, "leave off"] . . . cow."

If the child is confused by this, examiner repeats item, this time tapping the child's left knee, then right knee, in time with saying the first and second syllables of the word *cow-boy*.

*For a thorough description of the TAAS, see (4, pp. 46–49).

If the child remains confused, stop the test. If she responds correctly to items A and B, then administer 1. Do not teach from this point on.

2. If the child does not repond to a given item, repeat it once. If there is still no response, score the item "incorrect" and go on.

3. From items 4 on, a single sound is to be deleted. In identifying the sound to be deleted, say the sound the way it is spoken in the context of the test word.

4. Stop testing after two successive "incorrects" or after all 13 items have been administered.

TO SCORE THE TAAS

The score on the TAAS *is the number of the last item performed correctly*. For example, if items 1, 2, and 3 were passed, 4 failed, 5 passed, 6 and 7 failed, then the child's score is 5.

EXPECTEDS

Table 8.4 shows the TAAS scores expected of children from prekindergarten and above. If the child fails to score at the expected level, interpret it as signaling the possibility of an auditory perceptual skills disorder.

WHAT THE TAAS TESTS

First, one more definition. Visual perceptual skills were defined as the ability to identify the task-pertinent concrete features of a spatially organized array. Auditory perceptual skills* may be similarly defined: The ability to identify the task-pertinent concrete features of an *acoustical* array (4). The only difference between the two sets of skills, therefore, is in the nature of the sensory pattern that is to be analyzed. All else is the same.

The TAAS satisfies this definition. The acoustical array is a spoken word. The task: delete a unit of sound, as specified by the examiner. Hence, the features of the array that are pertinent to the task are the "phonological"—the sounds of the spoken word and their temporal sequence.

Words may be spoken softly or loudly, slowly or rapidly, at a high pitch or a low pitch, and so on. All of these refer to concrete features of the acoustical array. But, they are not pertinent in the TAAS; they are not task-pertinent features (6).

The ability to identify the phonological features of spoken words is developed (13). The organization of the TAAS items, and the test score-grade expecteds, reflect this. Formal lessons are not required; so long as the child's neuromotor system is functioning normally and he is provided with a reasonably nourishing and stimulating environment, the skills will be acquired. Furthermore, the rate of their acquisition is predictable. Somewhere before or during his fifth year of life, he is likely to become sensitive to the separate syllables in compound words

---

*The terms auditory perceptual skills, auditory analysis skills, and phonic analysis skills are used interchangeably in this volume. The first is better established, but not as accurate as the other two (9).

TAAS Score	Expected for Children in:
1	Kindergarten
2	Kindergarten
3	Kindergarten
4	Grade 1
5	Grade 1
6	Grade 1
7	Grade 1
8	Grade 1
9	Grade 1
10	Grade 2
11	Grade 2
12	Grade 3
13	Grade 3

From: Rosner J. Helping children overcome learning difficulties. New York: Walker Publishing Co., Inc. 1979, p. 42.

Table 8.4   TAAS Expecteds

(i.e., recognize them as separate units [26]. Within the following year, this will be extended to an awareness of separate syllables in polysyllabic noncompound words. Then, after his sixth birthday, he will display an awareness of the smaller unit, the phoneme, if it is positioned at the beginning of a spoken word.* Over time, this awareness will extend to final sounds and then, as the test suggests, to the point where he is able to isolate sounds even when they occur in the context of consonant blends.

Thus, as was noted before in the discussion regarding the development of visual analysis skills, as the child grows, he becomes more competent at identifying a greater variety of task-pertinent features even when these are embedded in complex and distracting contexts (27).

□ Alternative Auditory Perceptual Skills Screening Tests

The tests listed here are the ones cited most frequently on psychoeducational assessment reports that accompany children to the optometrist's office. There are fewer of these than in the visual perceptual skills category.

---

*Note: this is not analogous to *hearing* beginning sounds. Children discriminate between beginning sounds far earlier in life. The 3-year-old typically responds differently to the words "toe," "no," and "go."

WEPMAN AUDITORY DISCRIMINATION TEST (WADT)*

The WADT, as its name indicates, is a probe of the child's ability to discriminate between pairs of words that may differ from each other only slightly. The test contains forty items: thirty pairs of words that are "different" (e.g., pat-bat; tug-tub; pin-pen) and ten pairs that are "the same." The test has been normed for children between the ages of 5 and 8 years, and test outcomes are reported as "error rates" that fall within or below normal expecteds.

GOLDMAN-FRISTOE-WOODCOCK TEST OF AUDITORY DISCRIMINATION (G-F-W)

The G-F-W is designed for children age 4 years and older. It employs an audio tape that allows the examiner to compare the child's ability to discriminate words when they are spoken against a quiet background versus when the background is noisy and distracting.

ETC.

In addition to the tests described above, there are a number of auditory perceptual skills tests where nonverbal sounds comprise the sensory array. For example, there are tests that ask the child to repeat a (hand) clapped pattern (28), or to discriminate between Morse-code (long and short) tones (28).

These are valid tests of the child's ability to identify such features as temporal organization or relative length of tone in arrays of nonverbal sounds. Sensitivity to such features, however, is not a critical concern of the optometrist attempting to provide primary-care services. She is concerned about perceptual skills because of their impact in the classroom and, in that context, what she wants to rule out is a deficiency in the ability to identify the phonological features of spoken language. That counts in the classroom. Why this is so will be discussed next.

□ The Relationship between Perceptual Skills and Classroom Performance

The optometrist is not expected to become expert in pedagogy simply because she screens for school-related perceptual skills dysfunction, just as screening for high blood pressure does not imply the ability to diagnose and treat hypertension. It is useful, however, to have a general understanding of the connection between the screening test and the related conditions; in this instance, between visual and auditory analysis skills and what the child is expected to do in the classroom.

*J. Wepman, Western Psych. Services, Los Angeles, CA 90025.

RELATIVE TEACHABILITY

Children vary in how well they profit from standard classroom instruction.* Some children are very easy to teach. All they seem to need is the learning opportunity: exposure to situations that illustrate central principles and the challenge to accomplish certain reasonable goals. They generate pertinent questions, follow up on intuitions, profit from their errors, recognize how new information links up with what they already know, and go on from there. Or, when presented with a basic concept, they apply it in a variety of situations, refining their understanding of it as they do. In short, easy-to-teach children require very little explicit instruction in order to learn; yet they learn a great deal.

Most children, of course, are not that exceptionally easy to teach, but neither are they the opposite. They are not able to figure out as much on their own, they need more clarifying explanations, more explicit examples, more drill and practice. But, given these supports, they do learn. And because they represent the majority, their performance is characterized as "satisfactory" and "average."

Some children, however, are very hard to teach in one or more of the basic school skills. They do not identify fundamental principles intuitively or grasp how to apply general concepts effectively. A few explicit examples and some drill yields insufficient progress. This does not imply that they cannot be taught. It simply means that they are hard to teach, that they manifest "learning difficulties" when compared with the average child in a standard instructional setting (9).

Some illustrations, some sample "lessons," will help at this point.

Lesson I

Look at the geometric designs in Figure 8.14. Your teacher informs ("instructs") you that, in this lesson, each of those shapes represents a specific quantity. The small circle indicates the quantity 1. The large circle, 10. Going on, the small square stands for 4. Now a question: "What does the large square signify?" You, of course, respond, "40." By responding correctly, you demonstrate that you learned something that went beyond what you were "taught." Indeed, you could demonstrate this even more convincingly if you were now questioned about the quantities represented by the two hexagons.

How did you manage to learn so much from so little direct instruction? You employed a variety of abilities, but, in essence, your remarkable performance may be attributed to two basic, interrelated factors: first, your ability to identify the features in the geometric designs that are pertinent to this lesson; second, your coming to this lesson with appropriate prerequisite knowledge, factual information acquired previously and retained for subsequent applications.

---

*The word *standard*, as used here, does not mean inadequate. By standard, we refer to a situation where a teacher with average training, skills, motivation, and energy is given commercially published materials and the task of teaching 25 or so children a certain amount of information and skills within the space and time constraints of the school schedule (9, p. xxviii).

Figure 8.14
Symbols for sample
lessons.

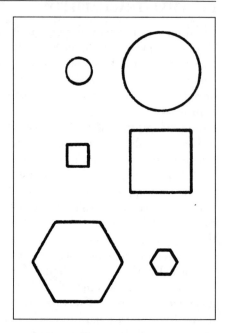

The first of these has been identified as a species-specific, naturally developed, general ability called *visual perceptual skills*. The second: the product of postnatal experiences; formal and informal instruction that reflects the individual's postnatal culture and experience, not her species.

As already noted, these two factors are interrelated. You could have chosen to focus on other spatial features in those designs: the *relative position* of the large and small shapes, for example. The reason you selected the number of lines that make up the designs and their relative size differences was that you "knew" that they were the appropriate ones in this context; they "made sense." How did you know that? You came to this lesson with sufficient relevant knowledge derived from previous experiences to identify the pertinent features of the visual array. Thus the linkup: you combined a general analytic ability with the specific knowledge that made it possible for you to select the features that were correct for this lesson, and, as a result, you learned; the lesson was effective. Had you selected the wrong features to pay attention to, the lesson would not have "made sense"; you would not have learned. Or, had you not previously learned the specific relationships between 1 and 10, and 4 and 40, information not "taught" in this lesson, once again the lesson would not have been effective; you would not have "learned."

Lesson II
Employing the same set of geometric designs, your teacher now instructs you that the small circle represents the spoken word "no," the larger circle, "note,"

the smaller square, the spoken word "go." And the larger square? "Goat," obviously. And, if you were now told that the larger hexagon represented the spoken word "wrote," there would be no difficulty in deciding what the smaller one represented.

Why is all of this so apparent to you? Because, once again, you are able to apply your naturally developed aptitude for analysis in combination with information brought forward from earlier experiences. This time, however, more than visual perceptual skills were needed. True, they were exercised in identifying the relative size differences among the designs. But certain auditory perceptual skills were needed to identify the pertinent (phonemic) components of the spoken words: "no," "note," "go," and "goat." And, since all of the words are already in your speaking vocabulary, it was easy to identify those features that were pertinent to this lesson.

The implication of these two lessons: the better one's perceptual skills, the more one learns from concrete experiences; and the more one learns from concrete experiences, the better his perceptual skills.

Suppose you did not learn from these lessons, yet your teacher was intent upon your learning. What then? You probably would be offered more explanation. Your teacher would point out specifically the features of the teaching examples that you were not noticing, and give you some drill in order to practice what you were to learn. If the lesson then worked, and if this modification was needed by most individuals, then you would be classified as "average," and not viewed as a learning problem.

But suppose, instead, that you needed more than the average amount of instruction, more than the average amount of explaining, more highlighting of pertinent features, more drill and practice? You would then be categorized as hard to teach or, more commonly, as having a learning problem. If you displayed this quality in all settings, not just in lessons devoted to learning one or more of the basic classroom skills, your ultimate classification would probably be "retarded." If, however, this were not the case, if your problem was evident primarily in the classroom—in tasks that involved learning how to use alphanumeric symbols as codes; if you appeared to be able to learn the many practical things that children learn outside the classroom, such as songs, games, how to operate various pieces of equipment (e.g., TV, record player)—then you would probably be described as having a "learning disability" or would be assigned one of the other labels used to describe such children.

Lesson III
There is another reason, of course, why Lessons I and II were so effective. Both were well designed; the salient information presented in each of the lessons was *apparent* rather than obscure, *unambiguous* rather than equivocal, and *systematic* (based on a "rule") rather than arbitrary. Now let us change conditions a bit and introduce some confusion factors into the situation. Imagine that the geometric designs in Figure 8.12 contained either horizontal or vertical, narrow, black and white stripes, assigned randomly; e.g., imagine horizontal stripes in both of the

circles and in the larger square, vertical stripes in the other three designs. If this revised figure had been used with Lesson I, a certain amount of confusion would have been experienced by all. The vertical and horizontal stripes are distractors. They make the lesson less effective because their use is not based on some orderly system (i.e., rule); hence, they tend to obscure and make ambiguous what was once apparent and orderly.

Despite this, however, it is very likely that you would have "learned" what the lesson was designed to teach, albeit a bit more slowly. Why? Because you have the analysis skills and related knowledge needed to learn from whatever errors the ambiguous stripes might have provoked, so long as you received appropriate feedback. You have the strategic skills needed to examine a problem, develop a reasonable solution, test the accuracy of that solution, and go on to generate an alternative, equally reasonable solution if and when your initial decision was wrong—to learn from your errors. Many school lessons present potentially ambiguous information. Not all children are able to overcome the confusion this generates. This is especially true of those who lack the fundamental analysis abilities defined here as perceptual skills. The outcome: They do not make satisfactory progress in school—they do not acquire information at the expected rate. This, in turn, compounds their school problems even further as the gap between what they are expected to know and what they actually do know becomes ever greater.

PERCEPTUAL SKILLS AND READING

Man spoke long before he invented a method for representing speech with graphic symbols. Reading is merely a by-product of that invention that enables one to acquire information by restoring symbolically coded language to its original state.

Visual Analysis Skills are related to learning to read in three ways. One, they affect the child's ability to master the directional conventions of reading. Second, they affect the child's ability to remember the printed letters, especially those that are easily confused, such as the *b* and the *d*. Third, they reflect the child's ability to retain what she had read. Children who are competent analyzers and organizers of concrete information also tend to be competent analyzers and organizers of abstract information (29,30,31,32).

Auditory Analysis Skills pertain to learning to read in a very direct and crucial way. They enable the child to identify what it is in spoken language that the letters represent; i.e., *what the code codes*. Hence, they ultimately affect the child's word-recognition skills (29,30,31,32).

PERCEPTUAL SKILLS AND ARITHMETIC

Arithmetic, like reading, enables one to acquire information by restoring symbolically coded information to its original state.

Thus, *visual analysis skills* are related to learning arithmetic in a very direct and obvious way. They enable the child to identify what it is that numerals represent; i.e., *what the code codes*. Hence, they ultimately affect her ability to remember number facts (29,31).

Auditory analysis skills do not appear to be related to learning arithmetic in any direct manner (32).

OTHER FACTORS THAT AFFECT CLASSROOM PERFORMANCE

Now a short step backward. Two interrelated factors have been identified that have a marked influence on a child's teachability. One, the competence of *her basic analytic aptitudes:* her visual and auditory perceptual skills; second, *her knowledge status:* how much she already knows relevant to the lessons she is to engage in.

There are, of course, other factors, in addition to the child's perceptual skills and knowledge status, that affect her relative teachability. Prominent among these, and worthy of some discussion, are the child's:

1. Physical status. It is obvious that a youngster will be relatively harder to teach if she is ill, undernourished (33), manifesting substandard hearing or sight, and so on. (Note: Worth mentioning at this point is the recently published evidence of the relationship between hyperopia and a delay in the development of visual analysis skills [34]. Cause and effect connections have yet to be established, but there is good reason to suspect that the ametropia—or, more exactly, the factor(s) that produced the hyperopia—is instrumental in the subsequent lag in visual perceptual skills development [35].)

2. Emotional status. Anxiety, motivation, social integration all affect teachability.

3. Process skills. This refers to the functional efficiency of the neuromotor systems that are critical to satisfactory achievement in the standard classroom; i.e., the ability to (a) control binocular functions efficiently (36,37,38); (b) speak intelligibly with ease; (c) manipulate a writing instrument efficiently.

4. Expressive skills. The ability to organize and express thoughts clearly and accurately.

These factors, in combination, determine a child's teachability. Most children, however, are physically healthy and adequately nourished; most children receive basic vision and dental care; most children are emotionally healthy; most have normal processing and expressive skills. Hence, we believe that the factors most influential in determining a child's teachability in the basic school subjects of reading, writing, arithmetic, and spelling are her visual and auditory analysis skills and the knowledge she brings with her as she engages in classroom activities (39).

However, not everyone shares our opinion. Some investigators argue that what we have identified above is insufficient, too simplistic; that we overlook some fundamental sensory-motor processes that have a profound effect on school learning. Some of the current and more intriguing of these are discussed below. (Note:

For an historical overview, which touches on "theories" that have been proposed over the past century and a half, see p. 450.)

OTHER PROPOSED CAUSES OF SCHOOL LEARNING PROBLEMS

Food Substance Allergies

The hyperactive, distractible behavior displayed by some children with school learning difficulties has been attributed to an allergic reaction generated by the ingestion of certain substances. Feingold, one of the chief sponsors of this idea, wrote and lectured extensively regarding the potential hazards of natural salicylates and artificial flavors and colors (40,41). Although he attracted a great deal of interest from anxious parents, his hypothesis has not been supported in any of the studies that were carried out to investigate its validity (42,43). As a result, believers continue to believe on the basis of what they perceive rather than scientific evidence. We do not necessarily agree, but we also readily admit that though we have no basis upon which to endorse Feingold's ideas, neither do we believe them to be harmful, in that they foster good dietary habits.

Dysmetric Dyslexia Caused by Vestibular Dysfunction

The term "dyslexia" deserves some discussion at this point. (For a fuller discussion, see Chapter 15.) It is one of those words whose meaning has changed over the years. At one time, *dyslexia* referred to a condition in which a once-literate individual demonstrated a marked deterioration in that ability because of a central nervous system lesion. The word has gradually become to mean a "reading problem," independent of cause—although the connotation of a medical etiology does persist.

The term *dysmetric dyslexia* appears to have been coined by two physicians, J. Frank and H. Levinson, who proposed that a significant number of reading problems stem from vestibular dysfunction, which also causes certain motor coordination problems. They devised a test that involves determining the rate of speed at which projected visual stimuli blur as they move horizontally (from left to right) across a screen. According to their postulations, children with dysmetric dyslexia demonstrate a significantly lower threshold in this activity. On the basis of this, they claimed that such problems should be treated medically, with anti-motion sickness drugs (44). Unfortunately, their hypothesis has not been supported by any research study that we have been able to identify; but it has been challenged by Brown et al, who found no differences between dyslexic and normal 12-year-old boys in vestibular function (45,46).

Scotopic Sensitivity Syndrome

This rubric, invented by H. Irlen (47), refers to a set of symptoms and behaviors that are often exhibited by children having difficulty in school. In essence, her thesis is that some children (and adults, as well) have a sensitivity to certain wave lengths of light that are revealed when they attempt to read—when they report that "the letters 'glare,' 'jump off the page,' " etc. She defined a test that empirically identifies (through the subject's responses to various filters) the offending wave lengths. She also proposed a treatment that requires the child to wear spectacles in which the lenses have been appropriately tinted. Unfortunately, Irlen's hypothesis has not been supported by any adequately designed research study that we have been able to identify (48). Hence, all claims as to its validity must be viewed with objective skepticism.

Unstable Dominance
The notion that ocular dominance has a unique influence upon how readily one learns to read has been around for a while. Orton (49) suggested it in his writings regarding strephosymbolia and dyslexia. Brod and Hamilton (50), and Delacato (51)—to name but two others—offered similar postulations.

In 1976, Dunlop and Dunlop described a test of ocular dominance that they believed to be effective in identifying a phenomenon that was directly related to dyslexia (52,53). Their test involves measuring the farpoint divergence (base-in) fusion range with a major amblyoscope, using a small (two-degree) stereo target in which there are "control marks"; i.e., certain parts of the target, when it is fused, are visible only to one eye *or* the other. As all optometrists know, when a fusion threshold is approached under these circumstances, the binocular patient will experience a disruption of binocular vision in the form of blur and/or unstable binocular fixation and, ultimately, diplopia or unilateral suppression.

The Dunlops' test focuses on identifying the eye that maintains fixation as this threshold point is reached. They termed this eye the *reference eye* and argued that the desired condition was when the reference eye corresponded with the individual's hand preference. In other words, a right-handed individual whose right eye was her reference eye was functioning optimally. The other conditions— i.e., the right-handed person with a left reference eye, or vice versa, or the person with "underdeveloped" dominance (when the targets of both eyes moved)—were much more likely to have difficulty learning to read.

Subsequent to the publication of the Dunlop test, a number of studies were carried out that employed the Dunlop test with some slight modifications (53,54,55). These used the Dunlop test to determine the *stability* of the individual's visual dominance and ignored its relationship with handedness. According to those reports (56), if the same eye maintains fixation in at least seven out of ten successive trials, the patient is classified as having *stable dominance*. If a less consistent pattern is shown, it is termed *unstable dominance*. These studies implicated unstable dominance with reading difficulties and attempted to explain this relationship by reasoning that the child with unstable dominance will—by definition— sometimes pay attention to the image from one eye, other times to the image from the opposite eye. As a result, this child will sometimes see letters in correct orientation, other times in reverse orientation, thereby generating the behaviors of visual dyslexia. They do not attribute all dyslexia to unstable visual dominance— only those that appear to relate to certain visual phenomena, such as reading/ printing reversals, losing of place on page, etc.

On the basis of this rationale, they then proposed a treatment method that employs unilateral patching to help the child establish stable visual dominance. Their results were remarkable; their data indicate that the patching produced stable dominance in most of their subjects and, more importantly, served to improve reading ability significantly.

Others have attempted, unsuccessfully, to duplicate the results reported above (57,58). Thus, the question continues to remain interesting but unresolved.

Faulty Eye Movement Skills

The proposition that a link exists between erratic eye movement patterns and reading difficulties is venerable, robust, and on the surface, reasonable (59,60). Few would argue with the statement that inept readers display irregular eye movements when they read. However, that hardly supports a cause and effect relationship. It is just as sensible to infer the opposite: that faulty eye movements stem from inadequate reading skills. Nonetheless, the proposition keeps reappearing.

One of the most recent proponents of this is Pavlidis (61,62,63), who reported that dyslexics display a less-than-satisfactory ability to execute saccadic eye movements, as tested by looking at a left-to-right sequence of lights. (Pavlidis differentiates dyslexia and poor reading ability, attributing the latter to a variety of exogenous and endogenous factors—e.g., socioeconomic class, IQ—and the former to some central processing deficit.)

Insofar as we have been able to determine, his eye-movement hypothesis has not been supported in any study that was carried out by an independent investigator. We have found the contrary: studies that replicated Pavlidis' methods but yielded different, less positive results (64,65,66).

Intelligence Quotient (IQ)

At this stage, the reader is likely to wonder why IQ has been ignored in a discussion regarding the relative ability of children to profit from standard instruction. After all, that is what inspired the development of the IQ test in the first place. The IQ test was not designed to measure an individual's intellectual potential, nor does it do that. The IQ test is designed to predict how well a child will succeed in school, and it fulfills that goal fairly well, sometimes for unfortunate reasons (see below).

In fact, the IQ has not been ignored here. Instead, it has been discussed in behavioral terms. If one takes the time to examine some IQ tests, it becomes obvious that, in essence, a child's IQ is an index of (a) her ability to solve problems that involve the analysis of spatially organized patterns and (b) her knowledge status: the two factors just discussed under the topic of teachability.

This is especially evident in the Wechsler Intelligence Scale for Children (WISC), which is designed to yield three IQ scores: a Verbal Scale IQ, a Performance Scale IQ, and a (combined) Full Scale IQ. The Verbal Scale reflects the child's knowledge status: what she knows about the world in comparison to other children of the same age; information she was not born with nor predestined to acquire but, rather, information derived from the culture in which she has lived. The Performance Scale reflects the child's analysis skills: how well she can solve different types of problems, such as reproducing a design with colored cubes (Block Design), jigsaw puzzles (Object Assembly), and so on, in comparison with other children of the same age; problems that are soluble on the basis of analysis rather than specific previous experiences. It is not coincidence, therefore, that children with visual analysis skills deficits also tend to display relatively low Performance Scale IQ scores on the WISC.

Other IQ tests, such as the Stanford-Binet and the Slosson, are similar to the WISC in the kinds of items they contain, but, in these tests, the items are mixed together. They yield but a single score and are not as useful to the optometrist who is concerned about the patient with a school learning problem. (Note: see [67] for an excellent, brief, clearly written description of the various psycho-educational tests typically administered to children with learning difficulties.)

What is the advantage, then, of using such terms as perceptual skills and knowledge status when a single, familiar, well accepted term such as IQ will do instead? The main advantage is that it avoids the pitfalls that are generated by the misconceptions regarding IQ. Despite popular belief, IQ is not immutable. But even recognizing that does not help eliminate a more devastating misconception: namely, that if the child's IQ is low, the only reasonable option available to the teacher is to lower the expectations regarding school performance; that is, teach less and expect less to be learned—the archetype of the self-fulfilling prophecy (68).

On the other hand, if one thinks not of IQ but of perceptual skills and knowledge status, then insights become available regarding how to eliminate or, at the least, alleviate the deficits and how to teach the child despite the deficits. It is information that may help the teacher teach. The IQ score serves just the opposite purpose. It is information that discourages the teacher from teaching; information that "explains" the learning problem without really explaining it.

VISUAL MEMORY

To learn in school means to remember what is taught. It is not unreasonable, therefore, to question why the screening procedure we suggest ignores other visual functions, such as visual memory. Visual memory testing is not suggested because, like IQ testing, it merely describes a behavior, it does not provide insights regarding treatment.

The typical visual memory test (e.g., Monroe V-III; Visual sequential memory subtest from ITPA) consists of showing the patient a pattern or a series of patterns (geometric designs, line drawings of objects, etc.) for a limited period of time (e.g., 10 seconds), and then comparing her ability to recall what she saw with other children of the same age—either by drawing, by selecting and arranging predrawn designs in correct order, or by naming.

It is safe to assume that the child with visual analysis skills deficits will also have inadequate visual memory. Consider what is involved. Figure 8.15 shows

Figure 8.15
Visual memory test
patterns.

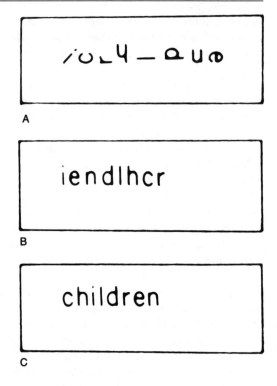

A

B

C

three patterns. If they were used as patterns in visual memory testing, it is obvious which would be the most difficult and which the easiest.

What does it require to remember pattern A? Admittedly oversimplifying, the patient has to identify pertinent (and memorable) spatial features of the separate rotated letters, *and* invent an effective system for coding these for storage in short-term memory, all within a short period of time. In other words, it requires competent visual analysis skills *and* knowledge.

Pattern B? It is much easier because the designs are readily recognized as lower-case manuscript letters. Visual analysis skills play a very small role because each letter is already stored in long-term memory and is recognized on the basis of minimal rather than extensive analysis. In addition, there is no need to invent a coding system. A standard one already exists: each letter has a name.

Pattern C? Easiest, so long as one can read and spell the language. Visual analysis skills play virtually no active part, and, once again, there is no need to invent a coding system. A remarkably efficient system, spelling and reading, serves well.

In short, it does not benefit the patient to document yet another inadequacy on her record form. It merely corroborates that she is hard to teach, that her deficient perceptual skills combined with her insufficient knowledge status do not provide her with the basis for identifying and applying the mnemonic strategies she needs in order to learn.

FIGURE-GROUND DISCRIMINATION

Figure-ground discrimination tests are yet another example of the great number of methods available for assessing individual differences in information processing skills without providing any constructive clinical data. They are of interest to cognitive psychologists who concern themselves with basic processes; they are of interest to some clinical psychologists because of what may be inferred from patient responses.* But, to the optometrist, they are best perceived as a measure of visual analysis skills in the presence of distractors.

SUMMARY

If a child is born with an intact neuromotor system and provided with reasonably adequate nourishment and experiences, she will acquire visual and auditory analysis skills on a fairly predictable schedule. She also will acquire the very complex process skills of vision, audition, speech, and manipulation. She will not require specific lessons. These are developed abilities. They are common to the species regardless of cultural background.

During those same years, the child will also acquire much knowledge about objects, people, and events, and the ability to express this knowledge in an organized way—but only if she has the necessary postnatal experiences. These are culture specific.

The two sets of abilities, those developed and those learned, are linked from the time of birth. The neonate exercising the innate preference for looking at black and white stripes instead of a detail-free luminous area (see discussion regarding preferential looking, Chapter 3) is "learning" something even though she is not yet able to express that knowledge in any measurable way. The next time she encounters this same stimulus, it is not as novel an event. She responds in a slightly more "educated" way. By the time she is 6 months old, she seeks other, more "interesting" things to look at. She makes decisions about what she will look at; no longer is she responding in a reflex-driven manner.

As she grows older, she gains experiences: visual, acoustical, tactile, and so on. She learns the spoken language of the culture in which she lives, and the universal, nonverbal language of space: the fundamental properties of magnitudes and relationships. Her constantly improving visual and auditory analysis skills aid her to understand the concepts of classification—of organizing information about people, objects, and events according to specific concrete features. This, in turn, serves to sharpen her analysis skills. And the cycle goes on, analysis skills subserving the acquisition of knowledge and the increased knowledge serving to improve the analysis skills (70).

All this presupposes that the cycle remains intact. If it does not, if a structural or functional deficit impairs development of process skills and analysis skills, knowledge acquisition is also impaired, which, in turn, has a detrimental effect

*See Witkin (69). He proposes that performance on a figure-ground test reflects one's psychological differentiation: the extent to which one is influenced (field-dependent) or not influenced (field-independent) by the environment.

on subsequent skills development. The cycle may also be interrupted by deprivation of experiences. In either case, the results are similar: delayed development of analysis skills and a knowledge deficit.

If the defect is in visual analysis skills, the knowledge deficit is likely to appear, generally, in the ability to produce neatly written (printed) papers and to organize information for application and retention, and specifically in arithmetic achievement and reading comprehension. If the problem is in auditory analysis skills, the knowledge deficit is likely to appear in the word-recognition aspect of reading.

If the cycle is reinstated early enough in the child's life—if her developmental lag is overcome, say, before she begins school—the knowledge gaps are likely to be eliminated. If, however, the cycle is not reinstated until well after the child has entered and begun to fall behind in school—if, say, her perceptual skills finally "catch up" when she is in the third or fourth grade—the knowledge gaps will have become difficult to eliminate. In a literal sense, it can be done. In a practical sense, it is exceptionally difficult to accomplish, because it requires the child to be sufficiently motivated to learn information that her classmates learned earlier and a teacher who is sufficiently knowledgeable and secure to make the decision to teach such fundamental information. And while all this is going on, the child's classmates continue to advance, meaning she continues to fall further and further behind.

Thus the importance of routine screening of perceptual skills development as early as possible. Late identification of a deficit is better than not at all, but in many ways it is analogous to finally discovering a reparable fault in a racing car long after the race has begun. The fault may be repaired, but it may be too late to catch up.

Time now to leave the topic of perceptual skills and move on to a description of one final screening test that should be administered under the general heading of developmental status (see D in Figure 8.1 flow diagram).

D. SCREENING FOR SPEECH DISORDERS

Here again is a primary-care obligation that can be fulfilled in very short order. It does not take the place of a professional evaluation conducted by a speech and language specialist, but it is far better than nothing.

Three aspects of speech should be screened (71): *articulation, voice,* and *fluency*. (These are part of a screening battery designed by Diana Phelps, Ph.D., ASHA/ CCC. In this context, of course, they cannot be used for diagnosis, but they are appropriate for screening.) The examiner should also be alert for signs of *language* disorders (e.g., inadequate vocabulary development and/or inappropriate use of language), but no testing method is described here, other than what was covered by the *Language* sector of the DDST.

□ Articulation

This component focuses on the child's ability to produce the speech sounds of the English language. Each item tests a specific sound within the context of a spoken word. The items are shown Table 8.5. Notice that they are ordered according to age, illustrating that the ability to express certain sounds is acquired through growth and development. When administering these items, pay special attention to the sounds that are represented by the underlined letters in each item.

TO TEST

1. Start with the first word in the 3-year-old category (see Table 8.5). Say to the child: "Say *knife*."
2. Pay attention to how the child produces the (underlined) "n" and "f" sounds.
3. Continue administering the test items until the child (a) repeats correctly all of the words through the level appropriate for his chronological age or (b) fails an item.
4. An inability to repeat correctly all of the words through the level appropriate for his chronological age constitutes reason for concern.

□ Voice

This refers to the quality of the child's speaking voice. It does not employ specific items. Simply listen for any of the following disorders:

1. Voice too high, low, or monotonous.
2. Voice too soft or loud.
3. Voice breathy, harsh, hoarse, raspy, scraping.
4. Voice nasal or denasal.

Age (years)	Items
3	knife, wing, how, money
3½	beep
4	yes, bacon, wagon, cow, go
4½	dishes, shoe, bird, radish
5	lunch, chin, sock, baseball
5½	valley, tent, cave
6	zoo, tooth, lazy, panther
6½	judge
7	beige, them, bathe

Table 8.5   Articulation Subtest from Speech/Language Screening Test

TO TEST

1. Listen to the child as he speaks.
2. Concern is justified if the voice sounds different enough to be considered "unusual."

□ Fluency

This component focuses on the rhythm of "flow" of the child's speech. Here, again, there are no specific items.

TO TEST

1. Listen to the child speak.
2. Consider any "unusual" hesitation, dysfluency, and/or stuttering as cause for concern.

■

REPORTING SCREENING TEST OUTCOMES TO THE PARENT

Once more the reminder: these are screening tests, not diagnostic instruments. Inadequate performance in any of them, however, constitutes reason for concern that is best translated into a professional referral. Specific comments regarding how to identify appropriate diagnostic and treatment resources are found in Chapter 15.

■

CONCLUDING THE EXAMINATION

In one sense, the answering of question 8 signals the end of the examination, unless there are some remaining, unanswered "keep-in-mind" questions that the optometrist has to address. Yet, in another sense, the visit may be over, but not the examination. Concern for the patient's well being does not commence when he enters the office and finish when he leaves. There is an ongoing commitment that bridges the intervals between visits. Thus, the examination—the formal process for accumulating information regarding the patient that may then be translated into useful recommendations—is also ongoing.

At any rate, it is now time to address the question of "So what?" Much information has been collected. How is that translated into useful recommendations? That is the topic of Part II.

■

PRACTICAL SUGGESTIONS

The information contained here is organized into three sections and presented in a question and answer format. The first section pertains to visual perceptual skills; the next to auditory perceptual skills; and the third to the types of questions parents and teachers often ask in regard to the links between vision, perceptual skills dysfunction, and school performance.

□ Questions Regarding Visual Perceptual Skills

8-1. Q: Everyone says that my child is very bright; I think so too. Her language is remarkable; she has always been able to express herself better than other children her age. Yet she has real difficulty when it comes to printing neatly, completing workpages, and other activities like that. Why is that, and what, if anything, should I do about it?

A: Barring the presence of some unique central nervous disorder, what you describe is best explained this way: Some children develop much more rapidly in one aspect of behavior than in another; e.g., some children are verbally precocious, yet lag in their visual analysis skills development—others, the reverse. Your child sounds like the former. Such children are always (and probably correctly) perceived as highly intelligent ("Just listen to her talk!"). The fact that they have trouble producing organized, neat-looking papers does not usually cause concern until they near entry into the first grade, by which time these youngsters— being bright—have learned to divert attention away from their shortcomings; i.e., when faced with a task they know to be difficult, they resort to what they know they can do well: *talk*. As a result, they get better at doing what they already do well (talking), but continue to lag in those skills that involve spatial analysis processes. Something should be done about it. (See Chapter 15 for specific treatment recommendations.)

8-2. Q: Can you test the visual and auditory analysis skills of my (3-year-old) preschooler?

A: Yes; but there are some qualifying statements that should be made. Two difficulties arise when testing this age group. One, the preschooler's response abilities are limited; there are very few geometric designs he can copy, very few puzzles he can solve. That creates a reliability problem. Second, preschoolers are notoriously independent test takers; some try hard—sometimes; some do not.

But none of this rules out testing a preschooler as long as the examiner recognizes that when the child responds satisfactorily, it should be viewed as reliable data; but when the child does not respond satisfactorily, it could be due to a true lacking *or* to the two factors cited above. (Two tests of visual analysis skills appropriate for preschoolers: the Gesell Copy Form Test [p. 305] and the fine motor-adaptive sector of the DDST [p. 285]. Some optometrists have devised their own informal tests, using such things as wooden cubes, form boards, jigsaw puzzles, or other materials that can be used to present a spatial analysis task to the child. Obviously, if this approach is taken, the optometrist has to use the task with enough children to develop "norms"—expecteds—that, in conjunction with clinical judgment, will enable the formulation of a reasonably valid opinion about this aspect of the child's development; and even then, the optometrist is restricted to clinical [qualitative rather than quantitative] terms when communicating with others.)

8-3. Q: My daughter is reputed to have visual perceptual skills problems. However, she is 17 years old and, as I understand it, the tests you customarily use are designed for younger children—up to about age 12. Do you have more difficult tests that can be used?

A: We do not need different, more difficult tests. Natural development of visual analysis skills (i.e., skills acquired independent of instructional experiences) tends to reach a maximum level at about age 10 to 12 years. But they can be tested at any age with these same tests—just as one's height can be measured with a standard ruler long after one has stopped growing.

This does not mean that some children do not acquire more sophisticated analysis skills as they grow older—but these are not the outcome of natural development; they are the result of specific learning. For example, optometrists exercise very precise visual analysis skills when examining patient's corneas with a biomicroscope. But this is not because optometrists have "developed" more precise analysis (perceptual) skills; rather, it is because they have "learned" a great deal about the eye, which enables them to use their basic analysis skills in a very sophisticated manner.

8-4. Q: Is it possible for a child "grow out of" his perceptual skills problems?

A: Yes, but the question is more complicated than that. Children develop at different rates. Some make very rapid growth during their early years, then slow down a bit; others, the opposite. Many (but not all) children with a visual and/or auditory analysis skills lag do grow out of their problem without any help; that is, by the time they are full grown, they have developed these basic analytic abilities. But, even so, there are two concerns one has to keep in mind when confronted with a child whose perceptual skills development is lagging: One, some children do not grow out of their problem; is this such a child? Second, given that the child will grow out of his problem, when will this happen? Will it occur *before* he falls significantly behind in school *because* of his problem? The answer to the first concern is best accomplished by ruling out possible etiologies that are known to have a detrimental effect on natural development—e.g., prenatal complications, premature birth, a traumatic occurrence at delivery, a postnatal event that caused a central nervous system disorder; general intellectual retardation. If these factors can be ruled out, then one may assume that the child will eventually "grow out of" his problem; but that still does not eliminate the concern about "when" and what that implies.

As noted above, progressing through elementary and secondary school is similar to engaging in a race. If the child falls too far behind during the early phase of the race because of some impairment (e.g., a pebble in his shoe), he will not catch up even though the impairment (the pebble) is ultimately eliminated. (See Chapter 15 for more discussion about this topic.)

8-5. Q: I think my child has "mirror vision"; she often prints some of her letters backward. Is this the same as a visual perceptual skills problem?

A: Many parents/teachers of children who manifest reading/printing reversals believe that such children "see backwards." The optometrist understands—and should explain—that this cannot be the case. Reversal problems are not due to seeing in reverse. If that were the case, the child would consistently reverse all letters—something she does not do. Hence, we must assume that (printing/reading) reversal tendencies are due to the child's (a) use of ineffective mnemonics for remembering the different letters; (b) exercising faulty habits that she established when she first learned to print/read. (This may be saying the same thing two different ways.)

There is little doubt that children display far fewer reversal tendencies if their visual perceptual skills are at about a 4- to 5-year-old level (or better) when they are first taught the lower case manuscript alphabet. If their visual perceptual skills are not at the appropriate level when they are taught these letters, they fail to identify and use effective strategies for remembering the different letters—and this becomes particularly evident with those letters that are very similar, such as the "b" and "d." It is conceivable, therefore, that the first grader who "prints backwards" did not have the necessary visual perceptual skills *at the time when she was taught the letters*, but subsequently acquired them. However, she continues to display the effects of that earlier skills lag by employing the ineffective memory strategies (the bad habits) she used early on—and by continuing to be confused by those letters.

8-6. Q: Does the child (who produced distorted drawings on the TVAS, the VMI, or the Rutgers) really see the designs the way he drew them?

A: No. These tests do not reveal what the child sees. Prove it to yourself. Show the child two versions of a pattern that he had trouble with: the incorrect one that he drew, and one that is drawn correctly. Have him select the one that matches the test item. Most children will select the correct pattern, a clear indication of what they perceive. The problem is not in what or how the child sees; the problem is that the child lacks the precise analytical skills needed to *duplicate* the designs. We all have had analogous experiences. Each of us, at one time or another, has attempted to draw something from nature—a person, an object— and not succeeded, not because we could not see it clearly or accurately but, rather, because we lacked the capacity/training/patience/etc. to work through the task, step-by-step, in an accurate, effective (analytic) manner.

8-7. Q: What about gross motor coordination? I have heard that that a child's perceptual skills problems often stem for inadequate development of lower-order gross motor abilities; yet you did not test these. Should we have someone else test them?

A: There is no need to test gross motor skills if the concern is inadequate classroom (reading, writing, arithmetic, spelling) performance and the factors that might influence it. Obviously, if the concern is the child's athletic abilities, then by all means have them tested—but that is a different problem. Visual analysis skills develop. If the child is fortunate, they develop "on schedule." General motor skills also develop, and once again this development is likely to follow some sort of predictable schedule. Some children who lag in visual analysis skills development also display lags in motor skills development. But it is not a cause and effect relationship; the lag in one did not produce the lag in the other. Therefore, testing and subsequently training a child's gross motor skills will not improve his visual analysis skills, unless the training activities also incorporate spatial analysis activities. And that is a roundabout way to address the problem.

□ Questions Regarding Auditory Perceptual Skills

8-8. Q: Are my child's inadequate auditory analysis skills indicative of impaired hearing?

A: It is possible, of course, but not probable. However, just as it is advisable to have the child's vision tested, even when you believe she sees well, so too is it a good idea to have her hearing tested.

8-9. Q: My child had chronic ear infections when he was younger. Did this cause his auditory perceptual skills deficit?

A: It could have. Many children with auditory analysis skills dysfunction have a history of chronic middle-ear infections. But, in any event, this question is academic. It should not influence our decision regarding treatment, so long as we are certain that he has no residual hearing impairment.

8-10. Q: Your tests show that my child has adequate auditory perceptual skills. Yet her teacher tells me that she has a very poor auditory memory and faulty "auditory processing skills"; she cannot remember spoken information as well as she should. When her teacher asks her to do something that involves more than one step, she simply is not able to complete the activity. Why is this; how can there be such disagreement about her auditory skills?

A: What her teacher has identified should not be attributed to inadequate auditory analysis skills. In all probability, these difficulties are due to the fact that (a) your child does not pay adequate attention when her teacher speaks to her, and/or (b) she does not understand the meaning of all the words being stated or what they refer to, and/or (c) there is just too much information being offered—it is more than she can memorize, and she has not yet developed the ability to organize information effectively for storage in short-term memory.

If it is the last—and most often it is—you should suspect visual analysis skills dysfunction, not auditory, even though the information is spoken and heard. This may sound paradoxical, but consider for a moment the normal brain; it does not function as a compartmentalized organ—there are a great number of "association pathways" that link up the different sections. Children who lack visual analysis skills, by definition, lack organizational ability—the strategies one employs when categorizing information based on identifying salient similarities and differences. Clearly, when this is lacking, remembering information becomes exceptionally difficult, regardless of how that information is produced: acoustically or visually.

8-11. Q: Do children with auditory perceptual skills dysfunction grow out of their problem in time?

A: Yes. But, as with visual analysis skills, that does not mean that they also grow out of the academic problems that were produced because of the poor auditory analysis skills. (See Practical Suggestion 8.4, above.)

□ Questions Regarding Learning Disabilities

8-12. Q: What is the difference between a "learning disability" and "dyslexia"?

A: For all practical purposes, there is no difference between the two. At one time, the term *dyslexia* applied to a reading problem that was caused by specific damage to the central nervous system. Now the word is used to describe reading problems that are not attributable to a general cognitive deficit; in other words, reading problems in individuals who should not be experiencing them.

8-13. Q: To what extent does hand preference (dominance) influence a child's school performance?

A: There is a lot yet to be learned about the influence of hemispheric (sensory and motor) dominance on cognitive functioning. At present, the honest and most practical approach is to acknowledge that although there are relatively more left-handed children in "learning disability" populations, there are also many left-handed children who do very well in school. In that same vein, a great many children who have difficulty in school are right handed. Hence, hand preference, in itself, does not seem to be a significant factor.

8-14. Q: My first grader is ambidextrous; that is, sometimes she uses her right hand for printing, sometimes her left. Do you think that her printing reversals are connected with this in some way?

A: Yes, if by "ambidextrous" you mean that she has not yet established a preferred hand for printing, etc. (Usually, it is more accurate to describe such children as "nondextrous.") Hand preference develops; very few children settle on being right or left handed until they are about four years old. Sometimes they eat, draw, throw, etc., with their right hand, sometimes with their left. But this should all be resolved by the time they reach their fifth birthday. Children who are late in establishing consistent handedness are demonstrating a "developmental lag"— one that will affect their ability to remember spatial relationships. Obviously, the child who does not remember spatial relationships will display confusion when it comes to remembering which is the "b" and which the "d," etc. In other words, it is highly likely that the child who does not develop a consistent hand preference at the expected age will also reveal a (related) lag in visual perceptual skills. (See Practical Suggestion 15-19 for treatment suggestions.)

8-15. Q: What about mixed hand-eye dominance; does that cause learning problems?

A: No, it does not appear to cause learning problems. Granted, over the years this notion has surfaced many times, only to be rejected when studied scientifically. There is no apparent validity to the proposal that the child who "sights" with his left eye and prints with his right hand is more at risk to school learning problems than the child who is "right eye dominant," and right handed.

REFERENCES

1. Rosner J. Screening for perceptual skills dysfunction: an up-date. JAOA 1979; 50(10):1115.
2. Frankenburg WK, Dodds JB. The Denver Developmental Screening Test. J Pediatr 1967; 71:181.
3. Frankenburg WK, Goldstein AD, Camp BW. The revised Denver Developmental Screening Test: its accuracy as a screening test. J Pediatr 1971; 79(6):988–95.
4. Frankenburg WK, Sciarillo W, Burgess D. The newly abbreviated and revised Denver Developmental Screening Test. Behavioral Pediatrics 1981; 99(6):995–99.
5. Harris DB. Children's drawings as measures of intellectual maturity. New York: Harcourt, Brace & World, Inc. 1963.
6. Goodenough FL. Measurement of intelligence by drawings. New York: Harcourt, Brace & World, 1926.
7. Gesell A, Amatruda CS. The embryology of behavior. New York: Harper, 1945.
8. Hetherington EM, Parke RD. Child Psychology. New York: McGraw-Hill Book Co., 1975.
9. Rosner J. Helping children overcome learning difficulties. 2nd ed. New York: Walker Publishing, 1979.
10. Rosner J, Fern K. A new version of the TVAS: a validation report. JAOA 1983; 54:603–606.
11. Thomas CB, Ross DC, Freed ES. An index of Rorschach responses: studies of the psychological characteristics of medical students. Baltimore: Johns Hopkins Press, 1964.
12. Rosner J. Perceptual skills development in children with learning disabilities. In: Gottlieb J, Strichart S, eds. Developmental theory and research in learning disabilities. Baltimore: University Park Press, 1981.
13. Rosner J. The development of a perceptual skills curriculum. JAOA 1973; 44(7):698.
14. Terman LM. The measurement of intelligence. Boston: Houghton Mifflin, 1916.
15. Dong D, Lee R, Sanchez-Salazar J. Relationships among copy form tests. Unpublished thesis, School of Optometry, University of California at Berkeley, 1978.

16. Bender L. A visual motor gestalt test and its clinical uses. New York: Am Orthopsych Assn, 1938.
17. Watkins EO. The Watkins Bender-Gestalt scoring system. San Rafael, CA: Academic Therapy Publications, 1976.
18. Koppitz EM. The Bender-Gestalt test for young children. Vols. 1 & 2. New York: Grune & Stratton, 1975.
19. Frostig M, Maslow P. Learning problems in the classroom. New York: Grune & Stratton, 1973.
20. Olson A. Factor analytic studies of the Frostig Test of Visual Perception. J Spec Ed 1968; 2:429, S-F.
21. Beery NA. Relative contributions of auditory and visual perception to first grade language learning. Ph.D. thesis, University of Chicago, 1966.
22. Ilg FL, Ames LB. School readiness. New York: Harper & Row, 1965.
23. Roach E, Kephart N. Purdue perceptual-motor survey. Columbus, OH: C. E. Merrill Publ. Co., 1966.
24. Denton A. Slosson drawing coordination test. Review in: Buros O, eds. Seventh mental measurements yearbook. Highland Park, N.J.: Gryphon Press, 1972.
25. Maccoby EE, Bee HL. Some speculations concerning the lag between perceiving and performing. Child Dev 1965; 36(2):367–77.
26. Rosner J, Simon D. The auditory analysis test, an initial report. J Learn Dis 1971; 4(7):384–92.
27. Rosner J, Cooley WW. Changes in perceptual skills and early academic achievement. Pittsburgh: LRDC, University of Pittsburgh, 1971.
28. Rosner J, Richman V, Scott R. The identification of children with perceptual-motor dysfunction. Pittsburgh: LRDC, University of Pittsburgh, 1969 Working Paper 47.
29. Rosner J. Testing for teaching in an adaptive educational environment. In: Hively W, Reynolds M, eds. Domain-referenced testing in special education. Reston, Va.: Council for Exceptional Children, 1975.
30. Weaver PA, Rosner J. Relationships between visual and auditory perceptual skills and comprehension in students with learning disabilities. J Learn Dis 1979; 12(9):617–21.
31. Rosner J. Language arts and arithmetic achievement, and specifically related perceptual skills. Am Ed Res J 1973; 10(1):59–68.
32. Rosner J. Individual differences in perceptual skills: identification, modification and effects. Proceedings Am Psych Assn 80th meeting. Published by LRDC, University of Pittsburgh, 1972.
33. Evans D, Hansen JDL, Moodie AD, van der Spuy HIJ. Intellectual development and nutrition. J Ped 1980; 97(3):358–63.
34. Rosner J, Rosner J. Differences in the perceptual skills development of young myopes and hyperopes. AJOPO 1985; 62(8): 501–504.
35. Rosner J, Rosner J. Some observations of the relationship between the visual perceptual skills development of young hyperopes and age of first lens correction. Clin & Exper Optom 1986; 69(5):166–68.
36. Chernick B. Profile of peripheral visual anomalies in the disabled reader. JAOA 1978; 49(10): 1117.
37. Ritty JM. Assessing and alleviating visual problems in schools. Reading Teacher April 1979, p. 796.
38. Hoffman LG. Incidence of vision difficulties in children with learning disabilities. JAOA 1980; 51(5):447–51.
39. Rosner J, Rosner J. The management of perceptual skills disorders in a primary-care practice. JAOA 1986; 57:56–59.

40. Feingold B. Why your child is hyperactive. New York: Random House, 1975.
41. Feingold B. Cooking for your hyperactive child. New York: Random House, 1977.
42. Connors CK, Goyette CH, Southwick DA, Lees JM, Andrulonis PA. Food additives and hyperkinesis: A controlled, double-blind experiment. Pediatrics 1976; 58 (2):154–66.
43. Harley JP, Ray RS, Tomasi L, Eichman PL, Matthews CG, Chun R, Cleeland CS, Traisman E. Hyperkinesis and food additives. Testing the Feingold hypothesis. Pediatrics 1978; 61(6):818–27.
44. Frank J, Levinson H. Seasickness mechanisms and medications in dysmetric dyslexia and dyspraxia. Academic Therapy 1976; 12:133–52.
45. Brown B, Haegerstrom-Portnoy G, Yingling CD, Herron J, Galin D, Marcus M. Dyslexic children have normal vestibular responses to rotation. Arch Neurol 1983; 40:370–73.
46. Brown B, Haegerstrom-Portnoy G, Herron J, Galin D, Yingling CD, Marcus M. Static postural stability is normal in dyslexic children. JLD 1985; 18(1):31–34.
47. Irlen H. Successful treatment of learning disabilities. Unpublished paper presented at APA, August 1983.
48. Rosner J, Rosner J. The Irlen treatment: a review of the literature. Optician 1987; 194(5116):26–33.
49. Orton S. Reading, writing and speech problems in children. New York: WW Norton & Co., Inc. 1964.
50. Brod N, Hamilton D. Binocularity and reading. JLD 1973; 6:47–49.
51. Delacato C. The diagnosis and treatment of speech and reading problems. Springfield, Ill.: CS Thomas, 1963.
52. Dunlop P. Orthoptic management of learning disability. Brit Orthop J 1979; 36:25–35.
53. Dunlop DB, Dunlop P. A new orthoptic technique in learning disability due to visual dyslexia. In Moore S (ed). Orthoptics: past, present, future. New York: Stratton Intercontinental Med Book Corp., 1976.
54. Stein J, Fowler S. Effect of monocular occlusion on visuomotor perception and reading in dyslexic children. Lancet 1985; July 13:69–73.
55. Stein JF, Riddell PM, Fowler MS. The Dunlop test and reading in primary school children. Brit J Ophthal 1986; 70:317–20.
56. Stein JF, Fowler S. Diagnosis of dyslexia by means of a new indicator of eye dominance. Brit J Ophthal 1982; 66:232–36.
57. Newman SP, Karle H, Wadsworth JF, Archer R, Hockly R, Rogers P. Ocular dominance, reading and spelling: a reassessment of a measure associated with specific reading difficulties. J Res in Reading 1985; 8(2):127–38.
58. Bigelow ER, McKenzie BE. Unstable ocular dominance and reading ability. Perception 1985; 14:329–35.
59. Solan HA. Eye movement problems in achieving readers: an update. AJOPO 1985; 62(12):812–19.
60. Olson RK, Kliegl R, Davidson BJ. Dyslexic and normal readers' eye movements. J Exp Psych 1983; 9(5):816–25.
61. Pavlidis GT. Eye movements in reading. Nursing Mirror 1980; Jan:22–26.
62. Pavlidis GT. Do eye movements hold the key to dyslexia? Neuropsychologia 1981; 19:57–64.
63. Pavlidis GT. Eye movement differences between dyslexics, normal, and retarded readers while sequentially fixating digits. AJOPO 1985; 62(12):820–32.

64. Stanley G, Smith GA, Howell EA. Eye-movements and sequential tracking in dyslexic and control children. Brit J Psych 1983; 74:181–87.
65. Stanley G, Smith GA, Howell EA. Eye-movements in dyslexic children: comments on Pavlidis' reply. Brit J Psych 1983; 74:195–97.
66. Brown B, Haegerstrom-Portnoy G, Yingling CD, Herron J, Galin D, Marcus M. Tracking eye movements are normal in dyslexic children. AJOPO 1983; 60(5):376–83.
67. Klein SD. Psychological testing of children. Boston: Exceptional Parent Press, 1977.
68. Rosenthal R, Jacobson L. Pygmalion in the classroom; teacher expectation and pupils' intellectual development. New York: Holt, Rinehart and Winston, 1968.
69. Witkin H et al. Psychological differentiation. New York: Wiley, 1962.
70. Simon H. Science of the artificial. Cambridge, Mass.: MIT Press, 1969.
71. Phelps D, Rosner J. Screening for speech disorders in a primary care practice. Unpublished paper presented at the annual meeting of the American Academy of Optometry, Chicago, December 1979.

II

THE
POSTEXAMINATION
PROCESS

■
■
■
■

9

The Postexamination Process

□

THE POSTEXAMINATION CONFERENCE

The postexamination conference may take various forms, ranging from a brief summing up of what has been discussed continuously throughout the examination to a separate, formal session where all data are thoroughly reviewed.

In any instance, it is important to remember that the patient's/parent's motivation for seeking professional services was concern: perhaps anxiety regarding a specific problem, perhaps routine precaution, but concern nonetheless.

As such, the optometrist's ultimate goal goes beyond the reporting of examination outcomes. That is but a step in the process. Her ultimate goal is to express an informed opinion and to prescribe—to "specify with authority" (Webster's New Collegiate Dictionary, 1974). This is so even if the prescription is reassurance that no clinical problem exists.

The eight-question format of this book provides an effective method for organizing the postexamination conference. For example, the conference could proceed along these lines:

"Your concerns regarding your child's eyes/vision are/are not well founded."
"His eyes do/do not appear to be healthy and normally formed."
"He does/does not see clearly."
"He does/does not need glasses."
"His two eyes are/are not aligned accurately."
"His two eyes do/do not work together efficiently."
"His developmental status/perceptual skills are/are not appropriate for his age/ grade."
"The problem does/does not appear to be related to the events noted in the case history."
"In consideration of all this, I recommend the following. . . ."

This portion of the book (Chapters 9 through 15) is devoted to those recommendations. The format is consistent. Each chapter addresses a specific clinical condition and discusses prescription options for that condition.

The list of clinical problems is limited to those that present with some degree of regularity: ametropia (Chapter 10), strabismus (Chapter 11), amblyopia (Chapter 12), nystagmus (Chapter 13), substandard vergence and accommodation facility (Chapter 14), and perceptual skills dysfunction (Chapter 15).

In all instances, the list of prescription options is limited to those that are exercised with some degree of regularity: (a) remedial therapy; (b) compensatory therapy; (c) reassurance therapy; (d) refer for consultation. And, although the specific procedures and practices vary according to clinical problem, the general formats of the treatment regimens are more or less the same for all clinical conditions. The goal of this chapter is to define those formats in the form of flow diagrams, thereby providing the basic organization for the subsequent chapters.

I. REMEDIAL THERAPY

The general goal of remedial therapy is to alter the course of the diagnosed condition; to eliminate it totally or in part, or perhaps only to halt its progression. The remedial treatments discussed in this book vary with the condition, but none conforms with the so-called medical model of employing a drug to attack the cause of the disease while doing as little damage as possible to the patient. Rather, the treatments we propose take the form of instructional processes, skills training programs that are intended to teach the patient. As such, even the simplest treatments require planning as well as precise and clear communication between the optometrist and the patient/parent.

A. DESIGN AND DESCRIBE THE TREATMENT PROGRAM

The first decision point in the Figure 9.1 flow diagram is B, where the likelihood that the patient/parent will follow the program as directed is questioned. The treatment program must be designed and described before the decision can be made. Hence, the first step in the remedial process: provide the patient/parent with the information needed in order to decide whether or not the obligations to the program can be fulfilled. It is an important step. The ultimate benefit: fewer treatment programs that were destined to failure from the onset.

Four related topics should be discussed when the treatment program is proposed:

1. What outcomes the patient/parent can reasonably expect if he follows the program; i.e., the probable ultimate (maximum and minimum) benefits to be derived from the remedial program.

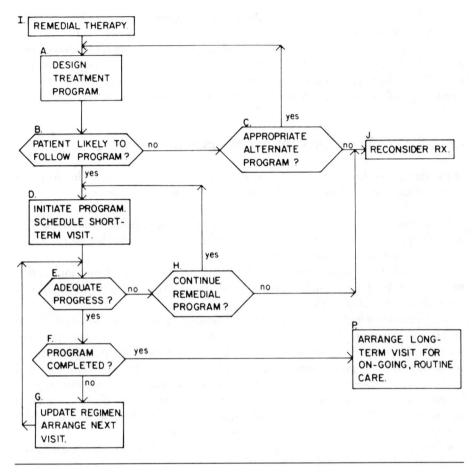

Figure 9.1   Remedial therapy.

2. What the patient/parent will be expected to do; i.e., Wear glasses? Bifocals? Wear a patch? Undergo surgery? Engage in office-based treatment sessions? In home-based treatment sessions? Doing what? How often? Etc.

3. What the patient/parent can expect if the recommendations are not followed; i.e., the probable consequences of ignoring the condition. Will it get worse? Will the opportunity for improvement be lost forever, if delayed now? What alternatives are there, if the patient is not able to engage in a full-scale treatment program at this time?

4. Costs; i.e., time? (How long will the program take?) Effort? (How much time each day? How much supervision?) Money?

Obviously, these topics cannot be discussed in great detail at a single postexamination conference. It would consume an unreasonable amount of time, and, even if time were not a concern, detailed discussion would require the mapping out of the separate steps of the program, from beginning to end. That is not a reasonable undertaking; often, at this stage, even step two cannot be determined with certainty until after the patient has taken step one and its effects have been assessed. The point: a remedial program is not analogous to a recipe for baking a cake. True, there is a certain structure—a predictable sequence of events—but greater specificity than that is rarely possible before the program gets underway.

□ Objectives of the Clinical Management Plan

How, then, does the optometrist deal with the topics listed above? She develops a clinical management plan by analyzing the case along these lines (1,2):

1. *Define the ultimate goals of the therapy program in behavioral terms;* i.e., what the patient will be able to do at the end of the treatment that he could not do at the beginning and/or vice versa.

2. *Identify the abilities that are subordinate to the terminal goal and define their hierarchical interrelationships;* i.e., which are prerequisite to which; which are independent of the other?

3. *Determine which of the subordinate abilities the patient has already achieved and which remain to be accomplished.* This does not present much of a problem once steps 1 and 2 are accomplished. If the hierarchy is valid, the patient's position within it is established by employing appropriate placement tests—tests designed to determine not so much what the patient cannot do but, more importantly, what he can do. This is a crucial step in the management of an effective remedial therapy program; it is impractical to attempt to teach something to someone until you determine what he already knows about that topic.

4. *Identify activities/procedures that will facilitate attainment of the yet-to-be-mastered subordinate abilities;* i.e., the methods that will close the separation between the patient's present status and the status defined as the ultimate goal of the treatment.

□ Instructional Principles

In identifying appropriate treatment activities/procedures, four instructional principles should be followed:

1. *The activity should be designed to aid the patient acquire an ability that he currently lacks, is prepared to learn, and now needs if he is to make progress.* A placement test procedure is developed in accord with this principle. The patient should not be assigned activities that are intended to teach an ability he has already acquired, or an ability that is far too difficult or, worse yet, an ability that is not directly related to the stated goals of the treatment program. It not only is a waste

of time; it also tends to destroy motivation. The patient should work on goal-related skills that stem from his already acquired abilities.

2. *The activity should be designed so that its difficulty may be regulated on the basis of the amount of support provided.* The tasks should be difficult enough to provide a challenge, but if the patient requires some extra assistance in order to get started in an activity, that aid should be available and then gradually reduced as it becomes less essential. For example, if the patient cannot obtain binocular fusion unless aided by prism, he should have the prism and work toward obtaining fusion without it.

3. *The activity should be quantifiable; it should be possible to "keep score"* e.g., speed, accuracy. This will provide concrete goals for the patient to aspire to surpass as the therapy proceeds. It is useful motivating device.

4. *The activity should be self-instructional. It should be designed so that the patient is able to monitor his own performance.* An external (feedback) signal that reinforces correct performance should be built into the activity; a tangible, extrinsic signal that the patient will be able to relate to intrinsic (somatic) signals, so that he can learn to match what he "feels" with what he "sees." Over time, and with sufficient practice, the patient will be able to assess his performance exclusively on the basis of intrinsic signals, thus creating the proper conditions for transforming a newly acquired behavior into an habitual pattern.

This fourth principle highlights a pivotal issue. As already noted, remedial training is not analogous to drug therapy. Neither is it a form of calisthenics in the sense that the goal is stronger muscles. The patient engages in activities that are best described as instructional. Therefore, he must be reasonably "instructable"; i.e., teachable (see Chapter 8). In fact, the key to success in a remedial skills training program is the patient's ability to "teach himself": to relate how he feels with what he sees and does. It is an abstract task, not easily accomplished by the patient who lacks the ability to learn inductively.

In addition, the patient must be prepared to engage in these activities for an extended period of time. And in the case of children, the parent must be willing to supervise the home-based portion of the program over that extended period of time. Reeducating the neuromotor responses that control the eyes and what they perceive is not a quick and easy thing, even though the activities may appear to be uncomplicated. Along with the self-instructional aspect, there is the need for prolonged, repetitive practice. If the therapy is to succeed, old habits must be replaced by new behaviors that must then be repeated until they become habit—performed automatically, without conscious thought or effort.

Remedial skill therapy is a challenging undertaking, and the goal is worthwhile. However, it is not the best approach for every patient; it constitutes a professional error to presume otherwise. It therefore constitutes a second professional error to extol remedial skills therapy to a patient who will not profit from it. It is important to remember this while designing a treatment regimen; the treatment should suit the patient.

The central point in all of this: the optometrist should make her selection of a treatment program not only on the basis of what is *best*, but also on the basis of what is *feasible*.

___■_____

B. IS THE PATIENT LIKELY TO FOLLOW THE PROGRAM?

Once the therapy program has been proposed it becomes the patient's privilege to accept or reject the recommendations.

☐ If Yes

Initiate the remedial therapy program (see D in Figure 9.1 flow diagram and below).

☐ If No

Consider the possibility of a reasonable alternative that *is likely* to be followed (see C in Figure 9.1 flow diagram and below).

___■_____

C. IS THERE AN APPROPRIATE ALTERNATIVE PROGRAM?

If the alternative program is sought because the *optometrist decides* that the child/parent is not equipped to engage in a full-scale program (which she therefore does not recommend), then the "alternative" program will be the initial recommendation. If the alternative program is sought because the *child/parent decides*, after hearing the initial recommendations, that it is more than they can deal with, then the optometrist is well advised to make clear that the alternative will not be optimal (unless it will); that, in her opinion, it is second best and must be viewed in that way. (Indeed, some clinicians might even take the position in this situation that "second best" is unacceptable to them, and advise the patient/parent to seek a second professional opinion.)

In any event, the alternative program must have clinical purpose and value. It must not simply be "busy work" that satisfies anxieties and does little else. In essence, an alternative program is appropriate only if it is designed to achieve the same goals as the full-scale program, albeit at a slower rate.

□ If Yes

Describe that alternative program to the patient/parent (see A in Figure 9.1 flow diagram).

□ If No

Reconsider the original decision and select a different treatment approach (see J in Figure 9.1 flow diagram).

___

D. INITIATE THE THERAPY PROGRAM

A key characteristic of an effective therapy program is structure. This is especially so in respect to the home-based aspects of the program. The patient/parent must fully appreciate the need for regularly scheduled, thoughtfully conducted home sessions. One does not become proficient with a complex neuromotor skill by engaging in erratically scheduled, casually conducted instructional sessions—be it learning to play the piano or maintaining bifoveal alignment or enhancing vergence facility.

It is wise to organize the training activities into levels, arbitrarily defined if necessary, each with its own goals. This provides the patient with attainable stepping stones that bridge the distance from his existing performance level to where he hopes ultimately to be (3).

Regular reassessment by the optometrist is also essential. It was stated earlier that the program cannot be fully predetermined. The goals, yes; but not the process. It is designed as progress is (or is not) made, as improvement is (or is not) observed. If the program is to be home-based, office visits should be scheduled on at least a twice-per-month basis. If the program is to be office-based, with a supplemental home component, then the frequency of visits will be greater, of course.

Continuous monitoring is important. It cannot be overly stressed that a properly conceived treatment program is truly an educational process and that the decisive ingredient is the patient's ability to learn—to "catch on." How this will occur cannot be predicted. The optometrist implements procedures that are designed to facilitate it, but her procedures are not infallible. Unless she also maintains a careful watch on changes as they occur, she is apt to miss critical opportunities which, once passed by, may be a long time in reappearing.

■

E. HAS THE PATIENT MADE ADEQUATE PROGRESS?

The purpose of a follow-up visit is to determine what has occurred since the previous visit and to lay out the assignment for the next block of time. Have instructions been followed? Has progress been achieved?

If the treatment program is valid, the first question is answered by the second question, and the second question is answered in two ways: first, by report. If the assigned activities were organized into levels, the patient/parent should be able to report the child's present status in those terms; i.e., identify the level he has achieved. Second, by measurement. If the child has made progress in his home assignments, it should be apparent in the office measures, so long as what he was making progress on at home is directly related to what is measured in the office. (And, if it is not, then some reconsideration should be given to why he is being asked to do the home activities.)

☐ If Yes

Determine whether the program is completed (see F in Figure 9.1 flow diagram).

☐ If No

Attempt to establish why this is the case. If it is due to misunderstanding, remedy the situation and arrange for the next visit. If it is due to a lack of participation at home, attempt to determine whether there is any reason to anticipate something different in the future, and act accordingly; i.e., give it another try (see H in flow diagram) or reconsider the original recommendation (see J in Figure 9.1 flow diagram).

■

F. PROGRAM COMPLETED?

Literally translated, that question asks whether the goals defined at the beginning of the program have been achieved. In practical terms, however, it may be that these were reconsidered and redefined. In any event, a properly designed remedial training program has an ending as well as a beginning, and when that terminal has been achieved, it should be acknowledged.

□ If Yes

Arrange for routine, ongoing care (see P in Figure 9.1 flow diagram).

□ If No

Make a new assignment and arrange for the next visit (see G in Figure 9.1 flow diagram).

II. COMPENSATORY TREATMENT

The general goal of compensatory treatment is to enable the patient to perform satisfactorily despite the diagnosed problem. Ordinarily, compensatory treatment is indicated when the prognosis for remedial therapy is distinctly unfavorable. Compensatory treatment tends to be less complicated than remedial treatment, although there are cases where it may become quite involved (e.g., in the management of adolescents with perceptual skills dysfunction). The process begins with the selection and dispensing of the treatment (see K in Figure 9.2 flow diagram and below).

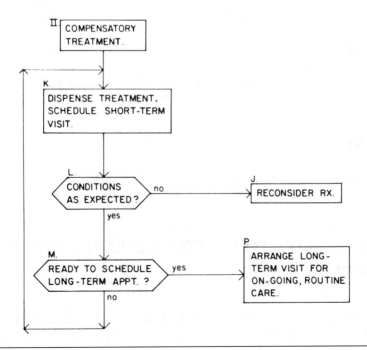

Figure 9.2 Compensatory treatment.

K. DISPENSE TREATMENT, SCHEDULE SHORT-TERM VISIT

In some cases, there is but one compensatory treatment; in others, there may be a number of options. In the latter, it is important to include the patient in the decision process. They will be the users, after all. Once the treatment has been dispensed (or put into effect in those cases where the treatment involves communication with school teachers and others), arrange for the patient to return within a relatively short period of time (see L in Figure 9.2 flow diagram and below).

L. CONDITION AS EXPECTED?

Ordinarily, the compensatory treatment accomplishes what it was expected to accomplish, but not always. It is useful to confirm expectations by means of a follow-up visit.

□ If Yes

Determine the need for additional short-term visits (see M in Figure 9.2 flow diagram and below).

□ If No

Reconsider the original recommendation (see J in Figure 9.2 flow diagram).

M. READY TO SCHEDULE LONG-TERM APPOINTMENT?

The long-term appointment is scheduled when there is evidence that the compensatory treatment is fulfilling its designated purpose. In some cases, this is easy to determine (e.g., when the correct compensatory lens prescription has been given to the five-diopter hyperope); in some cases it is not (e.g., the previously mentioned adolescent with perceptual skills dysfunction).

□ If Yes

Do so (see P in Figure 9.2 flow diagram).

□ If No

Continue short-term visits (see K in Figure 9.2 flow diagram and above).

■
III. REASSURANCE THERAPY

Reassurance therapy is dispensed when the clinical data indicate that (a) the patient's concerns are unfounded or (b) the patient's concerns are justified, but the clinical data show that action is not called for at this time; the disease is benign (4) (see Figure 9.3).

In addressing the question: *What to say to symptomatic patients with benign diseases?"* Sapira defines six steps:

1. *Elicit a detailed description of the symptoms.* This is usually accomplished as the case history is acquired.
2. *Elicit the affective meaning of the symptoms;* i.e., the kinds of feelings that are associated with the symptoms. Such feelings are communicated not only in

---

Figure 9.3
Reassurance therapy.

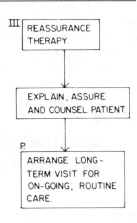

words, but also in nonverbal ways that indicate the patient's unstated anxieties and fears (e.g., tone of voice, manner of speech, posture). Sapira suggests that to insure achieving this second step, the clinician should make a direct request: "Tell me more about the way this worries you." He also suggests that the query be followed by silence so that the patient has time to think before responding.

3. *Examine the patient.* Sapira points out that the "laying on of hands" increases the effectiveness of subsequently stated opinions.

4. *Make a diagnosis,* and just as important, state what was ruled out; i.e., *what it is not.*

5. *Explain the pathophysiology of the symptoms.* More important than making clear the technical aspects of the examination and test outcomes, the patient should be made to recognize that:

    a. The clinician understands the origin of the symptoms.

    b. The clinician, although concerned about the patient as a person, is not worried, anxious or frightened by the symptoms.

    c. The clinician is sympathetic. In effect, she gives the patient "permission" to have the symptoms and, indeed, to present with them again if need be.

6. *Reassure the patient.* For example, in a case of irreversible strabismus, the patient/parent should be assured (if it is the case) that:

    a. A problem (e.g., strabismus) has been diagnosed.

    b. The problem is not trivial, but neither is it actively threatening.

    c. There is no value in initiating a treatment program *at this time,* because:

    (1) treatment will be ineffective, or

    (2) treatment will be too demanding for the patient. ("The cure will be worse than the disease.")

    d. There is no significant risk in "leaving well enough alone" at this time.

    e. The patient should return in _____months, the goal then to reassess the situation.

In brief, the optometrist seeks to assure the patient that (a) she—the optometrist—knows that a problem exists; (b) her recommendations are the best that can be made at this time; (c) conditions change over time, and new treatments come along once in a while; hence, assessment should be repeated at some specifically identified future date.

This entire process requires very little time. It is far more important than the time and effort it consumes would indicate.

INFORMING A PATIENT/PARENT OF "BAD NEWS"

In some situations, the patient/parent will have to be given bad news, which can range from advising that the child's cognitive deficits appear to derive from central nervous system involvement and are immutable, to informing that the child appears to have a sight- (or even life-) threatening condition. In such instances, the optometrist must do more than simply inform. She must plan how that information will be delivered, recognizing the emotional trauma it will cause. Klein and Klein, in a recently published report (5), suggest the following:

- Avoid using "protective" euphemisms when discussing the condition; use specific terminology.
- Try to help the patient understand the condition so that they may begin to carry out the proper steps that should follow; suppressing the emotions consumes much psychic energy and does little good.
- Try to encourage the patient to verbalize their distress and worry.
- Some patients become angry at these times about their fate. Encourage them to express that anger, explaining that it is a reasonable emotion under such circumstances. Repression of the anger is likely to result in depression.
- Try to identify key support people (family/friends) who will be available to help the patient and the clinician in the mourning and rehabilitation processes that are to come.
- Try to help the patient/parent identify counseling resources and self-help groups, to be called upon as needed.

IV. REFER FOR CONSULTATION

The general goal of a referral is to obtain the opinion of someone who is competent to diagnose and treat a condition that the optometrist has detected. In all cases, it is the obligation of the optometrist who recommends the consultation to assist her patient in selecting the individual who will provide that consultation.

N. CONSULTATION ACCOMPLISHED; DIAGNOSIS MADE; TREATMENT RECOMMENDED; REPORT RECEIVED; COUNSEL PATIENT

No explanation is needed, other than to point out that recommending a consultation does not remove the referring clinician from the scene. On the contrary, she should continue to play an important role in the process. Many patients depart from a consultation visit confused and anxious, uncertain about what they heard and too intimidated to ask questions. The optometrist, as the primary-care clinician in the case, owes her patient the explanation and advice they need in order to make correct decisions.

■

O. PATIENT'S NEEDS SATISFIED?

☐ **If Yes**

Arrange for long-term visit (see P in Figure 9.4 flow diagram).

☐ **If No**

Reconsider the initial recommendation (see J in Figure 9.4 flow diagram).

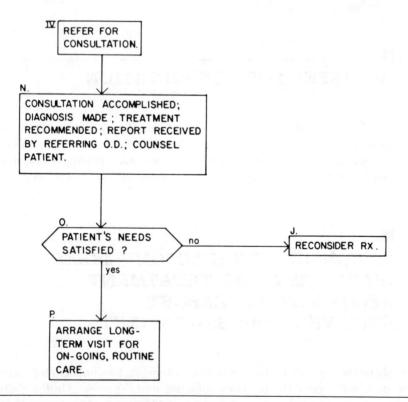

Figure 9.4   Refer for consultation.

■

PRACTICAL SUGGESTIONS

9-1. It is usually best to avoid using technical terms when communicating with parents about the outcomes of an examination. There is no need to provide a short course in optometry. It is also advisable to instruct your office assistants in how to explain the various conditions that present in an optometric practice. The following are offered as suggestions:

When discussing refractive status, lay persons are usually better able to understand 'myopia,' 'hyperopia,' and 'astigmatism,' if they are described functionally; e.g.:

"The '*near-sighted*' or myopic eye has *too much* built-in optical power for its size; as a result, it is in focus for near objects and blurred for things in the distance—somewhat like trying to see far away through a magnifying glass. Nearsighted persons therefore need lenses that reduce some of the eye's focusing *power*—concave or "minus" lenses."

"The '*far-sighted*' or hyperopic eye has insufficient built-in optical power, not as much as it needs, for its size, to see clearly at distance. But normally, young persons have the ability to overcome this deficiency by using extra power obtained from the focusing muscles that are inside their eyes—muscles they ordinarily should use only when looking at something up close. This enables them to see clearly at distance without glasses, but it creates a different problem when they then have to do some desk work or read. This requires that they place extra demands on those focusing muscles—again, something they often can do, but not without cost: fatigue, discomfort, etc. It is much like having to carry about a twenty-five-pound weight all day long. You can probably manage it, but you will certainly feel the weight and demonstrate the effects as the day goes by. For this reason, farsighted children need lenses that *add* focusing *power* to the eye—convex or 'plus' lenses."

"The *astigmatic eye* is an eye in which the front surface (the cornea) is 'out of shape'; something like what you would have if you squeezed a round ball (the 'optimal shape' of the front of the eye) from top to bottom, or from side to side, so that is was egg-shaped rather than round. This, of course, causes some of the rays of light that come into the eye to be out of focus, like looking through a cylindrical (long and narrow) drinking glass. Eyesight may be blurred, but not always; it depends upon the amount of distortion. Sometimes, if the astigmatism is not too great, the eye may have enough extra focusing power available to focus these rays as well; but when it does that, the opposite direction rays go out of focus. This causes the focusing muscles of the eye to work extra hard, shifting back and forth, focusing one set of light rays and then the other, but never the two at the same time. As a result: fatigue, headaches, and other discomfort symptoms. The astigmatic eye needs a lens that is *stronger in one direction than it is in the other,* so that all light rays are in focus at the same time—a 'cylindrical' lens."

When discussing binocular status and function with a parent, remember that lay persons are more apt to understand the terms accommodation and vergence, if they are described behaviorally, as follows:

"The normal eye has two sets of muscles. One set controls *direction:* where the eyes are 'aimed' or 'pointed'; up, down, to the left, right, at something close up, far way, and so on. The other set controls the *focusing power* of the eyes. A properly performing eye has just the right amount of 'built-in' optical power so that when these focusing muscles are relaxed, things far away (farther away than 20 feet) will be seen clearly; no extra muscle effort will be required. Seeing close up, however, will require this extra focusing power; reading, for example. Hence, the focusing muscles adjust the power of the eye for different distances. It is much like using a pair of binoculars. You have to 'aim' them and then turn the knob to focus what you are looking at to make it clear."

"The aiming muscles and the focusing muscles are linked together as a reflex. When one set goes to work or relaxes, so does the other, automatically. When you look at something up close, the aiming muscles turn the eyes 'in' so that they line up precisely on what you want to look at, and the focusing muscles provide just the correct amount of extra power needed to see it clearly. Then, when you decide to look at something far away, the aiming muscles pull the eyes into proper orientation and the focusing muscles relax (thereby reducing the power of the eyes) so that the distant object will be clear— presuming that the relaxed eye is in focus for distance; that it is not nearsighted, farsighted, or astigmatic."

"This reflex hook-up between the focusing and aiming muscles gets out of balance sometimes. When that happens, the eyes do not automatically aim at and focus for the same distance. The result: if the two functions—focusing and aiming—are not too far out of balance, the eyes continue to look normal but the child experiences lots of eyestrain. Glasses (to readjust the balance) and/or vision therapy (to teach the child how to cope with the imbalance), will usually remedy the situation."

"If the condition is left untreated, and if the two functions are significantly out of balance, the eyes may go out of alignment (intermittently or constantly) so that only one eye aims accurately while the other turns in (toward the nose) or out (away from the nose). This not only makes the child 'look different'; it also produces double vision, unless one eye stops working. In young children, it is the latter that usually happens; this is called 'suppression,' and if the cause is not eliminated, amblyopia—a lazy eye— will result." (But that is another subject; see below.)

When discussing vision training for patients with accommodation-convergence deficits (e.g., vergence or accommodation infacility, intermittent strabismus, constant strabismus that derives from innervational dysfunction), the above discussion about accommodation and vergence is effectively followed up by:

"Your child's ocular focusing and aiming muscles are not weak. Each set works very well, *on its own*. The problem lies in the fact that they do not work well *together*—they do not coordinate. Therefore, the therapy we recommend does not imply 'muscle building.' Rather, it will be devoted to improving binocular coordination—'teaching' his ocular aiming and focusing muscles to work together in a more accurate and efficient manner. It is much like the beginning, not-so-good golfer who becomes a good golfer by taking lessons and practicing what he is taught. His muscles really do not get any stronger; rather, he learns to *use* them in a more accurate, efficient manner. It is essential, therefore, that the activities we prescribe be engaged in regularly, and practiced to the point where they are something that the child can do automatically—without thinking. Only then can we expect the kind of results we seek."

You should demonstrate the difference between "weak muscles" and "binocular coordination." Show the parent how readily the child can accurately fixate at a distant or near object with either eye, as long as the opposite eye is covered; but not so readily when both are open. (This is easiest to demonstrate with children whose nearpoint of convergence is receded. Simply occlude the child's one eye and have him look nasally with the other; then move the occluder to the opposite eye.)

When discussing the use of bifocals as a method for managing myopia, consider the following:

> "Your child is nearsighted—i.e., her eyes are too strong; they have too much built-in optical power. Therefore, when she looks at something across the room, it is similar to what you experience when you look at something far away through a magnifying glass. The magnifying glass provides too much power for that distance. Hence, with the magnifying glass, you too are nearsighted."
>
> "Your youngster needs glasses only for distance—far off. She sees very clearly, without strain and without glasses, when she reads or does other activities that are within arm's reach. Hence, she is best off if she uses glasses for distance viewing only, doing close work without glasses."
>
> "But it is not reasonable to think that she will successfully deal with the obligation of putting on her glasses when she looks at the chalkboard or her teacher, then taking them off when she looks at something close up. This would be a real nuisance to her; she would have little time during the school day to do anything else but put on and take off her glasses. The solution: Lenses that provide her with good distance vision, yet are not too strong for near work. In short, bifocals. This does not imply that your child has the 'eyes of an older person.' On the contrary, in the typical bifocal of a person over 40, the upper (or 'distance') portion of the lens is weaker than the lower ('reading') portion. The type of bifocal we are recommending for your child is just the opposite; the lower portion of the lens is much 'weaker' than the upper. This will enable her to read and do other close work with her glasses in place."

When discussing amblyopia, stress that the condition rarely progresses, that the child is not in danger of 'going blind.' Rather, explain that amblyopia is the outcome of deprivation of clear sight, produced by strabismus, anisometropia, and/or marked bilateral ametropia that went unattended for too long. One useful analogy:

> "Amblyopia results from lack of use; it is similar to what would happen to your hand if you kept it in your pocket for a prolonged period of time. It would lose its capacity to function in a precise manner; it would not be 'rested'; on the contrary, it would be impaired. Similarly, if an eye does not experience clear sight for a prolonged period of time—and the younger the child, the shorter that period of time—it will lose its capacity to function in a precise manner; it, too, will not be 'rested'; it will be impaired."

9-2. *Written reports.* Because developmental lags/anomalies have such pervasive effects, written reports to other professionals are often a necessary follow-up. In many of these cases, the recipient will be a teacher, counselor, or principal in the child's school, but it also is not uncommon to communicate with a psychologist, the child's physician, and others. Such reports need not be long, exhaustive, and jargon-laden. They serve best when they present the pertinent information in as clear and succinct a way as possible.

A written communication should reflect the individual who produces it. Prepackaged reports may not do that; but it often helps the inexperienced report writer to have an idea about how others communicate, if only to get started on developing her own methods and styles. We therefore offer the following examples. The first is a structured, preprinted form in which the optometrist simply fills in the blanks, crosses out the inappropriate words, and adds a few personalized words (see Figure 9.5); the second is less structured, although its format does follow a specific organization that is explained below and illustrated in Chapter 16.

Vision Evaluation Report Form. The Visual Evaluation Report Form might very well be used for *every* young patient who presents in the optometrist's office, not just those who display a problem of one sort or another. It requires very little time and effort to prepare, and it serves the optometrist as a communication device as well as indicator of her interest in providing comprehensive professional services to children, including an assessment of their perceptual skills.

Notice that there is space for remarks at the bottom of the form. The following is typical of what might appear in that space:

> "In our opinion, Joe's learning difficulties do not stem from an ocular or sight problem, but *are* related to his visual perceptual skills deficits. Hence, we recommend that he (a) engage in activities specifically designed to improve his visual perceptual skills and (b) be provided with instructional conditions that take his perceptual skills deficits into account. Both approaches will help him perform better in school and, as the effects of the former become evident, the requirements of the latter will ease."
>
> "We are available for telephone consultation, should additional discussion/information be desired."

Personalized reports. Personalized reports require more effort than the preprinted form discussed above, but they need not be too demanding if a structured format is followed. The reports shown in Chapter 16 (filed for Patients 2, 9, 12, and 13, respectively) all follow the same organization, even though they deal with different conditions and recommendations.

Each of these reports commences with a paragraph that identifies the parent's stated chief concern and some pertinent information regarding the child's early general health and development.

The second paragraph centers on ocular health and visual functions: eyesight, refractive status, binocular status, and so on.

This is followed by a paragraph that reports the child's developmental status—perceptual skills with school-aged children; performance on the DDST with preschool youngsters.

The report then concludes with a summarization that leads to a diagnosis and treatment recommendations. Obviously, these could very well have been made

VISION EVALUATION REPORT

Patient _____ Date(s) of visit (s) _____

The following is a highly condensed summary. Additional and/or more detailed information is available.

OCULAR STATUS: Currently does/does not wear spectacles or contact lenses.

VISUAL ACUITY:	at distance;	at near:
Without Rx	Right eye _____	Right eye _____
	Left eye _____	Left eye _____
	Both eyes _____	Both eyes _____
With present Rx	Right eye _____	Right eye _____
	Left eye _____	Left eye _____
	Both eyes _____	Both eyes _____

OCULAR HEALTH: Evidence of disease and/or abnormality was/was not observed.
REFRACTION: A new spectacle prescription is/is not indicated.
BINOCULAR STATUS: The two eyes do/do not "team" adequately.
FUSIONAL AND ACCOMMODATIVE RANGES: Are/are not within expected limits.
PERCEPTUAL SKILLS: Visual: At/below expected level
                   Auditory: At/below expected level

RECOMMENDATIONS:
___ no action indicated
___ spectacles for: __ constant wear __ distance only __ reading only
___ vision training
___ referred to _____ for consultation and additional testing
___ additional testing in this clinic
___ other (see below)

COMMENTS:

Figure 9.5 Vision evaluation report.

longer and more detailed. But, for all practical purposes, there is no need, nor justification, for elaboration.

9-3. Develop a list of professionals to whom you may wish to refer patients; e.g., internist, neuroophthalmologist, pediatrician, psychologist, communication disorder specialist, tutor, etc. Obviously, you should keep this list current, adding new names as you learn of them and their respective professional competencies, and deleting those who have not served your patients as you would wish. Remember, a referral is no less a prescription than any other recommendation you may offer.

9-4. When offering recommendations regarding glasses or when dispensing home-based vision therapy for a young child, consider informing the youngster that when her parent insists that she wear her glasses, or when they administer a vision therapy session at home, it is not because they—her parents—wish to do it but because you—her optometrist—insist that it be done. We sometimes give the youngster one of our business cards and suggest that should she wish to register a complaint, she is to telephone us instead of complaining to her parent. There are instances where this is a very effective strategy.

■

REFERENCES

1. Gagne R. The conditions of learning. 2nd ed. New York: Holt, Rinehart and Winston, 1970.
2. Rosner J, Rosner J. Vision therapy in a primary care practice. New York: Professional Press, 1988.
3. Glaser R, Rosner J. Adaptive environments for learning: curriculum aspects. In: Talmage H, ed. Systems of individualized education. Berkeley, Calif.: McCutchau Publishing Corp., 1975. National Society for the Study of Education.
4. Sapira JD. Reassurance therapy: what to say to symptomatic patients with benign disease. Mimeograph, Birmingham, Ala., 1979.
5. Klein SD, Klein, RE. Delivering bad news: the most challenging task in patient education. JAOA 1987; 58(8):660–663.

10

Ametropia

□

The clinical management of ametropia customarily involves a compensatory treatment. It is the method of choice for most optometrists in most cases. Determining the lens prescription that will improve visual acuity to an optimal level is a clearcut task, and the effects of that improved acuity are apt to be immediately evident and gratifying, even when the patient is very young—chronologically or developmentally (1).

A remedial approach, when attempted, is likely to be multifaceted. It might involve the use of lenses, vision training activities, a visual hygiene regimen, sight-improvement exercises, reshaping or restructuring a portion of the globe, and an assortment of other practices.

■

MYOPIA

□ Compensatory Treatment

Once the decision to use compensatory lenses has been made, the central question becomes *when*, at what age should compensatory lenses be prescribed? In recent years, with recognition of the impact of early visual experiences on the subsequent development of the visual system (2,3,4,5), the tendency has been to recommend lens application for the very young.

This has not been emphasized quite so much for the young myope, however. The major effect of uncorrected myopia is reduced visual acuity at farpoint. Unless the myopia is exceptionally great and/or significantly different in the two eyes, the child will have many episodes of precise, clear visual resolution, albeit at a very close range. This is sufficient to prevent erosion of her capacity to discriminate high spatial frequencies. Early application of lenses is therefore not so critical in such cases. The child will display good visual acuity at distance when she is supplied with the proper lenses, regardless of how early or late they are prescribed and how steadily she wears them. Parents should not be led to believe otherwise.

Obviously, the optometrist will also have to be mindful of such factors as the child's awareness of and interest in her environment beyond the very close range, and her ability to interact effectively with people and objects in that environment. If her impaired eyesight seems to be creating difficulties in these aspects of her development, then lenses should be prescribed and their importance stressed.

When lenses are prescribed, should they represent a "full correction"? Should they fully compensate the myopia? If the goal is clear visual acuity and if the optometrist has no reason to consider factors that relate to halting the progression of myopia (see below), then compensatory lenses that provide 20/20 visual acuity at distance should be prescribed. These may be designed either as spectacles or as contact lenses, although the latter usually create too many management problems to make them worthwhile for the young patient.

□ Controlling the Progression of Myopia

LENSES

Most myopes are not born myopic (6). Most myopes are not myopic when they enter school at the age of 6 (7). The picture begins to change, however, during the elementary school years. With each grade, more children show the first signs of myopia, and a significant proportion of those who already were myopic show an increase in refractive error (8).

The progression of myopia has been a clinical concern for well over a century. Cohn (9) was among the first to point out a connection between the degree of myopia among school-aged children and their grade level, and to speculate on the powerful influence of reading. Over the years, many others have taken up support of this notion, but none has succeeded in providing sufficient evidence to validate unequivocally the relationship between reading and myopia.

At the root of this, of course, is the fact that the etiology of myopia has never been established. Today, the most popular and enduring theories cluster under one of three general headings: genetic, use-abuse, or a combination of the two (see Chapter 5). All three have their advocates, although currently the proposition that both nature and nurture are influential as joint forces, neither being the exclusive determinant, appears to be gaining more followers.

Those who subscribe to the notion that genetics is the sole determinant of refractive status do not concern themselves with ways to control the course of myopia. They assume a fatalistic attitude, usually going on to point out that a little myopia is not such a bad thing, since it allows the presbyope to read without glasses; and besides, they remind us (especially if they themselves are myopic), myopes have been shown to be more intelligent, better students, higher achievers, and so on (10,11,12).

The use-abuse group argues vigorously that myopia is caused by excessive sustained near work. Therefore, they reason, it can be controlled if proper steps are taken, and it is worth doing because myopia is not an inconsequential condition. At this point in the discussion, they are inclined to cite the data regarding retinal detachment among myopes as compared with nonmyopes; and those data are impressive (13).

The third group bridges the two propositions. Myopia, they argue, is the outcome of an interaction between certain genetic influences in combination with certain environmental factors, including nutrition, systemic health, and excessive close work. A number of recent investigations seem to add some support to their arguments, if only by implication. For example, it has recently been shown that myopes tend to display lower levels of tonic accommodation than do emmetropes and hyperopes, and that within the myopic population, those who did not manifest their ametropia until after the age of 15 ("late-onset myopia") have lower levels of tonic accommodation than those who became myopic earlier in life (14,15). In addition, myopes have been found to demonstrate a greater degree of accommodative hysteresis than do hyperopes and are slower in returning to their baseline levels (16). This information, in conjunction with evidence that the sympathetic nervous system does have an influence on the accommodative tonic state (17,18), tends to provide substance to the notion that, for some myopes at least, lens prescriptions should be designed in a way that takes these differences into consideration.

A variety of methods has been suggested for controlling the progression of myopia with lenses. Since the use-abuse theory centers on near work, it is not surprising that accommodation and/or convergence are often identified as the key factors in proper clinical management. This has spawned a number of hypotheses, all of which stress the importance of controlling the demands on accommodation and/or convergence. But they vary in approach; from overcorrection, to full correction, to undercorrection, to undercorrection only at nearpoint.

Full Correction
Donders himself was a supporter of this approach (19). Early in this century, Straub (20) published some data to support the hypothesis that full correction of myopia halted progression. The data were not convincing. The approach has not attracted many supporters, although a report relevant to that theme does appear occasionally.

Overcorrection
Goss investigated the potential benefits of overcorrecting myopia in order to slow the rate of progression (21). He identified 72 myopic subjects, ranging in age from 7 to 15 years. Half of these (18 males, 18 females) constituted the experimental group; the other half, the control group. Subjects in the two groups were matched according to sex, beginning (of myopia) age, beginning refractive error, and duration of time covered by their case records. The experimental group wore lenses that overcorrected their myopia by 0.75D. The control group wore full, single vision corrections. Outcomes indicated that the rates of progression for the two groups were not significantly different.

Undercorrection
(With or without base-in prism.) Undercorrection of myopia is sometimes suggested in connection with base-in prism, sometimes not.

The rationale for the base-in prism is that it reduces the need for convergence during close work (22). This is not only desirable for its own sake, but also because it reduces the stimulus to accommodation that would be present if full convergence were exercised.

The rationale for undercorrecting myopia is obvious: the patient is spared the need to accommodate fully while doing near work. There is also a drawback, however: Undercorrection results in less than 20/20 visual acuity at farpoint, something that may not annoy the patient (who, after all, presumably sees far better through her undercorrecting lenses than without lenses), but often does annoy school nurses, teachers, parents, and others who may informally assess the child's farpoint visual acuity and become concerned because it is not what it "should be."

Bifocals

Application of the bifocal lens was seen as a sensible solution to the inherent drawbacks of undercorrection. With it, full correction and 20/20 visual acuity could be supplied for farpoint, and the nearpoint prescription could be modified without causing inconvenience.

This approach has its advocates (23,24), its opponents, and a good number in between who are skeptical but willing to be convinced. As usual, the arguments of the extreme groups are based more on "theory"—more correctly, on rationalizing—than on solid data.

Among those who support the use of bifocals as a means for controlling the progression of myopia, Young has persisted the longest. He has published a number of studies regarding the development and the control of myopia in monkeys (and chimpanzees) and humans (24,26,27). He argues that the stretched globe of the myope is produced by sustained elevated intraocular pressure, which, in turn, is generated by sustained accommodation from prolonged near work. In this respect, he reports a study wherein bifocals (ranging from adds of +1.00 to +1.50 diopters) were found to reduce the annual rate of progression to 1/20 of a diopter, while those subjects who were not wearing bifocals progressed at an annual rate of a little over 0.50 diopter (28). Goss lends some support to this notion. In a retrospective study of the effect of bifocal lenses on the rate of childhood myopia progression, he observed that myopic esophores who wore bifocals (i.e., reduced minus at near) had a slower mean rate of progression than did single vision wearers (29).

Holding opposite views, Mandell (30) and Baldwin (31)—as cited by Borish (32)—examined the records of optometrists who sometimes used bifocals and sometimes did not, and concluded that bifocals do not appear to slow the progression of myopia.

Most recently, Grosvenor et al reported on the outcome of a longitudinal study designed to test the efficacy of bifocal lenses for the control of juvenile myopia (33). Each of 124 children, between the ages of 6 and 15 years, wore either single vision lenses, a +1.00D add, or a +2.00D add for a period of 3 years. They observed no significant between-group differences in refractive changes over that period of time.

Contact Lenses

The initial method of fitting hard corneal lenses was to use a lens with a relatively flat base curve—at or slightly less than the flattest corneal meridian. The effect of this, if the measurements were made not long after the lens was removed, was a flattening of the cornea and reduction in the amount of measurable myopia. This led certain early investigators to postulate that hard corneal lenses prevented or, at the least, retarded increases in myopia (34,35,36,37,38,39). Longitudinal studies have not supported this hypothesis. No such claims have been made for soft contact lenses. In fact, one report indicates small increases in myopia following soft contact lens wear (40).

Summary Comments Regarding the Control of Myopia with Lenses

The argument over the control of the course of myopia through the manipulation of the lens prescription goes on. The skeptics scoff. The believers believe and sometimes publish reports that profess their faith. They see value in what they prescribe for their patients, and accept this as substantive evidence, ignoring the scientific principles that have to be satisfied if the evidence is to convince those who do not share their faith.

There is a clear need for continued scientific inquiry. The notion that the course of myopia is influenced at least to some degree by the amount of close work a patient engages in is not absurd. Many optometrists are convinced of a cause-effect link between prolonged close work and myopia. The empirical evidence provided by their patients is too compelling to ignore, and the implications of the above-cited reports regarding dual innervation to the ciliary muscle, and differences in tonic accommodation between hyperopes, emmetropes, and early- and late-onset myopes seems to lend support to their speculations.

How this new information will eventually translate clinically, if it does in fact hold up, is hard to predict. It seems to us that what has been learned regarding the innervation of the ciliary muscle and the apparent influence of that on tonic accommodation, accommodative hysteresis, CA/C, AC/A, and the effect of cognitive effort on those functions hints at something promising. One could reason, as van Alphen did (see Chapter 5), that the child whose ciliary muscles have low tonicity *and* who has the cognitive abilities and temperament to do well in school is subject to myopia because of at least two reasons: (a) when her ciliary muscles are at rest, her sclerae are more vulnerable to stretching than are eyes with ciliary muscles of normal or high tonicity; (b) when engaging in close work—and such children usually do lots of close work—she experiences excessive accommodative hysteresis (i.e., she is prone to greater accommodative aftereffects than are emmetropes and hyperopes) and does not relax accommodation as rapidly as nonmyopic children when she ceases the nearpoint activity. This generates an increase in her tonic vergence state—esophoria—which serves to exacerbate the accommodative hysteresis. All of this, in the aggregate, may provide the visual centers that influence the emmetropization process with inconsistent information: The excessive accommodation and hysteresis during near work may be "read" as a signal that the eyes should increase in axial length, with a "pseudo-emmetropia" (and stability) being registered when the tonic state of the (uncorrected) myopic eye simulates that of the normal emmetropic eye—that is, when the uncorrected myopic eye is required to accommodate no more (from its baseline "resting state") than normal emmetropic eyes (with normal ciliary tonicity) when engaged in a nearpoint task. This status, of course, is obtained only after the myopia has increased a substantial amount without a change in lenses. Then, because acuity has dropped, another vision examination takes place, an increase in concave lens power is prescribed, and the cycle commences again—continuing until the eyes lose sufficient plasticity to stop increasing in length.

We acknowledge that much of this is fuzzy speculation, but empirical evidence makes it "feel" correct. For this reason, we suggest that serious consideration be given to the use of reduced lens powers for near work—i.e., bifocals—especially for the myopic children with esophoria. (See Practical Suggestion 9-1 for one way of explaining to a parent why a bifocal might be prescribed for a myopic child.)

OTHER METHODS OF CONTROLLING MYOPIA PROGRESSION

Visual Hygiene

Many young myopes are inclined to position themselves very close to the book or desk surface when they read or write. This has led many optometrists to recommend to those patients that they (a) maintain reasonably erect posture while doing near work (e.g., sit up, book on lap, good illumination); (b) take frequent rest periods during nearpoint activities (e.g., look at some distant point after every paragraph or page); (c) maintain awareness of peripheral visual fields; i.e., avoid restricting attention to the near task, ignoring all else.

Such notions are not new. Cohn, mentioned above as a pioneer in relating prolonged close work with myopia, proposed a chinrest type of device to be used when reading, so as to guarantee correct posture (41). He also incriminated bad lighting and inadequate ventilation.

Others have added to this list: "Myopia progresses because of exposure to too much light" (42). "Myopia is caused by too much strenuous physical effort" (43). And so on. Each of these was linked with an antidotal treatment, with some kind of apogee achieved when it was suggested that " . . . since close work produces myopia," the traditional school should be abolished; instruction should be mediated by touch and sound instead of sight (44).

It is difficult to argue against visual hygiene—except, perhaps, for the suggestion regarding the mode of schooling. After all, what reasonable argument can be made against good lighting, proper ventilation, and so on? None of these, however, has been shown to have any significant direct impact on myopia—its development or its subsequent course. Therefore, if a regimen of visual hygiene is recommended, it should be done in a way that does not delude the patient or her parents into expecting much in the way of remediation.

Vision Training

Vision training is sometimes recommended as a means for controlling the course of myopia (45,46). As one investigator characterizes it, the goal of the therapy is "to create a more efficient visual system which can more easily withstand stress" (47). Therapy regimens typically include monocular and binocular accommodative rock procedures that are intended to improve the patient's facility in exercising and inhibiting accommodation independent of vergence (see Chapter 14 for descriptions of procedures).

Once again, there is insufficient evidence available to assess the efficacy of these regimens. The optometrists who employ them do so because they believe that they are effective. That is not the equivalent of scientific validation, but neither should it be arbitrarily dismissed.

Drugs

A number of investigators have examined the effects of drugs, especially cycloplegia, on the course of myopia (48,49,50,51,52,53). Although their outcomes and conclusions vary, the majority opinion is that "atropine and tropicamide have been found to affect the evolution of the disease [myopia] favorably . . . but . . . the improvements are small" (55). Most of these studies also involve methodological difficulties that force one to temper the enthusiasm with which they interpret the results.

A host of other drugs (in addition to atropine and tropicamide) have also been found to have "some beneficial effect" on the progression of myopia. These include phenylephrine hydrochloride, pilocarpine, autonomic blocking agents, pituitary hormone, calcium chondroitin, and various vitamins (54).

DIET

Diet and myopia have been the subject of speculation and investigation for at least the past 50 years. Myopia has been linked with calcium deficiency (56), insufficient consumption of animal protein (57), excessive sugar and bread intake (58), and simply the lack of a balanced diet (59). Thus far, there has been insufficient evidence provided to support any of these hypotheses.

ULTRASOUND

Yamamoto (60) advocates holding a small, ultrasonic device on the eye for brief periods during the day, purportedly to reduce "congestion of the eye." He does not provide any data to support his contentions.

CHINESE EYE EXERCISES

It has been reported that Chinese school children engage in daily eye exercises designed to prevent or reverse myopia (61). This involves short periods of massaging four acapuncture points located in the neck and face. This method has been described as very effective, but thus far, no reliable documentation is available.

☐ Remedial Therapy

VISUAL ACUITY TRAINING

This approach has attracted prophets and followers for many years (55). In addition to "ocular calisthenics," a psychological component is incorporated into the training. This may take the form of a "mental set" or "blur interpretation" or a hypnotically induced psychic effect.

Here again, there is a distinct lack of validation data, counterbalanced by a cluster of enthusiastic disciples.

BIOFEEDBACK

Another treatment method that has attracted some attention in recent years has been the use of biofeedback to teach myopic persons voluntary control of accommodation. One supporter of this method states " . . . biofeedback of accommodation treatment to reduce myopia is effective when used in combination with proper generalization techniques and seems to be long lasting" (62, p. 642). Gallaway et al appear to disagree. They reported that this same biofeedback technique resulted in slight improvements in visual acuity with some subjects, but "it is not clear whether the improvements were due to the biofeedback training alone, or to a learning effect observed during repeated measurements of visual acuity. There were no changes in refractive errors" (63, p. 62).

STRUCTURAL MODIFICATIONS OF THE GLOBE

A variety of methods have been developed for altering the refractive status of the eye by modifying one of its optical components: cornea, crystalline lens, axial length.

CORNEA: ORTHOKERATOLOGY

During the past few decades, many optometrists have observed that corneal contact lenses often alter corneal curvature (64,65,66,67). What has not been studied until more recently is the possibility of altering corneal curves precisely and permanently so that the patient's eyes could achieve a permanent emmetropic state.

Procedures have now been defined for that purpose. Orthokeratology, as the field is known, is too new to evaluate. Or, stated more correctly, there are too few studies available to make it possible for the interested, unbiased optometrist to determine whether the procedures are as harmless to the cornea and as permanently effective as their proponents claim. But, clearly, the notion is interesting and not farfetched.

SURGERY

A number of surgical methods have been reported. In general, they rarely are justified because of their complexity and the inherent risks of surgery; the treatment may be worse than the disease.

Surgeons have attempted to alter corneal curves (a) by injecting a silicone fluid lens into the cornea (68); (b) by removing a button from the anterior cornea, freezing it, reshaping it on a lathe, an then returning it as a flatter corneal surface (69); and (c) by making a series of very small incisions around the limbus of the cornea that, when healed, will cause the cornea to flatten. This procedure, known as radial keratotomy, was pioneered in Japan and Russia, and depends upon computer calculations to determine the location and nature of the incisions. It is reputed to be effective, but the data are not conclusive (70,71,72,73,74).

CRYSTALLINE LENS

Extraction of the crystalline lens will certainly have an immediate effect on the optics of the eye. In theory a 13- to 18-diopter myope will be emmetropic (or close to it) once the crystalline lens has been removed. Once again, however, the potential risks that accompany ocular surgery tend to counterbalance the potential benefits. The procedure is rarely used.

AXIAL LENGTH

Initially developed in Germany (75), the procedure involves shortening the globe by excising a ring of sclera and then rejoining the two hemispheres (76). It is an heroic treatment, justified in extreme cases only. A second, somewhat less radical procedure entails strengthening the posterior globe by surgically attaching strips of sclera to it (77).

■

PSEUDOMYOPIA

Duke-Elder (41) defines two types of pseudomyopia: (a) a functional increase in ciliary tonus that occurs intermittently, particularly after close work; (b) a prolonged and severe spasm of accommodation that in some cases has exceeded 20 diopters (see also [78]).

□ Compensatory Treatment

Compensatory lenses are usually contraindicated for pseudomyopia, except to the extent that the patient is ametropic independent of that pseudomyopia. Lenses to compensate for the ametropia are justified, especially for hyperopia.

☐ Remedial Therapy

LENS THERAPY

This is almost invariably effective with the first type of pseudomyopia referred to above, but significantly less successful with the second. In essence, the goal of lens therapy is to reduce ciliary tonus. Borish (32) lists three approaches: (a) fogging lenses for all distances; (b) plus lenses for near only; and (c) base-in prisms.

The first of these tends to be counterproductive. It is a rare adult patient who will voluntarily tolerate a constant blur; there is no reason to expect a child to be any more accepting.

The second treatment is feasible, particularly if the lenses are designed in bifocal form so that the glasses may be prescribed for full-time wear.

The third method, base-in prism, is also reasonable, unless it introduces fusional difficulties. An effective method for employing base-in prism is in conjunction with a bifocal. This is readily accomplished with a Fresnel prism.

The impact of lens therapy on a prolonged and severe spasm of accommodation is less satisfying. It may help, of course, but it is usually insufficient.

VISION TRAINING

The focus of vision training in the management of pseudomyopia is on accommodative facility, convergence facility, and the linkage between the two (see Chapter 14). It is often effective where the ciliary spasm is not severe.

DRUGS

Donders (19) took a vigorous postion in this respect, suggesting leeches as well as drugs. Today, only the latter are used, with atropine being the most frequently applied. (This assumes that the spasm is due to an overstimulation of the parasympathetic innervation to the ciliary muscle. If the spasm is due to reduced sympathetic stimulation, then the drug of choice would be a sympathomimetic such as epinephrine hydrochloride [79]).

PSYCHOTHERAPY

Pseudomyopia has often been linked to hysteria. In those cases, the optometrist should seek appropriate consultation.

---■————————————————————————————————

HYPEROPIA

☐ Compensatory Treatment

In contrast to myopia, it is important to prescribe compensatory lenses for the young hyperope, even when the amount of refractive error is moderate. This, for two reasons: (a) the detrimental effect of uncorrected hyperopia on the development of normal binocular vision; (b) the possible retarding effect of uncorrected hyperopia on the development of normal visual perceptual skills.

In regard to the former, Ingram and Walker (80), in a study involving 215 children, found that "the presence of 2 or more diopters of spherical hypermetropia in both eyes . . . was significantly associated with the child being identified two or more years later as having either squint or amblyopia or both" (p. 238). They then conclude " . . . these observations suggest that, in man, blurred vision caused by an uncorrected refractive error may be more important than an inborn neurological lesion in causing squint and/or amblyopia" (p. 241).

This position is not universally held, however. Other authorities state that "in general, equal hyperopic refractive errors in patients with straight eyes need no prescription, if the refractive error is under 3 or 4 diopters" (81, p. 29).

It seems evident that both arguments are valid to a degree. Not all young children with 2 diopters of hyperopia will subsequently display significant binocular anomalies. On the other hand, some will, and that is probably sufficient reason for the prudent optometrist to prescribe compensatory lenses in *all* such cases—knowing that his action are likely to be misconstrued and criticized by certain prejudiced and/or uninformed observers.

This does not imply that hyperopia of less than two diopters should be ignored. On the contrary, moderate amounts of uncorrected hyperopia may produce significant discomfort symptoms. In those instances, the same guidelines followed for adults should be followed for children. Specifically, if there is evidence that at least some of the patient's clinical signs and symptoms stem from uncorrected hyperopia, prescribe lenses. Indeed, even a very modest lens prescription, such as +0.75D spheres, may produce highly desirable effects in some cases.

In respect to the impact of uncorrected hyperopia on the development of normal visual perceptual skills, two reports pertain. In the one, it was shown that elementary school-aged, hyperopic (>2.00D) children are much more likely to manifest substandard visual analysis skills than are their emmetropic and myopic age-mates (82). Following up on this observation, it was also shown that the age at which hyperopic (>2.00D) children obtained their first glasses had a significant effect. In the sample of elementary school-aged children referred to above, there was a much smaller incidence of vision perceptual skills dysfunction among those who started to wear compensatory lenses before the age of four than among those who did not obtain their first glasses until after their fourth birthday (83).

□ Remedial Therapy

LENS THERAPY

Most children are born moderately hyperopic and become less hyperopic as they grow and develop. Few children, if any, develop hyperopia postnatally.

There are some reports that contradict this statement. Brown (84) reported a tendency for hyperopia to increase up to about the age of 8 years, but these data are confounded by the fact that a higher-than-normal percentage of the children included in the study were esotropes. This suggests, of course, that their hyperopia did not increase; rather, it shifted from a latent to a manifest status. And, even ignoring that factor, the amount of change in refractive error reported by Brown was small.

It comes down to this: (a) there does not appear to be a way to control the development and progression of hyperopia with lenses; (b) this is not a serious problem because hyperopia does not develop or progress. In other words, there is no easily managed cure, but then there is no disease, either.

SURGICAL

There have been some experimental surgical methods attempted in cases of high hyperopia. These include (a) the implantation of a plastic lens in the corneal stroma; (b) radial incisions in the corneal epithelium that are designed to cause the cornea to pucker as it heals, thereby increasing corneal curvature; (c) placement of a silicone band around the equator of the globe that is tight enough to constrict it and thereby elongate the eye.

None of these has been used sufficiently to comment on their value.

ASTIGMATISM

☐ Compensatory Treatment

Recent studies (see Chapter 5) indicate a much greater prevalence of unstable astigmatism among very young children than was once believed (85,86) and a tendency for the astigmatism to diminish when the child reaches age 2 years or thereabouts (87). It seems reasonable, therefore, to avoid prescribing compensatory lenses for young astigmats, at least until after they have celebrated their second birthday.

On the other hand, Ingram and Walker (80) identify 1.5 or more diopters of astigmatism in 1-year-olds as a significant predictor of subsequent amblyopia and Helveston and Ellis (81), cited above as conservatives in prescribing compensatory lenses for hyperopia, state, "It has been our practice to correct 1.5 diopters or more cylinder for most children" (p. 29).

What, then, is the correct recommendation for the young child (15 months old, say) with 1.5 diopters of astigmatism in each eye? The evidence seems to argue *for* prescribing compensatory lenses (88). Perhaps if the child were younger (9 months old, for example), then the argument would we weaker, all things considered—that is, not only the purported temporary nature of the astigmatism at that age, but also the management difficulties of keeping glasses on the baby's head. But, once the child passes the 15- to 18-month-old mark, management of glasses is no longer a major problem, especially when viewed against the alternative of a possible lifelong meridional amblyopia.

None of this precludes the prescribing of small amounts of cylinder for older children, where indicated. Similar to hyperopia, moderate amounts of uncorrected astigmatism may produce significant discomfort symptoms. Hence, the same guidelines cited in that section prevail here: If there is evidence that at least some of the patient's symptoms are related to uncorrected astigmatism, prescribe cylinders. There is no surefire way of prejudging.

□ Remedial Therapy

What was stated above about controlling the course of hyperopia may be rightfully repeated in regard to astigmatism. A number of children display astigmatism at birth and no astigmatism a year or two later. Beyond the second birthday, the rate of change is very slow. Moderate changes may be noted throughout the individual's life but, unlike myopia, it does not cause concern unless there is an active pathological component. So, to paraphrase and repeat, there is no cure, but neither is there much of a disease.

ANISOMETROPIA

□ Compensatory Treatment

The management of anisometropia does not seem to be a debatable issue. The general consensus is that anisometropia in the amount of one or more diopters in young children is significant; that neglect will have long-term impact (80,81,89,90,91). Full lens correction is usually recommended, but there are two qualifying concerns. First, an attempt should be made to determine the lens prescription that will support binocular vision; i.e., if possible, use binocular refraction procedures (see Chapter 5). Second, in establishing binocular vision, be watchful for anisekonia. In this regard, consider the relative merits of spectacles as compared with contact lenses and prescribe accordingly.

□ Remedial Therapy

Relatively few persons manifest significant anisometropia, although the condition does become more prevalent with age. (Criterion used to define significant anisometropia = a between-eye difference of one diopter or more.)

Hirsch (92) reported less than 1 percent prevalence among a group of 5- to 6-year-olds, with this rising to 2.4 percent among 13- to 14-year-olds. Blum, Bettman, and Peters, reporting on the Orinda study (93), corroborate Hirsch when they observe that the prevalence of anisometropia does increase very slowly with age, but the change never reaches statistical significance.

More recently, Hirsch (94) reported data from a group of children who were initially examined (Time 1) at the age of 5 to 7, and again (Time 2) at the age of 16 to 19. He found approximately 6 percent prevalence (21 out of 359) at Time 2. Twelve of the 21 had developed their anisometropia since Time 1, and one youngster no longer displayed the anisometropia at Time 2 that had been present at Time 1. He had "grown out of it."

Hence, although the numbers are not great, anisometropia apparently does develop. However, no accompanying therapeutic methods have been proposed. It appears, therefore, the guidelines for the therapeutic management of anisometropia are the same as for the compensatory approach: Prescribe what will enable the patient to obtain comfortable, clear, single, simultaneous binocular vision.

———■————————————————————————————————

PRACTICAL SUGGESTIONS

10-1. *Prescribing first glasses for a hyperopic child.* Prescribe full plus power (as determined by retinoscopy) for the hyperope who has never worn glasses before. This pertains not only to the very young, but also to school-aged hyperopic patients who often "reject" this amount of plus when tested subjectively—cases where prudence may suggest that something less than full plus be prescribed. Keep in mind that the retinoscope does not overestimate in the direction of plus; that the patient must be at least as hyperopic as the retinoscope indicates; and that prescribing insufficient plus may cause an increase in signs and symptoms.

For example, a child who shows high hyperopia (e.g., $+6.00$ or $+7.00$ D) with the retinoscope, yet "accepts" (subjectively) only about half of that power, is apt to display more difficulties with the partial lens prescription than she did before she obtained her first glasses. Some such children often do not attempt to accommodate without glasses, but will if they are given a partial prescription; e.g., $+3.50$D lenses. Thus, to the parent, the effect of the lenses will be to alter an apparently "comfortable," nonspectacle wearing child to one who experiences asthenopic symptoms; in fact, it is not inconceivable that this "straight-eyed" child will become an accommodative esotrope when she starts to wear the $+3.50$D lenses. Neither of these outcomes is desirable.

Do not worry too much about the blur persisting. The probabilities are exceptionally high that the blur produced by the lenses will disappear within the first day, *if* the child wears the glasses *and* moves about in normal style. Mobility facilitates adaptation. As she walks about, coming into contact with objects as she views them, the proprioceptive information provided by these actions will foster visual adaptation. The extent to which the child allows this to happen will, in turn, be determined by how effectively the optometrist explains to the child's parents the importance of her wearing the glasses even if, at the outset, they generate a blur.

As an extra precaution, consider instilling a drop of 1 percent cyclopentolate in each eye when the lenses are first dispensed. This should aid adaptation when blur persists because of accommodative spasm.

10-2. *Prescribing first glasses for an astigmatic child.* The same principles apply when prescribing cylinders for the first time. It is not unusual to have a child present for his first eye examination at age five or six, as the result of a school vision screening, demonstrating about 20/50 unaided visual acuity in each eye, and a refractive status of something like O.U.: $+4.50 \ -4.00$ cx 180. Lenses improve his visual acuity, but only somewhat, and the temptation is to reduce the power of the prescription, at least for the first lenses.

Do not succumb. Prescribe full lens power. If the child is to develop refined visual acuity, he needs to experience focused images on retina. If he does not have these experiences in the very near future, he will remain amblyopic (albeit moderately) for the rest of his life. A partial lens prescription will *not* provide him with focused images on the retina.

What is the likelihood that he will be disoriented by the high cylinder power? Very low, except perhaps for a very brief introductory period—*if* he is mobile. As mentioned above in regard to plus lenses, mobility will facilitate adaptation; sitting passively will not.

REFERENCES

1. Bader D. Performance changes in a young cerebral palsied child fitted with spectacles. Can J Opt 1979; 41(1):25–26.
2. Ikeda H, Tremaine KE, Einon G. Loss of spatial resolution of lateral geniculate nucleus neurons in kittens raised with convergent squint produced at different stages in development. Exp Brain Res 1978; 31:207.
3. Weisel TN, Hubel DH. Single cell responses in striate cortex of kittens deprived of vision in one eye. J Neurophys 1963; 26:1003.
4. Held R. Development of visual resolution. Can J Psych/Rev Canad Psychol 1979; 33(4):213.
5. Mitchell DE. Effect of early visual experience on the development of certain perceptual abilities in animals and man. In: Walk JD, Pick HJ Jr., eds. Perception and experience. New York: Plenum Publ., 1978.
6. Cook RC, Glasscock RE. Refractive and ocular findings in the newborn. Am J Ophthal 1951; 34:1407–13.
7. Sorsby A, Benjamin B, Davey JB, Sheridan M, Tanner JM. Emmetropia and its aberrations. London: Med. Res. Council Special Report Series, #93, 1957.

8. Hirsch M. The changes in refraction between the age of 5 and 14—theoretical and practical considerations. JAOA 1952; 29(9):445–59.

9. Cohn H. Untersuchen der augen von 10,060 schulkindern nebst vorsehlangen zur verbeswerung der augen nachteiligen schuleinrichtungl. Eineatiologische Studie. Leipzig, 1867.

10. Hirsch M. The relationship between refractive state of the eye and intelligence test scores. AAAO 1951; 36:12–21.

11. Young FA. Reading, measures of intelligence and refractive error. AAAO 1963; 40:257–64.

12. Grosvenor T. Refractive state, intelligence test scores and academic ability. AAAO 1970; 47:355–61.

13. Perkins EJ. Morbidity from myopia. Sightsaving Review Spring 1979, 11–19.

14. Bullimore MA, Gilmartin B. Aspects of tonic accommodation in emmetropia and late-onset myopia. AJOPO 1987; 64(7):499–503.

15. McBrien NA, Millodot M. The relationship between tonic accommodation and refractive error. Invest Ophthal Vis Sci 1987; 28:997–1004.

16. Ebenholtz SM. Accommodative hysteresis: Relation to resting focus. AJOPO 1985; 62(11):755–762.

17. Gilmartin B, Bullimore MA. Sustained near-vision augments inhibitory sympathetic innervation of the ciliary muscle. Clin Vis Sci 1987; 1:197–208.

18. Gilmartin B, Hogan RE. The role of the sympathetic nervous system in ocular accommodation and ametropia. Ophthal Physiol Opt 1985; 5(1):91–93.

19. Donders FC. On the anomalies of accommodation and refraction of the eye. Translated by WD Moore. London: The New Sydenham Society, 1864.

20. Straub M. Over de aetiologie der brekingsafwijkingen van het oog en den oorsprung der emmetropie. Nederlandische Tijdschrift voor Genesskunde. 1909. Eerste Helft, Nos. 7, 8, and 9:446, 533.

21. Goss DA. Overcorrection as a means of slowing myopic progression. AJOPO 1984; 61(2):85–93.

22. Hay M. Ophthalmoscope 12,20 (1914).

23. Young FA. Bifocal control of myopia. AJOPO 1975; 52:758.

24. Roberts WL, Banford RD. Evaluation of bifocal correction techniques in juvenile myopia. Opt Wkly 1967; 58(38):25–31, (39):21–30, (40):23, (41):27, (43):19.

25. Young FA. The effect of restricted visual space on the primate eye. AAAO 1961; 52(5):799.

26. Young FA. The effect of restricted visual space on the refractive error of the young monkey eye. Inv Ophthal 1963; 2(6):571.

27. Young FA. The transmission of refractive errors within Eskimo families. AAAO 1969; 46(9):676.

28. Oakley KH, Young FA. Bifocal control of myopia. AAAO 1975; 52(11):758.

29. Goss DA. Effect of bifocal lenses on the rate of childhood myopia progression. AJOPO 1986; 63(2):135–141.

30. Mandell RB. Myopia control with bifocal correction. AAAO 1959; 36(12):652.

31. Baldwin WR. Some relationships between ocular, anthropometric and refractive variables in myopia. Ph. D. dissertation (unpublished), Indiana University, 1964.

32. Borish IM. Clinical refraction. 3rd ed. Chicago: Professional Press, 1970.

33. Grosvenor T, Perrigin DM, Perrigin J, Maslovitz B. Houston myopia control study: a randomized clinical trial. Part II: Final report by the patient care team. AJOPO 1987; 64(7):482–98.

34. Barksdale CB. The attrition and control of myopia in some selected cases. Contacto 1960; 4:349.
35. Bier N. Myopia controlled by contact lenses: a preliminary report. Optician 1958; 135:427.
36. Carlson JJ. Basic factors on checking the progression of myopia. Opt J Rev Optom 1958; 95:37.
37. Otsuka J. Influence of contact lens on the causal mechanism of myopia. Orient Arch Ophthal 1968; 6:156.
38. Kelly TSB, Butler D. The present position of contact lenses in relation to myopia. Br J Ophthal 1971; 26:33.
39. Dobrec P. Influence of hard contact lenses on the progress of myopia. Klin Monatsbl Augenheilkd 1981; 181:355.
40. Barnett WA, Rengstorff RH. Adaptation to hydrogel contact lenses. variations in myopia and corneal curvature measurements. JAOA 1977; 48:363.
41. Duke-Elder S. Systems of ophthalmology. Vol. V. St. Louis: Mosby, 1970.
42. Junius Z. Augenheilk 1920; 44:262.
43. Edridge-Green. Lancet 1:469 (1921), 2:883, 3:1209 (1924).
44. Harman. Trans Ophthal Soc UK 1913; 33:202.
45. Harris DA. Accommodative-convergence control in myopia reduction. JAOA 1974; 45(3):292–96.
46. Hildreth HR et al. The effect of visual training on existing myopia. Trans Am Ac Ophthal Otolar March-April 1946; pp. 260–72.
47. Birnbaum MH. Management of the low myopia pediatric patient. JAOA 1979; 50(11):1281–89.
48. Gimbel HV. The control of myopia with atropine. Can J Ophthal 1973; 8:257.
49. Bedrossian RH. The effect of atropine on myopia. Annals Ophthal 1971; 3(8):891–97.
50. Abraham S. Control of myopia with tropicamide: a progress report. J Pediatr Ophthal 1966; 3(4):10–22.
51. Kelly TS, Chatfield C, Tristin G. Clinical assessment of the arrest of myopia. Br J Ophthal 1975; 59(10):529.
52. Vancea P. New concepts in the treatment of progressive myopia. Annals Ophthal 1971; 3(10):1105–1108.
53. Cress J, Maurice DM. An attempt at a chemical treatment of myopia. Arch Ophthal 1971; 86(6):692–93.
54. Curtin BJ. Myopia: a review of its etiology, pathogenesis and treatment, Surv Ophthal 1970; 15(1):1–17.
55. Bates WH. The Bates method for better eyesight without glasses. New York: Holt, Rinehart and Winston, 1981.
56. Walker JPS. Progressive myopia—a suggestion explaining its causation and for its treatment. Brit J Ophthal 1932; 16:485–88.
57. Gardiner PA. Dietary treatment of myopia in children. Lancet 1958; 1:1152–55.
58. Walkingshaw R. Control of progressive myopia through modification of diet. First International Conf on Myopia. Chicago: Professional Press, 1964.
59. Kappel KG. Myopia control and nutrition. Nutrition and Vision Series. Optom Ext Prog Papers 1980; 52:25–30.
60. Yamamoto Y. Ultrasonic treatment of acquired myopia. Gan 1964; 6:935.
61. Roy FH. Chinese eye exercises. J Ped Ophthal Strab 1980; 17(3):198–202.
62. Trachtman JN. Biofeedback of accommodation to reduce myopia. A review. AJOPO 1987; 64(8):639–43.

63. Gallaway M, Pearl SM, Winkelstein AM, Scheiman M. Biofeedback training of visual acuity and myopia: A pilot study. AJOPO 1987; 64(1):62–71.

64. Morrison RJ. Contact lenses and the progression of myopia. JAOA 1957; 28(12):711–13.

65. Dickinson F. The value of microlenses in progressive myopia. Optician 1957; 133:263–64.

66. Bier N. Myopia controlled by contact lenses: a preliminary report. Optician 1958; 135:427.

67. Policoff W. The effect of contact lenses on myopia retardation. First Int'l Conf. on Myopia, New York City, 1964.

68. De Almeida Rev bras Oftal 1963; 22:269.

69. Barraquer JI. An Inst Barraquer 1964; 5:206.

70. Sato A. A new surgical approach to myopia. Am J Ophthal 1953; 36:823.

71. Ruiz RS. Radial keratotomy: can you throw away your glasses? Herman Eye Center. Views and vision. 1981; 4(1):5.

72. Deitz MR, Sanders DR, Marks RG. Radial keratotomy: an overview of the Kansas City Study. Ophthalmology 1981; 88:729–36.

73. Bender PS. Four year postoperative evaluation of radial keratotomy. Arch Ophthalmol 1985; 103:779–80.

74. Neumann AC, Osher RH, Fanzl RE. Radial keratotomy: a comprehensive evaluation. Doc Ophthalmol 1984; 56:275–301.

75. Muller L. Klin Mbl Augenheilk 1894; 32:178.

76. Muller L. Kiln Mbl Augenheilk 1903; 41(1):459.

77. Borley WE, Snyder AA. Surgical treatment of high myopia. Trans Am Acad Ophthal Otolaryn 1958; 62:791–802.

78. Stetson SM, Raskind RH. Pseudomyopia: etiology, mechanism and therapy. J Pediatr Ophthal 1970; 7(2):110.

79. Cogan DG. Accommodation and the autonomic nervous system. Arch Ophthal 1937; 18:737.

80. Ingram RM. Refraction as a means of predicting squint or amblyopia in preschool siblings of children known to have these defects. Br J Ophthal 1979; 63:238.

81. Helveston EM, Ellis FD. Pediatric ophthalmology practice. St. Louis: Mosby, 1980.

82. Rosner J, Gruber J. Differences in the perceptual skills development of young myopes and hyperopes. AJOPO 1985; 62:501–504.

83. Rosner J, Rosner J. The effects of early lens correction of hyperopia on visual perceptual skills development. Australian J Clin Exp Optom 1986; 69:166–71.

84. Brown EVL. Net average yearly changes in refraction of atropinized eyes from birth to beyond middle life. Arch Ophthal 1938; 19:719.

85. Howland HC, Atkinson J, Braddock O, French J. Infant astigmatism measured by photorefraction. Science 1978; 202(20):331–32.

86. Mohindra I, Held R, Gwiazda J, Brill J. Astigmatism in infants. Science 1978; 202(2):329.

87. Atkinson J, Braddock O, French J. Infant astigmatism: its disappearance with age. Vis Res 1980; 20:891–93.

88. Mitchell DE, Freeman RD, Millodot M, Haegerstrom G. Meridional amblyopia: evidence for modification of the human visual system by early visual experiences. Vis Res 1973; 13:535–58.

89. Parks MM. Ocular motility and strabismus. New York: Harper & Row, 1975.

90. Griffin JR. Binocular anomalies. Chicago: Professional Press, 1976.

91. Noorden GK von. Binocular vision and ocular motilities. St. Louis: Mosby, 1980.

92. Hirsch MJ. Visual anomalies among children of grammar school age. JAOA 1952; 23(11):663.
93. Blum H, Bettman J, Peters HB. Vision screening for elementary schools: the Orinda study. Berkeley: University of California Press, 1959.
94. Hirsch MJ. Anisometropia: a preliminary report of the Ojai longitudinal study. AAAO 1967; 44(9):581.

11

Constant Strabismus

☐

The clinical management of constant strabismus* is multifaceted, both in terms of ultimate goals and the means by which those goals are sought. This is not surprising, considering the variety of clinical pictures that cluster under the general heading of strabismus and the variety of etiologies that spawn them.

The various clinical pictures have already been reviewed (see Chapter 6). There is no need to repeat that information here.

Etiologies range from (a) central nervous system impairment to (b) localized neurological and motor deficits to (c) anatomical anomalies to (d) innervational imbalance.

Treatment goals range from (a) the optimal: normal (clear, comfortable, single simultaneous, central) binocular vision with high-grade stereoacuity to (b) approximate binocular alignment with peripheral stereopsis to (c) apparent cosmetic alignment without any binocular function.

Treatment methods range from (a) application of lenses that neutralize ametropia to (b) remedial therapy employing various procedures (e.g., "vision training exercises," and/or lenses and prisms, and/ or remedial surgery) to (c) compensatory surgery and/or compensatory lenses/prisms to (d) reassurance: consolation accompanied by a recommendation to leave well enough alone.

The treatments described here are not all inclusive. The topic merits (and has) its own volumes (e.g., [1,2,3,4,5]).

As indicated in Chapter 6, the scope of the information presented in this chapter is guided by the assumption that *all* optometrists are competent in the detection and diagnosis of strabismus and should also be able to (a) identify and treat effectively those strabismic patients whose prognoses are *"very good"* or *"good"* — patients who are very likely to respond favorably to basic vision therapy regimens

---

*The term "constant strabismus," as used here, applies when the patient, despite reasonably good and equal visual acuity in each eye, is *never* able to display stereoacuity better than 120 seconds arc at distance, or 60 seconds arc at near. It follows, therefore, that the term "intermittent strabismus" applies *only* when the patient is also able to display "intermittent binocularity." In other words, the patient whose eyes appear to be in alignment sometimes, and out of alignment at other times, is not an *intermittent strabismic* unless the condition of apparent alignment can be documented by the stereoacuity criteria defined above. Rather, such patients are more accurately classified as *constant strabismics* with two angles of deviation. This is an important distinction; the concepts and suggestions offered in this book are valid only if this taxonomy is followed. As such, this chapter refers to the patient with constant strabismus; Chapter 14, to intermittent strabismus.

that depend mainly on office-guided, home-based activities that employ transportable, easy-to-understand equipment; (b) identify and refer appropriately those patients with *"fair"* and *"guarded"* prognoses—patients who display some potential for binocular function but need a therapy program that goes beyond what most primary-care practitioners are prepared to offer; (c) identify, refer, and counsel appropriately those patients with *"poor"* prognoses—patients who are likely to be served best by surgical treatment or by reassurance and nothing more. We also believe that all optometrists should provide on-going, long-term care to *all* their strabismic patients, even when short-term management is transferred to another clinician; e.g., an optometrist who specializes in vision training or a surgeon.

___■_____

REMEDIAL THERAPY

See flow diagram in Figure 9.1.

□ Design the Regimen

FINAL GOAL

The ultimate goal of a strabismus remedial therapy program is normal binocular vision.

An unrealistic goal for a strabismic? In some cases, perhaps, but not if care has been taken to formulate a valid prognosis that justifies such optimism. Obviously, a prognosis is a prediction, not a guarantee. Hence, there will be cases where this goal will not be achieved, but so long as all parties recognize this fact, there is no reason to avoid an attempt if the evidence supports a favorable prognosis.

SUBORDINATE GOALS AND THEIR HIERARCHICAL INTERRELATIONSHIPS

We noted earlier (Chapter 6) that normal binocular vision comprises a central (macular) and a peripheral (extramacular) component, and that peripheral single binocular vision may operate in the absence of central single binocular vision but that the reverse does not occur. We noted, also, that central single binocular vision is derived from two functions: *stereopsis* and *fusion*. (Fusion allows for the localization of stimuli in a two-dimensional plane; stereopsis, in the third dimension: depth.) Peripheral single binocular vision is made up of three functions: stereopsis, fusion, and simultaneous perception—the latter being the ability to perceive an object as doubled, seen simultaneously by each eye in a different spatial location, when it is projected on the retina beyond Panum's area (e.g., physiological diplopia in properly aligned eyes; pathological diplopia in strabismics [3]).

As such, the abilities that subserve central single binocular vision are *central stereopsis, peripheral stereopsis, central fusion, peripheral fusion, and simultaneous perception*. The interrelationships of these five are discernable through analysis. The last of the list is clearly the most basic. Simultaneous perception can exist in the absence of binocular fusion and stereopsis; its absence precludes the other two. Peripheral fusion can exist even when central fusion does not, and peripheral stereopsis may be found when central stereopsis is absent; but in neither instance does the reverse occur. Hence, peripheral binocular functions are subordinate to their counterpart central functions.* That leaves only the relationship between stereopsis and fusion. Here, again, the evidence is clear: stereopsis predicts fusion, but not vice versa. Therefore, the hierarchical interrelationships of the five, from top to bottom, appear to be *central stereopsis, central fusion, peripheral stereopsis, peripheral fusion,* and *simultaneous perception*.

☐ Placement Procedure

Determine which of these subordinate abilities the patient has already achieved and which remain to be accomplished.

This has already been accomplished in part; the patient's current status was determined during the diagnostic and prognosis processes defined by the flow diagram shown in Figure 6.14. That process determined that the patient under discussion in this section displayed constant strabismus when tested while wearing lenses that compensate fully for his ametropia and any existing (accommodative-convergence) innervational imbalances, manifests no related pathology nor significant (unilateral or bilateral) amblyopia, but is able to obtain central and/or peripheral stereopsis (on the basis of normal retinal correspondence) if aided with compensating prisms. (In other words: *what he can do;* see p. 221.) All that remains to be done in preparing for the postexamination-pretreatment conference is to identify the abilities the patient must acquire as treatment progresses and the method(s) for accomplishing this. When that is done, the optometrist will have sufficient information to describe the therapy program to the patient/parent in adequate detail and proceed accordingly.

The treatment program the patient should engage in is one that enables him *to improve on what he already can do;* one that teaches him the higher order

---

*It is obvious that the difference between what is termed central and what is termed peripheral fusion and stereopsis depends upon the size and detailed nature of the target. A problem arises from this: How small and/or detailed must a stimulus be in order to be classified as a central target rather than a peripheral one? If it were only a matter of size, the problem would be simple. But, the variable of detail complicates the process. For the present, the answer is: *Estimate*.

Level I: Patient* with constant strabismus displays single,
              simultaneous binocular vision (on the basis of NRC) at
              distance and/or near by using prisms that initially
              accommodated only 50 pecent of the misalignment.

Level II: Patient* is able to maintain normal binocular function for
              limited periods of time without the aid of any compenstory
              prism; i.e., strabismus changes from *constant* to
              intermittent.

Level III: Patient* is able to recover and maintain normal binocular
              function when a moderate amount (about 3 to 5 pd) of
              counter-compensatory prism is introduced abruptly; i.e.,
              binocular status changes from *intermittent strabismus* to
              vergence infacility.

Level IV: Patient* demonstrates the capacity to adapt quickly and
              easily to reasonable amounts of base in and base out prism
              while holding accommodation constant.

*Patient may continue to use as much compensatory sphere/cylinder as he needs. For
example, patient initially manifests 15 pd esotropia at distance and 30 pd at near. Use of a
+2.50D add reduces the near angle to about 15 pd. He functions binocularly when provided
with this add and 15 pd base out. Patient will have completed Level I when he can function
binocularly with the same +2.50 D add but no more than about 8 pd base out.

Figure 11.1   Binocular ability goals.

skills needed to fulfill the ultimate goal defined at the beginning of this section.
Figure 11.1 defines these skills in four levels.

It shows that the first major goal (level I), to be attained by developing adequate
fusional ranges, is achieved when the patient is able to demonstrate normal binocular vision with about half of the prism support that was found to be necessary
during diagnosis. (Keep in mind that the patients under discussion here have
good or *very good* prognoses; as described in Chapter 6, they demonstrated,
during the diagnostic process, that they were able to function binocularly when
appropriate compensatory prisms were provided.)

The patient's next major goal (level II) is to alter his status from *constant* to
intermittent strabismus—to expand his fusional ranges to the point where he is
able to function binocularly, if only for very brief periods of time, without any
assistance from compensatory prism. Having accomplished this, the patient's next
goal (level III) is to acquire the vergence ranges that will enable him to display
the binocular abilities characteristic of *vergence infacility* rather than strabismus.
Finally, having accomplished this, the patient's next (final) goal is to be able to
demonstrate the fusional ranges and facility that signal normal binocular vision.

Apparatus	This Instrument Is Appropriate If the Patient Is to Start Therapy At/With:				Prerequisites*
	Far	Near	Base-in	Base-out	
Aperture rule		X	X	X	A
Brewster stereoscope; adult base-out comfort series	X			X	B
Stereoscope; Keystone-View Children's Base-out Stories	X			X	B
Stereoscope; Keystone-View Children's Base-in Stories	X		X		B
Minivectogram		X	X	X	A
Vectotrainer; Quoit vectograms		X	X	X	A
Any nonvariable disparity Tranaglyph		X	X	X	A
Brewster stereoscope; Bernell Base-out Storybook Cards	X			X	B
Brewster Stereoscope; Bernell Base-in Storybook Cards	X		X		B
Any variable disparity Vectogram set		X	X	X	A
Any variable disparity tranaglyph set		X	X	X	A

*Prerequisites (accomplished with aid of full lens correction and whatever additional spheres/prisms are necessary):
A = Third-degree fusion (i.e., stereopsis) at near.
B = Third-degree fusion at far.
C = Second-degree fusion at near.
D = Second-degree fusion at far.

Table 11.1   Additional Instruments

☐ Identify Procedures That Will Facilitate Attainment of the Yet-to-Be-Mastered Subordinate Abilities

Selection of an effective procedure should be done empirically, taking into account the patient's entering strengths and weaknesses (e.g., whether it is preferable to commence therapy at near or at far fixation, exercising abduction or adduction, etc.), the cognitive requirements of the procedure (e.g., does it involve reading or simply looking at pictures), and such pragmatic factors as the optometrist's personal preferences and the office's inventory of available vision therapy instruments.

Notice that the basic characteristics of strabismus—direction (eso, exo, hyper, hypo), magnitude (small-angle, large-angle), and so on—do not influence the selection of remedial activities. What matters is the extent to which the patient is able to approximate normal binocular vision.

The procedures described below are organized according to whether they focus on central or peripheral stereopsis.* They represent but a small sampling of the nonmedical remedial approaches that are available for treating strabismus patients with good or very good prognoses. Many other instruments and procedures can serve just as effectively. (See, for example, Table 11.1.) The key concern in strabismus remediation is to provide conditions that make it possible for the patient to (a) obtain normal binocular vision—with compensatory aid as needed; (b) know that he has obtained it (through visual "feedback"); (c) learn how to sustain it as compensatory aid is withdrawn, and ultimately (d) learn how to sustain it as counter-compensatory conditions are introduced. How this is accomplished—the specific instruments and procedures employed—is not as important a concern.

To get started, select one of the procedures defined below, implement it, measure the patient's baseline abilities with the procedure, evaluate the patient's ability to use it independently, explain to the patient how, when, and why it is to be used at home, and arrange for a subsequent appointment at which time his progress will be evaluated and treatment updated accordingly.

PROCEDURES APPROPRIATE FOR PATIENTS IN LEVELS I AND II

If, during the diagnostic process, the patient displayed normal peripheral stereopsis when provided with compensatory prisms, use the following.

Red/Green Stereo Trainer
Position the Stereo Trainer (Bernell Mfg. Co.) at the distance that is easiest for the patient and supply him with a set of red/green filters and the compensatory prisms he needs to obtain binocular vision under these conditions.**

Have the patient report what he sees. If the patient's response is *optimal*, displaying single, simultaneous, binocular vision—if he reports seeing two large circles, with the smaller of the two appearing to be floating a bit in front of (closer to him) or behind the larger one (depending upon the orientation of the red/green filters)—it indicates that he is achieving normal binocular vision under these circumstances and, therefore, can be treated by engaging in activities that extend his fusional ranges from this starting point. If he also responds that he perceives

*This is a departure from the traditional orthoptic sequence, where the procedures were designed in accord with Worth's fusion taxonomy: simultaneous perception, second-degree fusion, first-degree fusion. The shift to an emphasis on stereopsis is fairly recent, with strong impetus provided by Brock (6) who was one of the first to recognize the critical role of peripheral stereopsis and the practical value of filters for teaching binocular skills in true space.
**The amount of prism needed to obtain fusion should be about the same as the angle of deviation measured objectively during the diagnostic process. If it is markedly different and/or if the patient appears to be able to obtain fusion without the aid of compensating prism, suspect ARC; reassess the diagnosis and prognosis.

an illusion of depth from the smaller circles located to the left and right of the larger ones, consider it to be an even more favorable sign and inform the patient to that effect. This response suggests central rather than peripheral stereopsis, particularly if the target is located beyond 3 meters.

If, instead, the patient reports no awareness of the stereo illusion, try other fixation distances. If this does not enable him to obtain binocular vision, then recheck the original diagnostic data—perhaps insufficient compensatory prism was used—and reconsider the prognosis. The patient who is able to obtain stereopsis during the diagnostic process should be able to do it again, subsequently.

If the patient's response was optimal, measure his fusional ranges as he fixates at far, midrange, and near. Use a prism bar (or loose prisms), or simply reduce the amount of the compensatory prism, a few diopters at a time. Record these (far, mid, and near) base in and base out ranges as baseline measures.

Supply the patient with a Stereo Trainer, a set of red/green filters, compensatory prisms of appropriate power, and written instructions for home use. The instructions should be designed to lead the patient from his baseline, as established above, to the point where:

(a) if, in level I, he is able to perform binocularly with about half-power compensatory prism;

(b) if, in level II, he is able to perform binocularly even when all compensating prism is eliminated.

Red/Green Nearpoint Target

Hold the target (e.g., plate #9 from the Keystone Basic Binocular Skills Series: the duck and black ring; available from Keystone-Mast Co.) about 40 cm from the patient. Have him report what he sees as he looks at it through red/green filters and whatever compensatory prisms he needs to obtain binocular vision under these conditions.

If patient's response is *optimal*, displaying single, simultaneous, binocular function—if he reports seeing a duck that appears to be floating in front of, or behind the ring (depending upon the orientation of the filters)—it indicates that he is achieving normal peripheral stereopsis (under these circumstances) and, therefore, can be treated by engaging in activities that extend his fusional ranges from this starting point.

If, instead, the patient reports no awareness of the stereo illusion, try other fixation distances. If this does not enable him to obtain binocular vision, then recheck the original diagnostic data—perhaps insufficient compensatory prism was used—and reconsider the prognosis. The patient who is able to obtain stereopsis during the diagnostic process should be able to do it again, subsequently.

Measure the patient's fusional ranges with a prism bar or loose prisms. Record these base in and base out ranges as baseline measures. Supply the patient with a red/green target, a set of red/green filters, compensatory prisms of appropriate power, and written instructions for home use. The instructions should be designed to lead the patient from his baseline, as established above, to the point where

(a) if, in level I, he is able to perform binocularly with about half-power compensatory prisms;

(b) if, in level II, he is able to perform binocularly even when all compensating prisms are eliminated.

If, during the diagnostic process, the patient displayed normal central stereopsis when provided with compensatory prisms:

Tranaglyph Trainer

Supply the patient with a Minitranaglyph Trainer (Bernell Mfg. Co.), a set of red/ green filters, and whatever compensatory prisms he needs to obtain binocular vision under these conditions. Compensatory prism effect can also be obtained simply by separating the red and green targets the required amount; additional lenses are not needed.*

Hold the target about 40 cm from the patient and have him report what he sees. If the patient's response is *optimal*, indicating single, simultaneous, binocular function—if he reports seeing two circles, with one (the larger or the smaller, depending upon the orientation of the red/green filters) appearing to be floating a bit in front of or behind the other one—it indicates that he is achieving normal binocular vision (under those circumstances) and, therefore, can be treated by engaging in activities that expand his fusional ranges from this starting point.

If, instead, the patient reports no awareness of the stereo illusion, try other fixation distances. If this does not enable him to obtain binocular vision, then recheck the original diagnostic data—perhaps insufficient compensatory prism was used—and reconsider the prognosis. The patient who is able to obtain stereopsis during the diagnostic process should be able to do it again, subsequently.

Measure the patient's fusional ranges by separating the red and green targets in both directions. Record these base in and base out thresholds as baseline measures—starting points.

Supply the patient with a Tranaglyph Trainer, a set of red/green filters, and written instructions for home use. The instructions should be designed to lead the patient from his baseline, as established above, to the point where

(a) if, in level I, he is able to perform binocularly with about half-power compensatory prisms;

(b) if, in level II, he is able to perform binocularly even when all compensating prisms are eliminated.

Variable Mirror Stereoscope**

Supply the patient with a Variable Mirror Stereoscope (available from Bernell Mfg. Co.), a set of stereo targets, and whatever compensatory prisms he needs to obtain binocular vision under these conditions. Compensatory prism effect can

---

*The amount of prism needed to obtain fusion should be about the same as the angle of deviation measured objectively during the diagnostic process. If it is markedly different and/or if the patient appears to be able to obtain fusion without the aid of compensating prism, suspect ARC; reassess the diagnosis and prognosis.
**This device is especially useful if the patient manifests a moderate vertical deviation in addition to his horizontal one; the targets may be positioned in the stereoscope so as to compensate for the vertical deviation.

be obtained simply by separating the stereoscope mirrors the required amount; additional lenses are not needed.*

Have the patient report what he sees. If the patient's response is *optimal,* indicating single, simultaneous, binocular function—if he reports seeing two circles, one appearing to be floating a bit in front of or behind the other one, it indicates that he is achieving normal binocular vision (under those circumstances) and, therefore, can be treated by engaging in activities that expand his fusional ranges from this starting point.

If, instead, the patient reports no awareness of the stereo illusion, recheck the original diagnostic data—perhaps insufficient compensatory prism was used—and reconsider the prognosis. The patient who is able to obtain stereopsis during the diagnostic process should be able to do it again, subsequently.

Measure the patient's fusional ranges by separating the mirrors in both directions (or by reducing the amount of prisms, if extra lenses were used) until the patient reports that he has lost binocularity. Record these base in and base out thresholds as baselines measures—starting points.

Supply the patient with a Variable Mirror Stereoscope, a set of targets, and written instructions for home use. The instructions should be designed to lead the patient from his baseline, as established above, to the point where

(a) if, in level I, he is able to perform binocularly with about half-power compensatory prisms;

(b) if, in level II, he is able to perform binocularly even when all compensating prisms are eliminated.

Other Instruments/Procedures
It should be evident that many different vision therapy devices will serve the patient who has earned a good or very good prognosis and is currently placed at levels I and II. All that is needed is an apparatus that has the capacity to inform (provide feedback to) the patient when his two eyes are functioning in the correct fashion and instructions that guide him from an entering level—where compensatory prisms are necessary—to the level where his condition warrants the diagnosis of intermittent rather than constant strabismus. The above examples illustrate this. Tale 11.1 lists a number of other devices that can be used in a similar manner.

□ Anomalous Retinal Correspondence

This topic has already been discussed to some degree in Chapter 6. However, a few more comments might be helpful, especially because many patients will respond inconsistently to different tests of retinal correspondence.

---

*The amount of prism needed to obtain fusion should be about the same as the angle of deviation measured objectively during the diagnostic process. If it is markedly different and/or if the patient appears to be able to obtain fusion without the aid of compensating prism, suspect ARC; reassess the diagnosis and prognosis.

ARC is a significant concern in the remediation of strabismus. In one sense, it is the antithesis of normal binocular vision. But, in a literal sense, it is an adaptation that allows the strabismic to achieve a form of single, simultaneous binocular vision despite the fact that only one fovea is functioning normally. As such, it is a useful adaptation; it is not given up easily (1,2,4).

As has already been observed, many patients will display ARC in certain situations (i.e.,) tests and NRC in others. The implications of this are pertinent: above all, it indicates that retinal correspondence is not like so many other functional adaptations that, in time, alter structure and become virtually irreversible. ARC appears to be a reversible condition except, perhaps, in a small subgroup of strabismics who have been strabismic for a very long time and show ARC responses in every test condition (7).

This suggests two possible treatment approaches for ARC: (a) eliminate all signs of ARC before attempting to develop the normal binocular functions; (b) train binocular functions in those conditions where ARC does not manifest on the assumption that, as progress is made, the ARC will give ground and eventually be eliminated. The second is the better choice: determine the highest level of binocular function (see above) at which the patient displays ARC and institute a regimen that attempts to improve performance on the basis of what already exists. Ignore the ARC; avoid placing the patient in treatment situations where it is elicited. As the performance level improves, these same conditions may no longer elicit ARC. In other words, do not treat the ARC, do not attempt to eliminate the maladaptation; try, instead, to improve those aspects of binocular behavior that are desirable, thereby removing the need for an adaptation.

There are times, of course, when ARC has to be dealt with directly, when it is impossible, or impractical, to identify a level of normal function from which to neutralize the ARC. A number of treatment methods have been developed. These include (a) training procedures that start off by placing the patient in a completely contourless visual environment (e.g., facing a blank wall while wearing very high plus lenses), which he views through red/green filters. The initial goal: blend the colors (7); (b) alternating monocular occulsion, which by definition eliminates the need for ARC because it eliminates binocular vision; (c) prisms of sufficient power to overcorrect the deviation (i.e., transform an esotropia into an exotropia) (8). All of these methods have their advocates and their critics, which suggests that they are effective sometimes, but not always.

SUPPRESSION

We intentionally have not devoted significant attention to this topic. Suppression, in the presence of strabismus, is a neurosensory adaptation that spares the patient from diplopia (1). Most often, it does not pervade the full visual field. Rather, it exists only in those areas of the visual field that are most vulnerable to strabismus-related diplopia; i.e., the central zone and that peripheral area in the deviating eye that is stimulated when the preferred eye fixates on an object (2,9).

Suppression may be unilateral or alternating, depending upon the patient's fixation pattern. In either instance, the suppression area can be mapped with binocular perimetry, wherein fixation is controlled by the preferred eye and only the deviating (suppressing) eye is able to see the probe (9). The suppression area, a facultative scotoma, may vary in both size and location (2).

Suppression varies also in "depth"; i.e., the extent to which the nonsuppressing eye must be inhibited before the suppressing eye will display more normal receptive abilities. This is usually tested with a series of filters that are graded in density; the darker the filter required over the preferred eye to elicit nonsuppressing behavior from the nonpreferred eye, the deeper the suppression.

As one considers these characteristics of suppression, it becomes evident that the phenomenon is more helpful than harmful to the patient with strabismus. It is analogous to the limp one demonstrates when he gets a pebble in his shoe. The adaptation—the "limp"—is an automatic modification in behavior that enables the individual to continue functioning in a reasonably effective way. How should the patient (with the pebble in his shoe) be treated? By ignoring the pebble and instituting "antilimp" (antisuppression) exercises? Hardly. Obviously, the way to treat him is to remove the pebble—to eliminate the need to maladapt. Similarly, the way to address the suppression displayed by the patient with constant strabismus is (a) to eliminate the strabismus—the suppression will then disappear without special attention; or (b) if the strabismus cannot be eliminated, to allow the suppression to remain undisturbed. Remember, the adaptation came about because the alternative—diplopia—was less desirable. To remove this alternative from the patient with constant strabismus is to cause him diplopia and continued strabismus, hardly an improvement.

This does not imply that amblyopia should be ignored. True, an eye that starts to suppress early in life is likely to develop amblyopia—reduced capacity to see clearly. Amblyopia should not be ignored, but that does not suggest that the way to treat it is to attack suppression. (See Chapter 12 for a more extensive discussion regarding amblyopia.)

☐ Supplementary and Alternative Remedial Procedures

There are cases where a treatment other than vision therapy may be desirable. These may include the use of certain optical devices (e.g., spherical lenses that go beyond what is called for because of ametropia, prisms), occluders, surgery, and/or drugs.

SPHERICAL LENSES BEYOND WHAT IS NEEDED TO COMPENSATE AMETROPIA

The strabismus diagnostic flow diagram (Figure 6.14) calls for an evaluation of the effects of additional plus/minus lenses on the magnitude of the deviation; that is, a probe of the potential linkup between the patient's strabismus and accommodation. Indeed, one group of investigators argue, on the basis of an impressive data set (N = 1006), that 90 percent of esotropia has an accommodative origin and is best treated with an "overcorrection of manifest hyperopia reaching gradually to the full correction of the total hypermetropia" (10, p. 757). The outcomes of their treatment (more-than-maximum plus combined with constant monocular occlusion so long as the esotropia is apparent) are too impressive to ignore.

There are different methods for determining how much additional lens power (i.e., beyond what is called for by ametropia) to prescribe. A simple, yet valid method is to observe the effects of the lenses: hold the lenses in front of the patient's eyes, take note of the change in the angle of deviation (11) and then observe the patient perform certain visual tasks with the lenses in place. The purpose of this last step is to avoid placing the patient in a second undesirable condition—"out of the frying pan into the fire." The optometrist should not prescribe so much plus (for the esotrope) that the child has to hold reading material very close to her eyes, or so much minus (for the exotrope) that she experiences blur and utter accommodative exhaustion after a short time. (Flom [12, p. 216] offers a formula for calculating optimal additional lens power, should a more precise method be desired.)

Bifocals have been accepted as a useful treatment device (1,2,13). When they are prescribed, make certain that they occupy a significant portion of the lens. Remember that the child *can* see without the additional plus power, something that the presbyope cannot do. Hence, she may not bother to use the additional power unless it is positioned in such a way that makes it unavoidable without conscious effort. In practical terms, this suggests that the top of the seg be placed near or at the *upper* edge of the pupil. Children tolerate this with no difficulty. They tend to be shorter than the presbyopes: the floor is not so far away from their eyes.

PRISMS

This is not an innovative idea (14,15). In theory, prisms appear to be an ideal treatment for strabismus. After all, they can cause the images to fall on both macula (in a strabismic). Then, "all that is needed" is to improve the patient's fusional vergence ranges while gradually reducing the power of the prism. It is more than a theory. It works—in some cases (16).

One long-standing deterrent to the use of the prism—its physical properties: weight and appearance—was removed when the Fresnel lens was developed (17). This very thin membrane prism, available in powers up to 30 prism diopters, has solved those problems. The Fresnel prism is lightweight, fairly inconspicuous, and easily applied; it "presses on" to the rear surface of any spectacle lens.

Another potential deterrent to the use of prisms: ARC. By definition, the patient with ARC perceives an object to be in the same place with each eye even though the images are projected on noncorresponding retinal points. Prism alters the retinal location of the projected images, which, to the patient with ARC under those conditions, will stimulate a realignment of the visual axes. The upshot: an increase in the deviation. Hardly a desirable treatment effect but, on the other hand, not enough of a concern to rule out completely the use of prisms.

In general, the most productive and reasonable attitude toward the prism as a therapeutic device is to use it when it is justified, to keep an eye on its effects, and to act accordingly.

OCCLUDERS

The occluder is included here as an optical device because it can be used to prevent images from being projected onto certain areas of the retina. This makes it useful in the therapeutic managment of strabismus (18).

Full Occlusion

This may be direct or indirect. In the former, the preferred eye is covered, thereby stimulating the deviating eye to assume a position of alignment. Indirect occlusion is typically applied when there is a desire to interrupt the visual behavior pattern of a deviating eye. Both direct and indirect occlusion are discussed in the section devoted to the treatment of amblyopia (see Chapter 12).

Partial Lens Occlusion

Some clinicians advocate partial lens occlusion: binasal, bitemporal, the upper or lower half of one lens, and so on (19). This may be accomplished in a number of ways; any material that stops the transmission of light will do. It is wise, however, to give some thought to cosmetic effect. Scotch Magic Tape (available in office-supply stores) attached to the rear surface of the lens serves very well. The patient's eyes are visible through the tape yet, from the patient's view, no details are perceptible.

Where the tape is positioned depends, of course, on what area of the retina the optometrist wishes to mask. Binasal occluders obstruct the passage of light to the temporal retinas (when the eyes are directed straight ahead), bitemporal occluders obstruct nasal retinas, and so on.

To date, no consistent rationale has evolved regarding the use of partial occluders to accomplish goals beyond what is mentioned above. Those who advocate their use do so on the basis of their own clinical experiences. Some express their views very convincingly (7), but it is not equivalent to the data that the interested clinician hopes to have.

SURGERY

Another controversial issue! Vigorous proponents; equally staunch opponents! Both groups are substantial in size. Both groups are committed to their respective positions, tending to play down the validity of any other. Both groups have their share of successful cases to which they may point with pride (20,21).

Where does this lead? Is surgery worth considering? If so, when is it useful, when should it be avoided? When, if ever, should the optometrist recommend a surgical consultation? When should she ignore that option?

Unfortunately, once again there is no clear-cut rule. The surgical approach to strabismus is direct. It is an effort to realign the visual axes by altering the influence of specific extraocular muscles on the orientation of the globes. The outcomes of surgery are strongly affected by many factors. Among the most important are (a) the sensory status of the two eyes at the time of the operation; (b) the accuracy with which the extraocular muscle alterations were calculated and carried out.

In respect to the first, the sensory status of the eyes at the time the surgery was carried out: If achieved, binocular alignment makes fusion more possible; it does not guarantee it. No reputable surgeon will promise (or be utterly surprised by not achieving) precise bifoveal alignment solely on the basis of muscle surgery. The eyes have to be *capable* of binocular function; that is, (a) reasonably good and equal visual acuity in the two eyes; (b) the ability to perceive the images on both retinas simultaneously; and (c) the ability to detect the disparity of certain pairs of retinal images within Panum's area. Unless these three are available, the most precise surgery will not yield normal binocular vision.

The implication of this: Remedial surgery is best justified in those cases where the prognosis for nonsurgical treatment is also good, but when, for some reason or other, nonsurgical treatment is not feasible.

The second factor: the accuracy of the calculations and surgery itself. It helps to remember that surgeons are, in fact, human; and humans vary. Some surgeons are better than others, and all surgeons do better work on some days than on others. True, there is an ongoing effort by all health professions to upgrade and maintain the minimum quality of care they provide, but there is no way of disputing the fact that human variance does and will continue to exist. The implications of this: in recommending a surgical consultation, take care to identify for the patient the most competent surgeons only. Avoid all the others.

It seems reasonable, therefore, to suggest that surgery should be considered as part of a strabismus remedial regimen in some cases, but its limitations should be recognized and its position in the sequence of actions timed appropriately. Remedial surgery should be considered when the sensory status of the two eyes is such that bifoveal alignment will have significant value, but where for some reason a nonsurgical approach is not possible. A good example: The young child, whose strabismus does not derive from uncorrected ametropia and/or an unusually high AC/A ratio, who is too young to participate in the kind of activities described above, will remain too young for at least a few more years, and whose parents are very upset by the appearance of the strabismus.

Granted, a maintenance program could be put into effect, so that remediation was put off without ongoing deterioration of the neurosensory processes. At least, in theory it could be put into effect. The reality of modern life suggests something different. It is one thing to design a maintenance program that will prevent sensory-motor deterioration until the child is old enough to participate in a nonsurgical therapy program, and another thing to induce the child and parents to follow it. The optometrist has the obligation to prescribe the course of action that she considers to be best, but she also has the obligation to avoid prescribing regimens that she knows will not (in a practical sense, cannot) be followed.

DRUGS

Miotics, cycloplegics, and, more recently, botulinum toxin have been used in the treatment of strabismus (22).

Miotics

The rationale for the use of a miotic in esotropia is based upon the impact that the drug has on accommodation. As the demand for accommodation reduces, so too does the stimulus to convergence reduce. There are drawbacks, however: systemic and local side effects. Among the former, the usual systemic effects of a miotic: perspiration, nausea, vomiting, diarrhea. Locally: iris cysts. Phospholine iodide, a long-acting cholinesterase inhibitor, continues to be popular among many professionals, but in general the treatment approach does not appear to be as popular as it was a decade or so ago. Many now prefer bifocals for the same purpose (2).

Cycloplegics

Atropine has been recommended as a treatment for strabismus for many years (22, 23). It never achieved great popularity and presently is not viewed as an effective treatment method.

Botulinum Toxin

Recently, a new and promising method for treating strabismus was introduced (24,25,26). It takes advantage of the fact that botulinum toxin (Oculinum), injected into an extraocular muscle, causes temporary paralysis (produced by chemodenervation) with a resultant change in the ocular alignment when the effect of the toxin has worn off. Oculinum therapy has been used experimentally by a number of ophthalmologists. The reports that have appeared indicate that the treatment has some value—more so with adult patients who have experienced recent-onset rectus muscle paralysis than with children. However, not enough is known at this time to make definitive statements about the drug's ultimate potential.

☐ Some Concluding Remarks Regarding Strabismus Remedial Therapy

Strabismus is a prevalent problem. If it is neglected, it is rarely outgrown. It is worthy of the optometrist's attention and concern; and it is worthy of remedial efforts. The view taken in these pages has been pragmatic: namely, in those cases where nonsurgical remedial treatment appears to be justified, it should be instituted, if the patient/parent is up to it. If the patient/parent does not appear to be capable (or willing) to engage in nonsurgical regimen, then the combined efforts of the surgeon and the optometrist should be applied in order to provide some aspects of care—even at the expense of achieving a less-than-optimum result.

COMPENSATORY (COSMETIC) TREATMENT

Compensatory (cosmetic) treatment (see Figure 9.2 flow diagram) is indicated when the prognosis for remedial therapy is very unfavorable and the strabismus constitutes a cosmetic problem; i.e., a horizontal deviation in excess of 15 to 20 prism diopters (depending upon I.P.D., angle kappa, width of bridge, and other facial features), a vertical deviation in excess of about 10 prism diopters. Smaller deviations may also take on cosmetic importance if the strabismus is accompanied by a head tilt or turn.

Two treatments are often possible: (a) surgical; (b) optical. Each has its practical advantages and drawbacks. Both should be considered and, where justified, presented to the patient/parent for consideration.

□ Optical

"People looking at a subject wearing prism see his eyes through the prism; each eye and its orbit appear displaced in the direction of the apex of the prism. Thus, placing a base-in prism before a blind esotropic eye will make the eye apprear to be more temporalward in the head" (12, p. 221).

The potential of Flom's observation is often overlooked. The procedure is not universally applicable, but when the conditions warrant it may provide the strabismic patient with a high degree of satisfaction.

The likely candidate for a cosmetic prism is the strabismic whose deviation is unilateral and constant. The visual acuity of the deviating eye should be depressed, the eye being either amblyopic or in a state of constant suppression.

The cosmetic prism must not elicit a movement from the nondeviating eye (27, p. 410). It therefore should be placed before the deviating eye only; placing a prism in front of the preferred eye will stimulate a movement of that eye and a conjugate movement of the nonpreferred eye.

Determining the power of the cosmetic prism is, for all practical purposes, a trial-and-error procedure. Start with a relatively moderate power, oriented appropriately, and work up in small increments until the optimal cosmetic effect is obtained. (Base in for esotropia; base out for exotropia; base up for hypertropia; base down for hypotropia.)

□ Surgery

The effectiveness of cosmetic surgery for strabismus is well established. One report claims that cosmetically satisfactory results (postsurgical deviations of 10 degrees or less) are obtained in almost 90 percent of procedures performed (25). Surely an impressive performance record. True, it is hardly the equivalent of a functional cure (nor do all reports confirm the 90 percent success rate), but it is no trivial accomplishment to the strabismic who is concerned about her appearance.

There does not appear to be a reasonable argument against cosmetic surgery, as long as the chances for functional improvement have been thoroughly assessed and judged to be very poor. However, the optometrist should exercise the same kind of concern in these cases as she does when she suggests surgery as part of a remedial approach: Recommend only those surgeons whom she knows to be first-rate.

■

REASSURANCE THERAPY

See flow diagram (Figure 9.3) and discussion in Chapter 9.

■

REFER FOR CONSULTATION

See flow diagram (Figure 9.4) and discussion in Chapters 6 and 9.

■

THE VERY YOUNG PATIENT

As was noted in Chapter 6, the very young patient requires special consideration. Although the same diagnostic probes are applied with young children as with older ones, it is obvious that vision therapy that exploits the principles of modifying behavior through feedback is not appropriate for the very young. As already acknowledged, the only type of nonmedical/nonsurgical remedial therapy that is of any use with the very young patient is (a) application of lenses that compensate for existing ametropia, (b) extra power lenses, if they facilitate binocular alignment by taking advantage of the link between accommodation and convergence, (c) prisms that make it possible for both foveas to be stimulated equally and simultaneously despite their misalignment (28,29,30).

In brief, then, the following guidelines apply with the very young strabismic patient:

1. Make certain that the child is provided with whatever lenses she needs to compensate fully for existing ametropia. This is particularly important if the child is esotropic and hyperopic, or exotropic and myopic.

2. Take whatever action is needed to reduce/prevent amblyopia.

3. Provide sufficient prism to compensate for the deviation, and whatever additional spherical lens power that appears to facilitate alignment; e.g., plus spheres—at near only (of course)—for the esotrope; minus spheres—at near and distance, or at distance only (depending upon the magnitude of the strabismus at those fixation distances)—for the exotrope. When prescribing a prism, it is usually best to begin with Fresnel prisms and spheres. If the patient does not adapt to them, if they continue to neutralize the deviation after a week or two of wear, have the prism/spheres incorporated into the lenses. If, instead, the patient does adapt, if her eyes return to a strabismic position despite the prisms, reassess and (a) prescribe newly determined prism power, or (b) discard all prisms.

4. Reassess the child's ametropia and binocular status on a regular basis, updating and expanding the treatment program when feasible.

5. If there is no evidence that the strabismus is linked, at least in part, with an innervational component (a situation more common among infantile—congenital—strabismics than those who do not manifest a deviation until after their first birthday), give serious consideration to recommending a surgical consultation. Many pediatric ophthalmologists suggest that the optimum time for surgery with congenital strabismics is between the ages of 12 and 24 months (31,32,33,34). It should also be pointed out that "successful surgery," in these cases, does not imply normal binocular vision. Typically, it means that the patient will have the appearance of "straight eyes" and, in some cases, be able to display some gross (peripheral) stereopsis. But, on the other hand, that is not an unsatisfactory outcome to the parents of a child with overt strabismus—and rightfully so. (This suggestion does not preclude the four guidelines that preceded it. On the contrary, there is evidence to support the notion that prism application in advance of strabismus surgery enhances the chances for successful [as defined above] outcomes [35].)

PRACTICAL SUGGESTIONS

11-1. Patient's often report that they find it easier to extend base-in vergence ranges if they "relax" and gaze upward. This translates to engaging in their vision therapy activities while settled in a comfortable chair and positioning what they are to look at above eye level.

Similarly, many patients observe that it is easier to exercise positive relative convergence when in downward gaze. Hence, it is advisable to suggest to the patient who is having difficulty activitating convergence that she sit erect and position what she is to look at below eye level.

11-2. The esotropic patient may benefit from being advised to "let the targets blur a bit—relax your eyes, as though you were daydreaming." This, of course, implies that she learn how to relax accommodation for the sake of acquiring binocular alignment. Her next step: clear the image (exercise accommodation) while maintaining that alignment.

11-3. Vision therapy is most effective if the patient is able to translate what she sees into "feelings." The strabismus patient who responds well to the vision therapy will be able to control the position of her eyes by feelings; she will "know" when her eyes are in and out of alignment even though she will not be able to express in words what it is that enables her to do this. Hence, encourage your patient to "think" about what her eyes feel when she is responding correctly and incorrectly to the various vision therapy activities you prescribe.

11-4. Accentuate the "bright side" when counseling a constant strabismus whose vision therapy prognosis is poor, but whose cosmetic appearance is acceptable. This does not imply being untruthful; if the patient is strabismic, she (and/or her parents) should be so advised. However, if the condition appears to be immutable, this also means that it will not worsen either. That is a point worth stressing. Perfection is a worthy goal, but most of us do not achieve it.

■

REFERENCES

1. Griffin JR. Binocular anomalies. Chicago: Professional Press, 1976.
2. Noorden GK von. Binocular vision and ocular motilities. St. Louis: Mosby, 1980.
3. Parks MM. Ocular motility and strabismus. New York: Harper & Row, 1975.
4. Hugonnier R, Hugonnier S. Strabismus, heterophoria and ocular motor paralysis. St. Louis: Mosby, 1969.
5. Guibor GP. Squint and allied conditions. New York: Grune & Stratton, 1959.
6. Brock FW. Visual training, part III. Opt Wkly 1/26/56, 6/7/56, 6/14/56, 6/28/56.
7. Greenwald I. Effective strabismus therapy. Duncan, Okla.:O.E.P. Foundation, 1979.
8. Fleming A, Pigassou R, Garipuy J. Adaption of a method of prismatic overcorrection of treating strabismus in children one and two years old. J Pediatr Ophthal 1973; 10(2):154–59.
9. Jampolsky A. Characteristics of suppression and strabismus. Arch Ophthal 1955; 54:683.
10. Rethy I, Gal Z. Results and principles of a new method of optical correction of hypermetropia in cases of esotropia. Acta Ophthal 1968; 46:757.
11. Raab EL. The +3.00 D test in esodeviations. J Pediatr Ophthal 1972; 9(4):207.
12. Flom MC. In: Hirsch MJ, Wick R, eds. Vision of children. Philadelphia: Chilton Books, 1963.
13. Helveston EM, Ellis FD. Pediatric ophthalmology practice. St. Louis: Mosby, 1980.

14. Donders FC. On the anomalies of accommodation and refraction of the eye. Translated by WD Moore. London: The New Sydenham Society, 1864.
15. Graefe A von. Uber musculare asthenopia. Von Graefe's Arch. Ophthal 1862; 8:314.
16. Pigassou R. Prisms in strabismus. Int'l Ophthal Clinics 1966; 6:519.
17. Jampolsy A, Flom M, Thorson JC. Membrane fresnel prisms: a new therapeutic device. In: Fells P, ed. The First Congress of the International Strabismological Assn. St. Louis: Mosby, 1971.
18. Allen M. Occlusion syllabus. JAOA 1973; 44(6):636–39.
19. Jacques L. A father's advice. Opt Wkly 1957; Vol. 58, p. 588.
20. Ludlum WM. Orthoptic treatment of strabismus. AAAO 1961; 38(7):369–88.
21. Weve HJ. The operative treatment of strabismus. Doc Ophthal 1954; 8:495.
22. Javal E. Manuel theoretique et practique du strabisme. Paris: G. Masson, 1896.
23. Laurence JZ, Moon RC. A handy book of ophthalmic surgery for the use of practitioners. Philadelphia: H. C. Lea, 1866.
24. Magoon EH. Botulinum toxin chemo-denervation for strabismus in infants and children. J Ped Ophthal Strab 1984; 21(3):110–22.
25. Metz HS. Botulinum injections for strabismus. J Ped Ophthal Strab 1984; 21(5):199–201.
26. Helveston EM. Botulinum injections for strabismus. J Ped Ophthal Strab 1984; 21(5):202–204.
27. Hirsch MJ. Prism in spectacle lenses for cosmesis. AJOPO 1968; 45:409–12.
28. Albouy RP. Prisms in strabismus management. Past, present and future. J Ped Ophthal Strab 1980; 17(5):325–30.
29. Shippman S, Cimbol D, Weseley AC. The preoperative use of prisms in esotropic children. Am Orthop J 1984; 34:72–76.
30. Berard PV. The use of prisms in the pre- and post-operative treatment of deviation in comitant squint. Congress of Internation Strabismological Assn. St. Louis: CV Mosby Co., 1971.
31. Zak TA, Morin JD. Early surgery for infantile esotropia: results and influence of age upon results. Can J Ophthalmol 1982; 17(5):213–18.
32. Lang J. The optimum time for surgical alignment in congenital strabismus. J Ped Ophthal Strab 1984; 21(2):74–77.
33. Ing MR. Surgical alignment for congenital esotropia. J Ped Ophthal Strab 1984; 21(2):76–77.
34. Kraft SP, Scott WE. Surgery for congenital esotropia—an age comparison study. J Ped Ophthal Strab 1984; 21(2):57.
35. Rubin W. Varieties of prism application in strabismus therapy. In: S Moore, ed. Orthoptics: Past, present, future. New York: Stratton Intercontinental Med Book Corp., 1976.

12

Amblyopia

□

The clinical management of amblyopia differs from the management of strabismus and ametropia, in two fundamental ways. First, in prescribing for strabismus or ametropia, the optometrist has to decide between a compensatory and a remedial approach; the two are not complementary. In the management of amblyopia, no decision is required. There is no conflict between the two approaches; each subserves the other. Second, optometrists are split in their opinions regarding the potential value of a remedial approach to ametropia and strabismus. Some believe it is useful; others see it as a waste of time and effort. In contrast, all optometrists agree that amblyopia therapy is effective—*in some cases*.

As such, the first step in formulating recommendations for a patient with amblyopia is to attempt to determine the prognosis for a remedial approach. This was discussed in the diagnostic section (see Chapter 6). Assuming that the decision is to try remediation, then the next step is to design the treatment program.

■

REMEDIAL THERAPY

See flow diagram in Figure 9.1

□ Design the Regimen

THE FINAL GOAL

The ultimate goal of an amblyopia remedial therapy program is 20/20 visual acuity in each eye. True, this may be overly ambitious in some cases, and something less will have to suffice. Nonetheless, it should be the designated goal at the outset.

SUBORDINATE GOALS AND THEIR HIERARCHICAL INTERRELATIONSHIPS

In order for the patient to be capable of attaining 20/20 visual acuity in each eye, she will have to display:

1. "functional" emmetropia; i.e., no refractive error, obtained with neutralizing lenses if necessary;

2. foveal alignment, each eye;

3. retinocortical pathway and visual center capacities necessary to process high spatial frequency visual patterns.

Having listed them, the next task is to order the three abilities according to their interdependence; i.e., the extent to which one can be acquired in the absence of the other two.

There is little doubt about which should head the list as the most fundamental. Making the ametropic eye emmetropic by introducing lenses is independent of the other two. In fact, it usually has already been accomplished by this stage. (This does not imply that the prescription determined during the amblyopia diagnosis will remain precisely accurate. The prescription may have to be refined as the patient's visual discrimination skills improve.)

What next? The establishment of foveal alignment or the rehabilitation of retinocortical function? Clearly, it is the former. Appropriate retinocortical stimulation depends upon foveal alignment; the opposite is not necessarily true. In other words, an aligned eye *may be* amblyopic; an unaligned eye *will be* amblyopic.

□ Placement Procedures

Determining which of the subordinate abilities have and have not yet been attained is a straightforward activity. The patient either does or does not display ametropia; lenses either have or have not been prescribed; the prescription either is or is not accurate. Foveal alignment either is or is not accurate. Only the third function, retinocortical function, presents a problem in that it cannot be measured directly. It has to be inferred from a behavioral or an electrodiagnostic procedure; or, in fact, by deduction on the basis of the status of the other two abilities in the list. In other words, if ametropia is neutralized by lenses, and if foveal alignment is obtained (and, or course, if there are no obstructions—observable or unobserable—within the media or along the visual pathways), then the only reasonable explanation for the patient's reduced visual acuity is inadequate retinocortical function.

□ Remedial Activities

Furthermore, the activities appear to sort into two categories: those that will lead to (a) accurate foveal alignment; (b) normal (or, at the least, improved) retinocortical function. There is no need to discuss activities that lead to making the eye functionally emmetropic. These optometric procedures are already well defined and established.

PROCEDURES DESIGNED TO IMPROVE THE ACCURACY OF MONOCULAR FOVEAL ALIGNMENT

The procedures described below are listed in the order of their dependence on office-based equipment and treatment. Those described first require no office-based equipment or treatment; those at the end, do.

Thus, when using this list as an aid in designing a therapy program, the activities described at the end of the list are representative of a full-scale treatment program while those at the beginning may serve, by themselves, as an alternative, scaled-down treatment approach. As such, they should not be considered as all that "different," just less extensive. (Some optometrists prefer to classify amblyopia treatment as *active* or *passive*. In that taxonomy, the first procedure—occlusion—is passive; those that incorporate hand-eye tasks with occlusion are active.)

Occlusion

Patching an eye is the foundation of amblyopia therapy. It is a well-established treatment (1), and for good reason. It requires little from the patient beyond tolerance, yet it is very effective—*in some cases*.

The basis for patching is self-evident. Amblyopia is typically accompanied by strabismus and/or anisometropia. In the former, a patch over the fixating eye forces the normally deviating eye to take up alignment, except perhaps in one type of deviation: eccentric fixation (see below); and even here it *may* work. In anisometropia without strabismus, the patch eliminates the inhibitory influence imposed on the amblyopic eye when the nonamblyopic eye is open and functioning (2). Hence, the patch is a formidable device in that it usually brings about the desired conditions for improved function.

Because it is so powerful, patching should not be done without close supervision. The wearing schedule must take into account the child's age. The younger the patient, the more susceptible the nonamblyopic eye is to the detrimental effects of the patch. *Occlusion amblyopia* may be produced in children up to about the age of five (3). The best method for dealing with this concern is to alternate the patch from one eye to the other, thereby providing the better eye some occasional visual stimulation but not so much as to neutralize the effect of the treatment on the amblyopic eye. The following guidelines appear to be effective and safe:

Age of patient	Patch on good eye/ poor eye	
birth–one	2 days	1 day
one–three	3 days	1 day
three–four	4 days	1 day
four–above	6 days	1 day

Notice that on those days when the patch is not occluding the nonamblyopic eye it is placed over the amblyopic eye. The rationale for this varies from: (a) psychological: it does not disrupt the child's acceptance of the patch; to (b) physiological: it prevents a slipping back into the former, faulty binocular condition wherein the nonamblyopic eye imposes an inhibitory influence on the amblyopic eye.*

Some optometrists elect to patch by occluding a spectacle lens, others by occluding the eye directly. The former may be accomplished by painting the lens with natural shade nail polish, or covering the inside surface with translucent Scotch Magic Tape, or simply wrapping it with a strip of cloth. In most cases—especially with younger children—we prefer direct patching of the eye. This, too, may be done in a variety of ways. Some optometrists suggest that an opaque contact lens be used because it eliminates the social discomfort that the patch may cause some children and/or their parents. For the less adventuresome, there are commercially produced occluders, including the (paper thin, semiporous, hypoallergenic) Opticlude eye patch and the Elastoplast Eye Occlusor.

Application of a patch has significant effects on the child's ability to function effectively. Hence, the optometrist must take into account how the patient is to spend her day. Preschool-aged children will encounter far fewer problems from full-time patching than will older patients. The school-aged child, whose visual acuity in the amblyopic eye is very poor (e.g., 20/200), will not be able to comply with the therapy yet meet the requirements of her classroom. A part-time regimen will be more suitable for her, at least until school vacation commences. (Indeed, there is a fair amount of published evidence that indicates that part-time patching produces good results, that constant occlusion is not essential [4].)

The patient should be rechecked often and regularly, more often if she is very young (e.g., twice a month with 1- to 2-year-olds, up to once a month with 5-year-olds and above). The visit is used to reassess visual acuity and fixation accuracy, probe for other treatment effects, obtain a report from the parent regarding observations and problems encountered, and revise the regimen if so indicated.

Ordinarily, initial changes are more dramatic than later ones. It is not unusual to record a change from 20/200 to 20/70 or so within the first few weeks of patching, and a subsequent improvement to 20/30 or 20/40 over the next 3 to 4 months.

Stop patching therapy after visual acuity has stopped improving; after visual acuity has remained unchanged for 3 months or so (5).

Alternatives to Patching

Drugs. Although there are variations in approach, the central concept in the use of drugs for the treatment of amblyopia is to substitute the patch with a drug-induced blur. Atropine is the drug cited most often (e.g., see [6]). The method became popular under the name *penalization*. Many reports were published documenting its value. These have since attracted counterarguments, and it appears now that the method is not sufficiently effective to warrant its use in place of a patch.

*Because the patch is used during waking hours only, the child will undoubtedly have some occasions, albeit brief, to look about with both eyes open. This is considered desirable by some authorities and irrelevant by others.

Plus Lens.   The principle behind this method is obvious. A plus lens of sufficient power will function much like a blur-inducing drug, but it avoids the problems that the drug might generate. Its drawback is also obvious: The child is able to avoid the blur by looking over the lens—something he cannot do if a drug or patch is used.

Light Filter.   This involves the reduction of light available to the nonamblyopic eye by application of filters. Wesson (8) reports successful use of the method (using a polaroid filter) with a 7-year-old anisometropic, eccentrically fixating amblyope; visual acuity improved from 20/100 to 20/26, fixation from 2 degrees eccentric to "unsteady central," and stereoacuity from 0 to 140 second arc.

Procedures to Supplement Patching

Listed below are a variety of activities (some suitable for children as young as age 2) that supplement occlusion therapy and may be particularly useful in cases where monocular foveal alignment is not accurate. All of the activities are similar in that they are designed to stimulate precise spatial localization in the amblyopic eye. They vary in regard to the materials/equipment employed, a factor that influences motivation and therefore is important to the endeavor.

The activities may be used interchangeably or in combinations. There is no order of efficacy implied in the listing, but this flexibility should not be reflected when the procedures are described to the patient/parent. Activities should be thoroughly defined, a daily schedule should be determined, and the necessary materials either identified or provided, depending upon availability. In other words, even though the activities and materials may reflect a casual approach to therapy, the attitude with which they are prescribed should not. The patient/ parent should be impressed with the need for regular practice and precision: *structure;* benign structure, but structure nonetheless.

Representative Activities.   The activity should be designed to aid the child develop the ability to localize objects precisely with his amblyopic eye. This takes precedence over the ability to discriminate fine detail. In other words, initially it is more important for the eye to become adept at determining the *where* of objects than the what.

The goal in each activity is to perform the prescribed task as precisely and effortlessly as the nonoccluded eye will allow. The list is not exhaustive. Very little imagination is needed to expand it significantly.

Follow a designated path. This may vary from a series of stepping stones in a public park to a path defined by foot-sized pieces of construction paper that meanders through a house.

Kick an object toward a specific target. This may vary from a large soccer ball kicked in some general direction to a ping-pong ball or marble kicked into a large drinking glass (positioned horizontally) by the big toe.

Fishing with a hook and eyes. This involves inserting "hook-eyes" into an assortment of objects (e.g., edible marshmallows work well). Supply the child with a "fishing pole" from which a line and hook (such as one used to suspend a plant from a ceiling) are suspended. The goal, obviously, is to obtain ("catch") the marshmallows. Variation is possible by using (a) different-sized hook-eyes; (b) poles of different lengths; (c) lines of different lengths.

Play catch. Initially, it is best to use an inflated balloon. In time, a large, then a small, ball may be introduced in place of the balloon.

Hit the ball. All sorts of apparatus may be used: e.g., baseball bat, tennis racket, ping-pong paddle, etc.

Draw, trace, color, follow-the-dots, cut out patterns, string beads or popcorn or various breakfast cereals, "spear" raisins with a toothpick, pound nails, duplicate letter sequences on a typewriter, reconstruct (copy) patterns with paper and paste, blocks, construction toys, pegboards, geoboards, etc. (A number of the visual perceptual skills activities described in Chapter 15 may be used here. The difference: In this context, the child works monocularly; the other eye is occluded. In the pursuit of improved spatial analysis skills, the patch would function as an extraneous distractor.)

Map reading and map construction. The basic map reading task may take the form of having the child position an assortment of kitchen utensils (e.g., knife, fork, spoon) in conformance with a drawn sketch. The beginning map construction task might follow the same format. In time, these activities might reach the stage where the child is able to produce a map (i.e., floor plan) that depicts objects within a defined space (e.g., furniture in a room; trees in a yard), illustrating clearly an awareness of spatial relationships.

Target practice. This may vary from "bowling" with a rubber ball and a paper towel tube to attempting to activate a photoelectric cell with a light gun.

Etc. It should be obvious that there are countless options: variations, and variations of those variations. Everything and anything is suitable so long as the previously defined instructional principles are kept in mind (see Chapter 9).

Other Procedures to Supplement Monocular Occlusion When the Patient Displays Eccentric Fixation

We noted above that monocular occlusion alone may not have sufficient impact on amblyopia that is accompanied by eccentric fixation. The activities described above are likely to be helpful, but there are a few other supplemental activities that should also be considered, particularly when the ones already described prove to be insufficient.

Red Filter. This calls for total occlusion of the nonamblyopic eye and constant use of a red filter in front of the amblyopic eye. The filter should obstruct wave lengths shorter than 640 μm (Kodak gelatin Wratten filter No. 92). There is disagreement regarding why (e.g., see 9,10), but there is consensus that the procedure is often helpful.

Prisms. A number of different approaches have been proposed that incorporate a prism before the eccentrically fixating eye. Some report good results with "reverse prism." For example, Pigassou and Garipuy (11) recommend the use of a base-in prism for nasal eccentric fixation, and a base-out for temporal eccentric fixation, with the power determined by the distance between the fovea and fixation point. Others disagree (12) and offer alternative suggestions. The concept continues to be explored and debated. The optometrist is well advised to monitor the literature and be guided accordingly.

Inverse Occlusion. The notion of occluding the amblyopic eye is linked specifically with the treatment of eccentric fixation, the rationale being that the eccentrically fixating eye should not be allowed to function except under controlled conditions, such as during treatment sessions (see pleoptics discussion, below). Inverse occlusion has yet to demonstrate its worth when compared with direct occlusion (13). Its popularity, never great, now appears to be waning.

Pleoptics. The essential rationale in pleoptics is that the eccentric fixator will use his macula if the area surrounding it is bleached out with a very bright light.

Two methods emerged during the decade following World War II. One employs a modified indirect ophtalmoscope (pleoptophor) to shield the fovea while dazzling the surrounding retina with bright light (14). The other (15) is an extension of this in that the patient is taught to take advantage of the afterimage produced by circummacular dazzling done with an instrument known as a euthyscope; to use the afterimage as a "tag," a method for knowing where to direct his gaze in order to gain optimal visual acuity. Both approaches use inverse occlusion except during treatment sessions until central fixation becomes established.

A number of hand-eye activities and instruments were produced to accompany the procedures, and in fact schools were founded in Switzerland (Sehschulen) so that the children would be in daily attendance, thereby allowing for high-intensity treatment schedules.

Pleoptics was never completely accepted in the United States. Many of its initial supporters have now dropped it (6). It appears that the central notion is well founded; that is, treatment of a sensory-motor deficit works best when the patient is provided with an external signal that enables him to monitor the accuracy of his performance. Pleoptics does this, but so too do any number of simple hand-eye activities done in combination with occulsion of the nonamblyopic eye (see above). The key ingredient, obviously is the patient's ability to "learn" from the procedure.

Entoptic Phenomena 1. *Haidinger's brushes.* This phenomenon was mentioned earlier, in regard to the assessment of fixation accuracy (see Chapter 4). It may also be used in therapy, and properly so, because (a) the patient will perceive the "brushes" if his macula is intact; (b) the brushes, by their very nature, emphasize spatial localization; they are external markers of foveal projection; (c) the patient monitors his own performance by noting the match between where he is attempting to fixate and where he perceives the brushes; (d) this match may be quantified.

Implementation is not complicated, but explaining the phenomenon and associated procedures to young children is exceptionally difficult; too difficult for most preschoolers.

The procedure calls for the patient to attempt to project the brushes onto various fixation targets by controlling where he fixates, using his finger or a hand-held pointer as an aid in monitoring his performance. A number of manufacturers produce instruments capable of eliciting this phenomenon.

2. *Maxwell's spot*. This is similar to Haidinger's brushes in that seeing the spot depends upon macular integrity, and where it is perceived—its location—on where the eye is fixating. It is used in much the same way as Haidinger's brushes, both in the testing and training of fixation accuracy. As such, it too is not useful with preschoolers. The quality of the visual illusion is too abstract to explain properly to that age group.

3. *Afterimage transfer*. This method calls for stimulating the fovea of the normal eye with an appropriate light source in order to evoke an afterimage in that eye; then effecting a transfer of the afterimage to the amblyopic eye. Once done, the patient is encouraged to project the afterimage in the amblyopic eye onto letters of decreasing size, thereby eliminating fixation errors (16).

Auditory Feedback. Although this approach is still at the experimental stage, it is sufficiently impressive to acknowledge. In essence, the patient is supplied an auditory signal that, by its pitch and position, informs him of where he is fixating. It has been found to be effective with adult, eccentrically fixating amblyopes in helping them maintain steady and foveal fixation (17).

PROCEDURES DESIGNED TO IMPROVE RETINOCORTICAL FUNCTION

The focus of this section is the patient who manifests unilateral amblyopia *despite* accurate foveal alignment. Hence, a basic difference between the procedures described here and those in the previous section is that the latter emphasized accurate localization: the *"where"* of a visual stimulus within a visual space. These stress visual discrimination: the *"what."* The connection between the two is obvious. Refined localization is prerequisite to refined discrimination.

In fact, of course, many of the procedures described in the preceding section are, with slight modifications, applicable here with certain patients. The determinant is the patient's binocular status.

The patient who lacks normal binocular vision even though she fixates accurately will benefit from the procedures described above so long as the emphasis is shifted from precise localization to precise discrimination. This is not the case with amblyopes who do have binocular vision. They need a different treatment approach.

For this reason, the material that follows is organized into two sections: (a) procedures for the amblyope with accurate foveal fixation who lacks binocular vision; (b) procedures for the amblyope who displays binocular vision.

FOR THE CENTRALLY FIXATING AMBLYOPE WHO LACKS NORMAL BINOCULAR VISION

As noted above, remedial therapy for the amblyope who lacks normal binocular vision, because of unilateral strabismus and/or anisometropia, is not radically different than therapy for the amblyope with eccentric fixation. The basic approach continues to be direct monocular occlusion in combination with supplementary activities, if the child is old enough to profit from the activities; if she is not, then patching alone will have to do.

Occlusion
See above. The same guidelines are applicable here.

Procedures to Supplement Patching
Once again, the list is not exhaustive. It may easily be expanded.

1. Follow a designated path. This has already been described (see p. 402). In this instance, however, use more demanding visual stimuli, such as a printed maze through which a path is to be drawn with a pencil.
2. Precise pointing. Insert a pointer (e.g., a knitting needle) into a straw without touching the side of the straw.
3. Precise tracing, coloring, filling in and/or counting all the letter "o's" in a newspaper column (or the "a's," or the "p's," etc.).
4. Define specific routes between two points on a road map.
5. Find and circle specific number/letter sequences in a newspaper or telephone book (e.g., circle the sequence "123" whenever you find one; or the sequence "321" or "adg," etc.).
6. Etc.

FOR THE CENTRALLY FIXATING AMBLYOPE WHO DISPLAYS SINGLE BINOCULAR VISION

There are advantages in avoiding occlusion with this group. The optometrist should attempt, instead, to institute a therapy program that stimulates the amblyopic eye while the nonamblyopic eye is open and functioning. In other words, the patient engages in monocular therapy under binocular viewing conditions.

Red Pencil and Red/Green Filters
Supply the patient with a pair of red/green filter spectacles* and a red pencil.** If a red line is drawn on paper, the eye behind the green filter will perceive it

*Available from Bernell Mfg. Corp.
**Eagle Prismacolor: Scarlet red #992.

as black. The eye behind the red filter will not see it at all. Hence, if the green filter is placed before the amblyopic eye and the patient is asked, say, to trace over a black line drawing with the red pencil, both eyes will perceive the black line drawing but only the amblyopic eye will see the lines drawn with the red pencil.

For variation, provide the child with follow-the-dots activities, mazes, "hidden pictures," the task of filling in all the letter "o's" she can find in a newspaper column, and so on. These are all useful if the visual target is printed in black (visible to both eyes) and she writes with the red pencil, which is visible to the amblyopic eye only. (These conditions may also be reversed: Draw o's with the red pencil and have patient fill them in with black pencil, etc.)

Another variation: Obtain (or make your own) *red* (rather than black) mazes, follow-the-dot patterns, and other activities. Have the child work through these with a black pencil. Again, the green filter is placed before the amblyopic eye, thereby limiting the red material to that eye while both eyes see what is drawn with the black pencil.

Cheiroscope Tracing

This refers to a condition wherein a stimulus is presented in a stereoscope to one eye: the eye opposite the patient's preferred drawing hand. The other eye views a blank sheet of paper. The patient with normal binocular vision will project the stimulus onto that blank space and be unaware of which eye is perceiving the stimulus and which is projecting it.

The patient is given a colored pencil and asked to trace over the projected stimulus. Because the space before her is blank (but covered with paper), it will appear to an onlooker as though the patient is drawing the stimulus, but in fact she is tracing over it—as long as she functions binocularly.

Start with simple line drawings and work up to complex ones.

The procedure may be varied in a number of ways. For example, play tic-tac-toe; one person marks X's on the drawn pattern that is in front of the patient's eye opposite her preferred drawing hand, while the patient draws O's on her apparently blank—but not to her—stage.

Both Wheatstone and Brewster stereoscopes have been adapted for this purpose.

Physiological Diplopia

The phenomenon of physiological diplopia also may be exploited usefully in the treatment of the amblyope who displays single binocular vision. Although a pencil or a finger will do, the so-called Brock string (18) has gained favor. It has the distinct advantage of not only eliciting physiological diplopia but, at the same time, providing the patient with a precise method for monitoring where her eyes are directed (see discussion regarding use of pointers, p. 421).

The basic procedure calls for a string to be stretched taut, one end held by the patient at the bridge of her nose, the other end attached to some distant point (e.g., the therapist's hand or a doorknob). The binocular patient fixating at the far end of the string should see two strings that converge to a point at the fixation target in the form of a horizontal "V." Obviously, the string that appears to be coming from the patient's left eye is, in fact, projected by her right eye, and vice versa (i.e., crossed diplopia).

If a small target (e.g., a paper clip or a pen) is suspended from the string at a point between the patient and her fixation point, she will perceive two suspended targets, assuming that both her eyes are fixating simultaneously. By varying the number of suspended targets and their relative locations, the patient is provided with a series of experiences that will aid in sensitizing her amblyopic eye, while the other eye continues to function normally.

Bar Reader
This is a simple apparatus. Actually, any vertically oriented object will do, if its width causes the fields of both eyes to be obstructed but not overlapped when it is held between the eyes and the object of regard. It may be used while the child reads sequences of letters, numerals, words, etc., arranged horizontally. Obviously, the demands on the amblyopic eye increase as smaller stimuli are introduced.

Bar readers are produced commercially, but there hardly seems to be any justification for purchasing them. A wooden tongue depressor or, for that matter, a 3/4-inch strip of paper will serve well.

TV Trainer
This device has already been described (see p. 225). In this instance, there is less concern regarding viewing distance and more on clarity of image perceived by each eye.

CAM
This procedure generated great interest when it was first reported. The patient views slowly rotating, high-contrast square wave gratings (black and white stripes) with her amblyopic eye, sometimes playing tic-tac-toe on a transparent plastic sheet that covers the rotating stripes. A treatment session lasts 7 minutes. The patient does not use an occluder except during the treatment sessions.

Initial reports regarding this treatment claimed significant effects after remarkably few (e.g., three) sessions (19). The rationale proposed by its authors was that all visual cortical neurones were stimulated by using the different spatial frequency square waves at varying rates.

Many researchers have investigated the CAM method. Their reports are not so enthusiastic and, in the main, tend to conclude that some improvement in visual acuity often does result from the treatment, but that it is probably attributable to the short-term occlusion and to improved visual acuity (VA) test-taking abilities rather than to the rotating gratings (20,21,22,23,24,25). The method undoubtedly will be investigated further. As of now, it must be viewed as an interesting idea, not a validated treatment.

BILATERAL AMBLYOPIA

Bilateral amblyopia has been ignored here, thus far, not because it is unimportant but, rather, because there is relatively little that can be done in such cases. The rule of thumb with bilateral amblyopia, usually associated with high hyperopia and/or astigmia, is to apply a correct and full compensatory lens prescription as early in life as is possible. Remedial therapy has not been shown to be of any value (26).

SUMMARY COMMENTS REGARDING REMEDIATION OF AMBLYOPIA

Amblyopia is a prevalent condition that is readily identified in very young children and often can be reduced, if not eliminated—*if remedial treatment is started early enough*.

Treatment programs tend to be uncomplicated, easily managed, and relatively quick acting. Obviously, there are cases where the amblyopia is intractable, but no case should be so labeled until significant efforts have been devoted to conclusive diagnosis and/or remediation.

■ COMPENSATORY TREATMENT

There are very few useful compensatory treatments for amblyopia. Obviously, the best of these is the same as the first step of a remedial effort: determine and prescribe lenses that will neutralize the patient's ametropia and maximize her visual acuity. Other than that, low vision optical aids and special placement in school or work may be useful; i.e., enrollment in a class for the visually impaired, if that is warranted, or perhaps simply a seat closer to the front in a standard classroom. However, these approaches are not usually needed. Most amblyopes manifest the condition in one eye only, thereby eliminating the need for special arrangements in school or work.

■ REASSURANCE THERAPY

There are three types of amblyopic patients who should be offered reassurance.

One, the patient with unilateral amblyopia who has already been correctly treated but did not benefit very much from that treatment. For example, a 10-year-old patient with congenital, unilateral strabismus who, when he was younger (five, say), engaged in an appropriate patching regimen for more than a year but showed only limited improvement in acuity (e.g., obtained 20/80 acuity fairly quickly but stopped there). It is not reasonable to expect different and better results now, unless there is a question about his compliance during the first attempt.

The second type: the patient with unilateral amblyopia who has never been treated, who is now well past the so-called "critical period" of vision development, who has made an acceptable adaptation to the condition, and whose amblyopia derives from a binocular anomaly that persists and is not likely to be eliminated. (Note: Just what the critical period is for humans has not yet been determined. Most authorities tend to agree that it extends from birth to about age six or seven (27). When the phrase is used in this book, it refers to that definition.) For example—and a fairly common circumstance—a 12-year-old whose amblyopia derives from marked anisometropia (O.D.): +0.50D sph; O.S.: +4.25 −3.50 cx 145). She was given her first glasses when in first grade, but did not wear them very much. "They did not help." Glasses were tried again a year later with the same outcome. No other treatment has been tried.

Why should she be reassured? Why not make another attempt at glasses and vision therapy? After all, no one can predict what might happen to her right (nonamblyopic) eye at some future date. What if something did occur that impaired the sight of that eye? She would then have to depend on the amblyopic left eye. All of this adds up to a strong argument for taking action now, albeit the poor prognosis—looking after the "spare tire," "just in case," rather than waiting until it is "too late."

The argument sounds reasonable. And, in fact, such patients sometimes do respond to vision therapy, even at this late date. The visual acuity of their amblyopic eye improves a line or two, evidence of the fact that their visual systems had developed somewhat during their early years. But, the fact is that the potential for improvement that exists now, at age ten, will continue to exist in the future. This patient, already past the developmental period, will respond the same to amblyopia treatment later on as she does now—even if treatment is held off for many years—so long as nothing alters the integrity of the visual system in the interim (e.g., cataract, corneal scar, central nervous system lesion, etc.). Should the latter occur, it will, of course, alter the above prediction, but the same negative effects would also be suffered by the patient who did receive amblyopia treatment now. In short, once the patient is past the critical period of vision development, the "spare tire" argument is not valid. What has developed will remain intact; what not yet developed will not develop now. Therefore, in most cases, reassurance is as good a treatment as is patching; and in some cases, it is preferred because it does not disrupt the (presumably) satisfactory adaptation that the patient has effected.

The third type: the bilateral amblyope. For example, a patient with significant bilateral hyperopic astigmatism (O.U.: +6.50 −2.25 cx 90) who did not begin to wear glasses until past the age of 5 years. There is very little to do for this type of amblyopia except to prescribe compensatory lenses (as early in life as possible), stress the importance of constant wear, alleviate whatever anxieties there may be about the long-term implications of the condition (i.e., that it will not get worse), and instruct the parents on the importance of early identification should others in the family have a similar condition.

___■_____

PRACTICAL SUGGESTIONS

12-1. Patches may be decorated to make them more attractive; e.g., use different colored materials, draw "smile" faces.

12-2. Active therapy may be carried out at mealtimes by having the child "spear" garden peas, raisins, and other small things with a toothpick. (This will not do much for table manners, but . . .)

12-3. Scotch (3-M) Magic Tape applied to the inner surface of a lens functions very well as a patch—so long as the goal is to produce complete blur rather than to prevent light stimulation. This tape has the characteristic of making the lens translucent from the wearer's point of view, but almost transparent to the external observer. Hence, it is less objectionable to the patient who is concerned by the attention a patch is apt to draw.

12-4. Keep an eye out for toys/activities that would be useful for amblyopia vision therapy. For example, mosaic blocks that are colored in a way compatible with the red/green filter glasses used in tranaglyph activities, etc.

___■_____

REFERENCES

1. De Buffon M. Dissertation sur la cause du strabisme ou des yeux louches. Hist Acad R Science 1743; p. 231.
2. Schor C, Terell M, Peterson D. Contour interaction and temporal masking in strabismus and amblyopia. AJOPO 1976; 53:217.
3. Noorden GK von. Experimental amblyopia in monkeys. Further behavioral and clinical correlations. Inv Ophthal 1973; 12:721.
4. Mitchell DE, Howell ER, Keith CS. The effect of minimal occlusion therapy on binocular visual functions in amblyopia. Invest Ophthal Vis Sci 1983; 24:778–81.
5. Gregersen E, Rindzuinski E. "Conventional" occlusion in the treatment of squint amblyopia. Acta Ophthal 1965; 43:162.
6. Noorden GK von. Binocular vision and ocular motility. St. Louis: Mosby, 1980.
7. Brack B. Penalisation and prism: new results obtained with the method of treating squint amblyopia with eccentric fixation. In Moore S, ed. Orthoptics: past, present, future.

8. Wesson MD. Use of light intensity reduction for amblyopia therapy. AJOPO 1983; 60(2) :112–17.
9. Brinker WR, Katz SL. New and practical treatment of eccentric fixation. Am J Ophthal 1963; 55:1033.
10. Adler FH. Foveal fixation. Am J Ophthal 1963; 56:483.
11. Pigassou R, Garipuy J. Traitement de la fixation excentrique strabique par le port d'un prisme et l' occlusion. Boll Mem Soc Fr Ophtal 1966; 79:367.
12. Aust W. The use of prisms in pre- and post-operative treatment. In: Fells P, ed. The First Congress of the Int'l. Strabismological Assn. St. Louis: Mosby, 1971.
13. Mackensen G et al. Untersuchungen zum problem der exzentrischen fixation. Doc Ophthal 1967; 23:228.
14. Bangerter A. Behandlung der amblyopie. Ophthalmologica 1946; 111:220.
15. Cuppers C. Moderne Schielbehandlung. Klin Monatsbl Augenheilkd 1956; 129:579.
16. Caloroso E. After-image transfer: a therapeutic procedure for amblyopia. AJOPO 1972; 49 (1):65.
17. Flom MC, Kirschen DG, Bedell HE. Control of unsteady, eccentric fixation in amblyopic eyes by auditory feedback of eye position. Inv Ophthal 1980: 19(11):1371.
18. Greenwald I. Effective strabismus therapy. Duncan, Okla.: O.E.P. Foundation, 1979.
19. Banks RV, Campbell FW, Hess RF, Watson PG. A new treatment for amblyopia. Br Orthop J 1978; 35:1.
20. Koskela PU. Contrast sensitivity in amblyopia, I: Changes during CAM treatment. Acta Ophthal 1986; 64:344–51.
21. Nathanson DR, Ciuffreda KJ. Results in intensive CAM grating treatment in a strabismic amblyope. AJOPO 1982; 59(6):511–14.
22. Schor C, Gibson J, Hsu M, Mah M. The use of rotating gratings for the treatment of amblyopia: a clinical trial. AJOPO 1981; 58(11):930–38.
23. Woo GC, Dalziel CC. A pilot study of contrast sensitivity assessment of the CAM treatment of amblyopia. Acta Ophthal 1981; 59:35.
24. Dalziel CC. Amblyopia therapy by the Campbell-Hess technique. AJOPO 1980; 57:280.
25. Tytla ME, Labow-Daily LS. Evaluation of the CAM treatment for amblyopia: a controlled study. Inv Ophth 1981; 20(3): 400.
26. Singh G, Schulz E. Bilateral deprivation amblyopia. Annal Ophthal 1984; 16 (1):86–88.
27. Banks MS, Aslin RN, Tetson RD. Sensitive period for the development of human binocular vision. Science 1975; 190:675–77.

13

Nystagmus

☐

The clinical management of nystagmus is much like the clinical management of strabismus and amblyopia. Again, the optometrist must decide on what to recommend once active pathology has been ruled out: remedial, compensatory, or reassurance therapy.

■ REMEDIAL THERAPY

As noted earlier, this is a fairly recent and untested area of endeavor. Five procedures have been reported. The order in which they are presented below does not imply relative merit.

1. Elicit an afterimage (e.g., with a strobe light) and urge the patient to control its movements. Clearly, this requires remarkable insights and abilities from the patient, but some success has been reported (1,2,3).

2. The patient engages in a variety of visual tasks (e.g., searching for specific letters in a page of print, tracing over drawings) while looking through a Kodak Wratten #92 (red) filter. Here too, the ultimate value of the therapy depends upon the patient's ability to invent a method for maintaining images on the central retina. The purpose of the red lens is to limit visual stimulation to the foveal area; this based on the rationale that only the cones will be stimulated by the light passing through the filter (4).

3. Auditory biofeedback has been shown to have some value (5). The patient is given tonal information about the relative location and stability of his eye. He attempts to exploit this information in acquiring control over the globe (6).

4. Strabismus therapy has been found to be useful in cases where the nystagmus appears to be secondary to strabismus (7) (see Chapters 6 and 11).

5. Atropine (1%) instilled daily in each eye has been reported to be helpful, especially in latent nystagmus (8).

A review of the information cited above corroborates what was stated initially. Relatively little has been validated. This does not rule out the possibility of employing one of the above procedures with a nystagmus patient. But, it does suggest that the treatment not be portrayed as anything but a "promising experiment."

■

COMPENSATORY TREATMENT

The nystagmus patient who has to tilt her head or cross-fixate in order to improve her visual acuity will be exceptionally grateful for any type of relief.

1. In cases where convergence is shown to reduce the nystagmus, consider:
   a. more minus (or less plus) than the farpoint refractive status calls for. This will stimulate accommodative convergence and therefore be helpful—to the extent that the benefit of the additional convergence is not counterbalanced by discomfort from the extra accommodation effort (9).
   b. base-out prism at farpoint (O.U.) to the extent that it reduces the nystagmus (and improves acuity) but does not exert excessive demands on the patient's positive fusional vergence abilities (10).
2. In cases where prism neutralizes the anomalous head position (see Chapter 6), prescribe the prism and/or recommend a surgical consultation to evalutate the potential benefit of extraocular muscle surgery in lieu of the prisms (11,12,13,14,15).
3. In cases where nystagmus is secondary to albinism or aniridia, consider a contact lens with an artificial iris to optimize visual acuity and control the transmission of light.

■

REASSURANCE THERAPY

See Chapter 9.

■

PRACTICAL SUGGESTIONS

13-1. Measure the nystagmus patient's visual acuity in primary gaze and again when she is in favored "head position." This provides useful baseline data.

13-2. Consider instituting some remedial therapy, based upon the patient's apparent ability to benefit from feedback.

REFERENCES

1. Cuppers C, Sevrin G. Le probleme de la fixation dans l'amblyopie et particularierment dans le nystagmus. Bull Soc F Ophthal 1956; 69:359.
2. Ciuffreda KJ. Jerk nystagmus; some new findings. AJOPO 1979; 56(8):521.
3. Mallett RFJ. The treatment of congenital idiopathic nystagmus by intermittent photic stimulation. Ophthal Physiol Opt 1983; 3(3):341–56.
4. Calcutt C, Crook W. A treatment of amblyopia in patients with latent nystagmus. Br Orthop J 1972;29:70.
5. Abadi RV, Carden D, Simpson J. A new treatment for congenital nystagmus. Br J Ophthal 1980; 64(1):2.
6. Ciuffreda KJ, Goldrich SG, Neary C. Use of eye movement auditory biofeedback in the control of nystagmus. AJOPO 1982; 59(5):396–409.
7. Healy E. Nystagmus treated by orthoptics: a second report. Am Orthop J 1962; 12:89.
8. Windsor CE, Burian HM, Milojevic G. Modification of latent nystagmus. Arch Ophthal 1968; 80:657.
9. Colburn EJ. Fixation of the external rectus muscle in nystagmus and paralysis. Am J Ophthal 1906; 23:85
10. Metzger EL. Correction of congenital nystagmus. Am J Ophthal 1950; 33:1796.
11. Goode-Jolly D. Larmande A. Nystagmus congenital. In: Les nystagmus. Paris: Masson, 1973.
12. Dell'Osso LF. Prism exploitation of gaze and fusional null angles in congenital nystagmus. In Moore S ed. Orthoptics: past, present, future. New York: Stratton International Med Book Corp., 1976.
13. Sandall GS. Surgical treatment of congenital nystagmus in patients with singular binocular vision. Ann Ophthal 1976; 8(2):227–38.
14. Scott WE, Kraft SP. Surgical treatment of compensatory head position in congenital nystagmus. J Ped Ophthal Strab 1984; 21(3):85.
15. Spielmann A. Congenital nystagmus: clinical types and their surgical treatment. Ophthalmologica 1981; 182:65–72.

14

Substandard Vergence and/or Accommodation Facility

□

The clinical management of vergence and accommodation infacility and intermittent strabismus* is not complex. Unlike constant strabismus, where the treatment is aimed at replacing a deviant behavior with a normal behavior, the goal in the treatment of inadequate vergence and/or accommodation facility is to enhance an already existing high-level, normal function.

As noted in Chapter 7, treatment may be remedial or compensatory, with the former being preferred if a choice exists. But, again unlike constant strabismus, there is no inherent risk in combining the two: providing an interim compensatory treatment and delaying the remediation effort until a more opportune time. Compensatory treatment of deficient vergence and/or accommodation facility does not include irreversible, surgically produced structural changes that often introduce their own complications, nor occlusion, with all the anxieties it may generate. It is not inappropriate, therefore, for the optometrist to incorporate into her recommendations an assurance that no harm will result from delaying remediation so long as compensatory treatment is provided in the meantime.

The treatment of vergence facility deficits is not markedly different, in principle, from the treatment of substandard accommodation facility. There is, however, sufficient difference in how these principles are applied in the two conditions to require that each be discussed separately.

■

DEFICIENT VERGENCE FACILITY

□ Remedial Therapy

See flow diagram in Figure 9.1.

---

*The treatment directives presented in this chapter pertain also to intermittent strabismus, as long as the patient, when her eyes are aligned, demonstrates precise binocular alignment: i.e., better than 120 seconds arc stereoacuity at distance and 60 seconds arc at near. See p. 206 for additional comments regarding this distinction between constant and intermittent strabismus.

FINAL (LEVEL IV) GOALS

Upon completion of treatment, the patient is able (and has practiced daily, for at least the past 3 months)* to execute fusional vergence "jumps" from:

At far: 6pd base-in *to* 12pd base-out, and vice versa;** *and*

At near: 12pd base-in *to* 14pd base-out, and vice versa.**

In both conditions (far and near), the treatment goals are far more demanding than the vergence facility screening test criteria stated in Chapter 7. The magnitude of the jump is greater (from base-in to base-out to base-in, rather than from plano to either base-in or base-out, then back to plano), the speed requirements are more stringent, and the patient must be able to sustain at the task for a much longer period of time. This is done to guarantee that the patient is *overtrained*, that the skills he is learning are developed to an automatic level of performance.

Notice, also, that the goals stress facility—fluent adaptability—more than magnitude. It is much more important to teach the patient the former than to foster the acqusition of inordinately high vergence and accommodation thresholds (1). This is especially true when treating intermittent strabismus.

SUBORDINATE GOALS AND THEIR HIERARCHICAL INTERRELATIONSHIPS

Defining subordinate goals for a vergence facility program is, in many ways, an arbitrary process. Because the patient already has normal single binocular vision, at least occasionally, the subordinate treatment goals are the same as the terminal goals in every way except their respective levels of difficulty.

One may designate many subordinate goals, each representing a small change in performance ability, or just a few levels, each one representing a substantial change. It is analogous to debating the merit of including 20/55, 20/45, and 20/35 lines of letters in a visual acuity chart. Both formats have their advantages, but practical considerations suggest that the best organization is something in between the two extremes.

The subordinate goals listed below represent a middle-of-the-road position. Three levels are defined (and listed in descending order of difficulty) as subserving the final (level IV) goals, stated above.

Level III: Patient is able to execute fusional vergence jumps from:

At far: 4pd base-in *to* 6pd base-out, and vice versa;†

and

At near: 8pd base-in *to* 8pd base-out, and vice versa.†

*A key factor in any skills training program is frequent and organized practice. As such, we recommend that remedial vision therapy be carried out at home, with office visits devoted to monitoring patient progress and modifying the treatment regimen accordingly; see Chapter 9 for additional comments regarding this topic.

**Sixty cycles within 5 minutes. Cycle = Start with fusion/clarity through base-in prism; then fuse/clear through base-out prism; then again through base-in. Test at far; then at near.

†Sixty cycles within 5 minutes; cycle = as defined above, for level IV. Test at far; then at near.

Level II: Patient is able to execute fusional vergence jumps from:
At far: 2pd base-in *to* 4pd base-out, and vice versa;*

and

At near: 4pd base-in *to* 6pd base-out, and vice versa.*
Level I: There are two goals for this level:

      a. Patient is able to execute fusional vergence jumps from:
      At far: 3pd base-in *to* plano, and vice versa;* 3pd base-out *to* plano, and vice versa;*

and

      At near: 6pd base-in *to* plano, and vice versa;* 6pd base-out *to* plano, and vice versa.*

      b. Patient experiences/reports physiological diplopia immediately upon being presented with appropriate stimuli and conditions (e.g., a row of letters at 6 meters and a penlight at 40 cm).

PLACEMENT TEST

Begin placement testing at level I. If the patient demonstrates mastery of those goals, test for level II goals, and so on, until failure is demonstrated. Patient is "placed"—i.e., is to begin vision therapy—in that level, the level in which she failed. (See case reports of Patients Arthur and Richard on pp. 504–510 for illustrations of this principle.)

During placement testing, pay special attention to relative differences in performance the patient may display as a function of:

1. *Fixation distance.* If she has significantly more difficulty at one fixation distance than at another (i.e., far versus near), therapy should begin with the least demanding condition, the other being introduced as progress allows. If no major difference is observed, then the patient may start where it is most convenient.

2. *Direction of the vergence adaptation.* Some patients have much more difficulty meeting the demands of base-out prism than they do base-in prism; others, vice versa. If the patient shows a marked difference, therapy should begin with the type of vergence demand that presents the least difficulty. If no major difference is observed, then she may start where it is most convenient.

REMEDIAL ACTIVITIES

There are numerous options (2,3,4,5,6). The essential aspect of a procedure should be that it provides the conditions for stimulating positive and negative relative fusional convergence: vergence that is triggered by pairs of disparate retinal images projected from a single object and occurs with no (or little) related changes in accommodation. If the procedure allows for that and if it can be carried out on a regular basis and independent of direct professional supervision (i.e., in the pa-

---

*Sixty cycles within 5 minutes; cycle = start with fusion/clarity without prism then fusion/clarity through base-in prism; then again fuse/clear when prism is removed. Repeat with base-out prism. Test at far; then at near.

tient's home), it is potentially useful; but some are more useful than others because of other factors.

One obvious reason why some procedures are more useful than others for a given patient relates to differences she displayed during placement testing in response to different fixation distances and different directions of vergence adaptation (see above). Another important factor is the spatial environment in which the activity is to be carried out and the instrument used to provide that environment. Earlier, a distinction was made between vision screening tests conducted in simulated space and true space (see Chapter 1). All else being equal, vision training procedures that are carried out in true space are preferred over simulated space conditions.

Devices that employ anaglyph or polarizing filters provide true space conditions, as do instrument-free procedures in which the eyes fixate at a point in space in front of (chiastopic fusion) or behind (orthopic fusion) a pair of matched targets and, by taking advantage of physiological diplopia, perceive a fused target. (This, of course, is exactly what occurs with a vectographic or anaglyphic device, except that when filters are not used the patient sees two additional, peripheral images; these are masked by the filters.)

Table 14.1 lists a number of instruments that may be employed effectively in treating vergence infacility. Each is identified with the fixation distance at which it is typically used, and the direction of vergence adaptation it presents.

Figure 14.1 defines one of these procedures, an activity that employs a minitranaglyph.*Notice that each task within the procedure has its own goal that enables the patient to monitor her own progress, and that these tasks may be made more or less difficult by amending the procedure (in the Special Instructions section) in accord with the patient's entering abilities.

For example, a moderately hyperopic patient will probably have less difficulty with base-out demand activities if she does not wear her glasses; hence, the procedure may be made a bit easier for her if the Special Instructions section advises her to start off without her glasses, then repeat the activities as she wears the glasses. Conversely, a myopic patient is apt to have relatively less difficulty with nearpoint, base-out demand activities if she wears her glasses, and more difficulty if she does not wear them.

Notice also that each task provides the patient with a means for assessing his own performance. The minitranaglyh targets, when correctly fused, provide a stereoscopic illusion. The patient knows he "is doing it right" when he perceives the stereopsis. In addition, the patient is taught a method for knowing where his eyes "are looking" when they "feel the way they do." This is accomplished by exploiting the phenomenon of physiological diplopia as was described earlier (see Chapter 11). Namely: a pointer held in the center of the visual field will appear to be single only when it is located at the plane of the perceived (fused) image— the point in space where the visual axes are crossing. If the pointer is held closer to the viewer than the fixation point, two pointers will be perceived in heteron-

*Available from Bernell Corp.

Apparatus	This Instrument Is Appropriate if the Patient Is to Start Therapy At/With:			
	Far	Near	Base-in	Base-out
[a]Aperture rule		X	X	X
[a]Eccentric rectangle cards		X	X	X
[a]Variable mirror stereoscope		X	X	X
Keystone stereoscope; Adult Base-out Comfort Series	X			X
Keystone stereoscope; Children's Base-out Stories	X			X
Keystone stereoscope; Children's Base-in Stories	X		X	
[b]Minivectogram		X	X	X
[a]Minitranaglyph		X	X	X
[a]Variable disparity vectograms (e.g., quoits, clown, spirangle)		X	X	X
[a]Fixed disparity tranaglyph		X	X	X
Bernell stereoscope; Base-out Story Book Cards	X			X
Bernell stereoscope; Base-in Story Book Cards	X		X	
[a]Variable disparity tranaglyphs		X	X	X
[a]Red/green Stereo Trainer	X	X	X	X
Brock string (physiological diplopia)	X	X		

[a]These may be used for vertical fusion training by using additional prism or controlling the height of the two targets.
[b]Also available in a model designed for increasing vertical fusion ranges.

Table 14.1   Vergence Facility Instruments

Vergence Facility

Minitranaglyphs

EQUIPMENT
1. Minitranaglyphs, holder, and pointer
2. Red-green (tranaglyph) filter glasses; red lens before the right eye

EQUIPMENT SETUP
1. See special instructions at the end of this procedure.
2. Insert the red target into the holder so that all the print is oriented in the same direction and the large red and green circles are superimposed perfectly (in register); the smaller circles will appear to be slightly out of register. This will place the pointer at the zero position on the holder scale.

Figure 14.1   Vergence facility training procedure (from Rosner J, Rosner J. Vision therapy in a primary care practice. New York: Professional Press, 1988).

3. Put on the red-green glasses, red lens over right eye. If you wear glasses, place filters in front of glasses.

4. Hold the targets about 16 inches from your eyes in such a way that the background beyond the targets reflects light but is free of extraneous or distracting details.

ACTIVITIES

1. Look at the target. You should see two circles, one large, the other small. The larger one should appear to be flat on the plastic holder; the smaller one, closer to you—floating in front of the holder. The print should be clear and single. If it is not, try to clear it by blinking forcefully while staring hard at the target.

Goal: To maintain a single, clear 3-D image of the target.

2. Separate the tranaglyphs to 2 on the scale. This will cause the entire target to appear to move closer to you, but it will not alter the relative positions of the two circles. The print should remain clear. If it blurs, blink forcefully as described above. When the target is single and clear, look at something across the room, then back at the target; try to recover fusion and clarity at once.

Goal: To recover and maintain a single, clear, 3-D image quickly and easily with the target set at 2.

3. Hold a pointer oriented vertically at the tip of your nose while continuing to look at the target. (Targets to be positioned as described in activity 2.) Even though you know there is only one pointer, it should look as though there are two, one before each eye. If you shut your right eye, the left pointer should disappear, and vice versa; check this. Slowly move the pointer toward the target, constantly looking at the target. The space between the two pointers will become smaller; ultimately the two will merge into one. That is the location in space where your two eyes are pointing.

In other words, if you are looking at the smaller of the two circles, the pointer will be single when it gets to the place where the small ring appears to be floating. If you are looking at the larger circle, the

Figure 14.1 (Continues on next page)

pointer will not be single until it is at the place where that circle is floating. Trace around the various landmarks of the target with your pointer: the large circle, the small circle, the letters, and so forth, being aware that the pointer is single only when it is positioned where your eyes are pointing.

Goal: To see the pointer as single or double, depending on where it is and where you are looking.

4. Rotate the holder (right to left) so that from your perspective without the filters the red circles are to the right of the green ones. This may cause you to see double. If it does, relax, look through the targets, and try to fuse them into one. When you have fused them, you will see the reverse effect of what you were seeing: the circles and letters will now look a bit larger and appear to be floating beyond the holder— away from you. When the target is single and clear under this rotated condition, look at something across the room, then back at the target; try to recover fusion and clarity at once.

Goal: To obtain and recover a single, clear image quickly and easily when the holder is reversed and the targets are set at 2.

5. Practice *rocking;* look at the target, see it singly and clearly, then rotate the holder (reverse the targets), regain fusion and clarity in this condition, then return to the original position, and so on. Separation between targets to remain set at 2.

Goal: 36 cycles within 3 minutes. (For one cycle, obtain fusion and clarity when targets are in original position, then in reverse orientation, then back to the original position.)

6. Gradually increase the separation between the targets (from 2, to 4, to 6, etc.), repeating at each step both the look-away-and-recover and rocking procedures described in activity 5. Work until you have the separation at about the 14 setting.

Goal: 60 cycles (original, reverse, and original positions) within 5 minutes when the targets are at the 14 setting.

Figure 14.1 (Continued)

SPECIAL
INSTRUCTIONS

When you do this procedure, follow the special
instructions checked below.

☐ Wear your glasses.

☐ Once you can perform the goal of activity 6, go
through it again with the targets at the _____
setting.

☐ Use the training glasses or prism we supplied
until you are able to achieve the goal of activity 6.
Then go back to activity 1 and work through all
the activities again, this time without the training
glasses or prism.

☐ Use the training glasses or prism we supplied
after you have achieved the goal of activity 6
without them. Wear them as you once more work
your way through all the activities, starting with
activity 1.

☐ Repeat all the activities while holding the
vectograms about _____ inches from your eyes.

Figure 14.1   (Continued)

ymous diplopia. If it is held beyond the fixation point, again two pointers will be
seen, this time in an homonymous diplopia orientation.

In all instances, the perceived fused image is to be clear. This can occur only
if accommodation is correct for the true position of the stimuli. Thus, the pointer
is a remarkably effective device for sensitizing the patient to the basic role of
fusional vergence (i.e., to fuse disparate retinal images), and at the same time, it
gives him a method for confirming the validity of his fusional vergence actions in
a very precise way (see Figure 14.2).

Figure 14.3 shows a procedure that links up with, and then extends beyond,
the goals of the minitranaglyph activities described in Figure 14.1. Here again,
as in the minitranaglyph procedure, the activities are organized into levels of
difficulty, each of which may be made more or less demanding via the Special
Instructions; here again, the illusion of stereopsis provides the patient an obvious
signal of correct performance; here again, the activity is carried out in true space,
with accommodation fixed at one distance (the plane of the stereograms) and
vergence manipulated in accord with the requirements of the task.

There are also differences between the minitranaglyph procedure and the one
described in Figure 14.3. The latter is "instrument-free"—no optical device is
used. The patient is taught to exercise positive and negative fusional convergence,
at distance and at near, quickly and easily, without the benefit of specially colored
targets and filters. Because there is no instrument, there is no setup time; the
patient may carry the eccentric rectangle targets (see Figure 14.4) with him and
engage in the procedure for brief periods of time throughout the day, as circum-

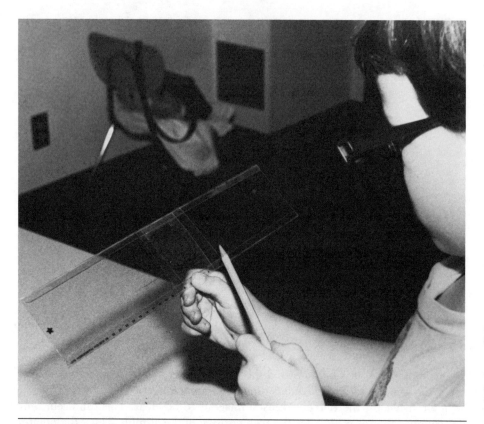

Figure 14.2   Using a pointer with the minitranaglyph.

stances allow. Indeed, once he reaches the point where he does not need the stereo effect as feedback to inform him when he has achieved fusion, he will no longer even need the eccentric rectangle targets; his thumbnails—or any other reasonably matching pair of stimuli—will suffice.

For these reasons, Figure 14.3 serves very well as the *final* procedure in the remedial treatment of vergence infacility. That is why the final task goal of the procedure calls for "daily practice session over prolonged periods of time;" it is only through such extended practice that the newly learned skills will be integrated to an automatic level of function.

SUPPLEMENTARY PROCEDURES

Of the two procedures discussed above, the latter is clearly the most versatile and effective. If used correctly and for a long enough time, it can remediate vergence infacility. No other procedure is needed *if* the patient is able to learn the behaviors this one requires. Most young patients, however, are not able to do this; they need some preliminary experience with an instrument that employs

Vergence Facility

Orthopic/Chiastopic Fusion at Near
with Eccentric Rectangles (Part I)

EQUIPMENT

1. One pair near-point eccentric rectangle targets
2. Pointer

EQUIPMENT
SETUP

1. See special instructions at the end of this section.
2. Hold the two targets in one hand or prop them against a wall so that they are about an arm's length away and at the same height, about chest level. Position the letter *A*'s next to each other and a center-to-center (or arrow-to-arrow) separation of about 2 inches.
3. Hold a pointer about halfway between you and the targets, positioned so that with only your right eye open, the pointer is centered on the left target; with only your left eye open, the pointer is centered on the right target.

ACTIVITIES

1. Open both eyes and look at the tip of the pointer. You should see three targets instead of two. The middle target will look different from the other two; it derives from fusing two images—one belonging to the right eye, the other to the left eye. (This is called *chiastopic fusion,* and is achieved by looking at a point in front of the targets.) Keep your attention on the middle target; ignore the other two; they are distractors. The rectangles should present the illusion of 3-D, with the smaller one appearing to be closer to you than the larger. Make a special effort to see the fused image clearly. It sometimes helps to move the pointer a trifle closer to you or farther away; it might also help to blink forcefully as you stare at the fused image.

Goal: To see three targets by exercising chiastopic fusion, with the help of a pointer if necessary. The fused target should be clear and present an illusion of depth, as described above.

2. Remove the pointer, but keep looking at the place where the pointer was; in effect, pretend the pointer is still there. You will know you are doing it correctly if you continue to see a fused, clear image which presents the illusion of depth (3-D).

Figure 14.3   Vergence facility training procedure (from Rosner J, Rosner J. Vision therapy in a primary care practice. New York: Professional Press, 1988). (Continues on next page.)

Goal: To see a fused, clear, 3-D image without the aid of a pointer.

3. Once the image is fused and clear without the pointer, look at something across the room. (Do not change your posture, but make sure to shift your focus.) Then look back at the targets and try to regain fusion and clarity instantaneously without the help of the pointer. If, at first, you need the pointer to do this, use it until you no longer need it.

Goal: 36 cycles within 3 minutes without the help of a pointer. (For one cycle, start with a fused and clear image, then look away, then regain fusion and clarity.)

4. Hold the targets closer to you (about 16 inches away) and repeat activities 1, 2, and 3. If you need the pointer at first, use it until you do not need it.

Goal: 48 cycles within 4 minutes exercising chiastopic fusion without the aid of a pointer.

5. Hold the targets so that the arrow-to-arrow separation is about 4 or 5 inches. Look through the space that separates the targets—across the room or out a window. You should see four targets, two with each eye. While holding your fixation constant, slowly bring the targets closer together until the four targets appear to merge into three—until the two middle ones blend into a single target. (This is known as *orthopic fusion* and is achieved by looking at a point beyond the targets.) Keep your attention on the fused middle target; ignore the other two; they are distractors. The rectangles in the middle target should present a 3-D effect, with the smaller one appearing to be farther away from you than the larger. Make a special effort to see the fused image clearly. It often helps to relax as you do this; try to adopt a daydreamlike attitude.

Goal: To see three targets (by exercising orthopic fusion, with the help of a pointer if necessary). The fused target should be clear and present an illusion of depth, as described above.

Figure 14.3 (Continued)

6. Once you have achieved the goal of activity 5, look away, then look back and recover fusion. Do this until you can accomplish it quickly and easily.

Goal: 36 cycles within 3 minutes exercising orthopic fusion.

7. With the targets positioned as described in activity 5, alternate between looking past the targets (orthopic fusion)—as you have just been learning to do—and looking in front of them (chiastopic fusion), as you did earlier (activities 1 and 2). Practice completing cycles with speed and ease, always maintaining clarity.

Goal: 60 cycles within 5 minutes. (A cycle now is fusion and clarity while shifting between orthopic fusion *and* chiastopic fusion.)

8. When you achieve this goal, you will have completed part I of this procedure. Do not go on to part II until we recommend it.

SPECIAL
INSTRUCTIONS

When you do this procedure, follow the special instructions checked below.
□ Wear your glasses.
□ Once you can perform the goal of activity 7, increase the arrow-to-arrow separation to about _____ inches.
□ Once you can perform the goal of activity 7, repeat activities 4 through 7 while holding the cards at **arm's length/as close as possible to your eyes.**
□ Once you can perform the goal of activity 7, repeat activities 4 through 7 while holding the cards **above/below** eye level and/or to the extreme **right/left.**
□ Use the training glasses or prism we supplied *until* you can perform the goal of activity 7. Then go back to activity 1 and work through all the activities again, this time without the training glasses or prism.
□ Use the training glasses or prism we supplied *after* you have achieved the goal of activity 7 without them. Wear them as you once more work your way through all the activities, starting with activity 1.

Figure 14.3   (Continued)

Figure 14.4
Eccentric rectangle
targets.

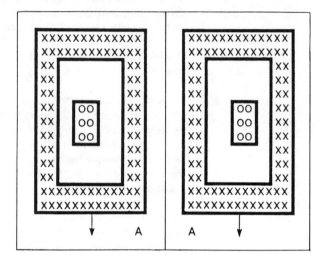

filters, or some other type of apparatus, that mask the extraneous images inherent in the instrument-free procedure. That is why we suggested the use of the minitranaglyph (or a similar) procedure as an initial step. It serves to sensitize the patient to physiological diplopia and teaches him how to exploit this phenomenon in order to determine where he is fixating; it teaches him to exercise vergence facility at a level within his capacity and then goes beyond that level; and it does all this without requiring the patient to deal with distracting, extra images, by using compatible red/green targets and filters.

As shown in Table 14.1, there are a number of different instruments that would serve just as well—or perhaps even better for some conditions—as the minitranaglyph. These are described below, organized into two categories: those that provide simulated space conditions and those that function in true space. As a rule of thumb, true space procedures are better because there is less of a transition from them to the ultimate, instrument-free procedure. However, some patients have great difficulty with true-space instruments and require simulated-space conditions, at least at the beginning of their therapy. Obviously, their treatment programs should commence with such instruments.

Simulated-Space Instruments
Stereoscopes. Both the Wheatstone and Brewster stereoscopes provide the conditions necessary for teaching fusional vergence skills. They are particularly useful for the patient who has little difficulty at farpoint and great difficulty at nearpoint.

There still are a few manufacturers who produce stereograms for this purpose. For example, Keystone View markets a number of different sets that appeal to children. Their Base-in and Base-out Children's Stories sets are useful because (a) they are carried out under farpoint viewing conditions, (b) they employ printed materials that require accurate, fixed accommodation while positive or negative

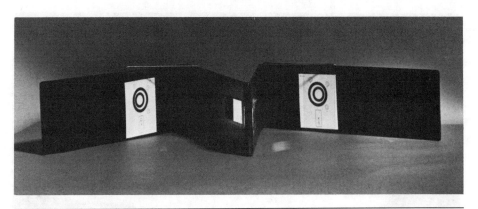

Figure 14.5 Variable-mirror stereoscope (Bernell).

relative convergence is stimulated. Nonreaders can use them if they are able to name the letters: they spell rather than read. And rapid readers may be slowed down by having them spell the words in reverse, or by skipping every other letter.

The Brewster stereoscope also has the unique characteristic of being able to make increasing demands on positive accommodation while, at the same time, requiring the patient to exercise more negative relative vergence. This is accomplished by what is known as "tromboning." To start, the patient obtains fusion with a given stereoscope card, at the appropriate (far or near) position. Then she moves the card holder closer to her eyes or farther away. The former requires more positive accommodation in order to maintain clarity and, in contrast, less convergence in order to maintain fusion. The latter, the opposite.

Variable Mirror Stereoscope (see Figure 14.5) (Bernell Mfg. Co.). This is a modest version of the major amblyoscope, not so versatile but far less expensive. It is accompanied by a number of fusion targets that appeal to children. Both farpoint and nearpoint conditions may be simulated by using spherical lenses to control accommodation. In addition, moderate vertical deviations may be accommodated with this device by placing the right eye and left eye targets at different heights in the target holders.

True Space Instruments
Vectogram Series (Stereo Optical Co., Inc.). This consists of variable and fixed disparity polarized stereograms, some with pictures that appeal to children; e.g., nursery rhyme characters; a clown. The quoit stereogram (shown in Figure 14.6) is in this series. Vectograms may be used at all distances: hand-held for nearpoint; with an overhead projector for farpoint. If the latter is desired, a nondepolarizing screen is necessary.

Orthofusor (B & L Co.). These are similar to the vectogram series but the targets are much more detailed. This may or may not be desirable, depending on the age of the patient.

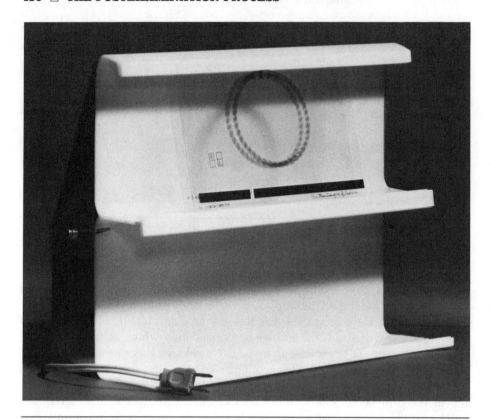

Figure 14.6 Vectogram #2: Quoit.

Tranaglyphs. These are red/green variable and fixed-disparity stereograms that resemble the vectogram series. They are inexpensive and very transportable. In addition, they are far less susceptible to deteriorating from exposure to light than are the polarized targets.

Aperture Rule Trainer (Bernell Mfg. Corp.). This unique device teaches chiastopic and orthopic fusion without employing filters. A mask with a strategically positioned rectangular aperture (or two apertures for orthopic fusion) performs the chore that is accomplished by the filters in the vectogram and anaglyph devices: it eliminates the physiological diplopia produced by chiastopic and orthopic fusion (see Figure 14.7).

Loose Prisms. Certainly one of the simplest methods for enhancing vergence facility is to provide the patient with prisms of increasing power and instruct her in their use, starting with a prism power that is just within her performance level and working up to the higher powers. Its negative feature is that it does not provide the feedback information that is so useful to effective treatment.

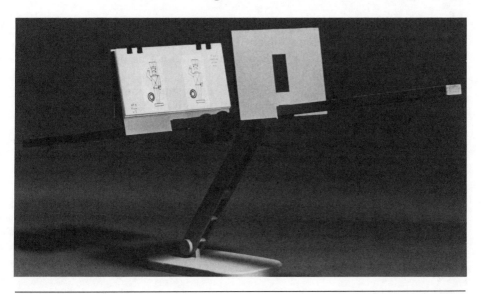

Figure 14.7   Aperture rule (Bernell).

Plus and Minus Spheres.   These are used primarily as adjuncts to any of the basic procedures described above. Chiastopic fusion requires positive relative convergence. Chiastopic fusion through plus spheres requires even more positive relative convergence because accommodation relaxes in accord with the lenses. The same but opposite effect is obtained from minus spheres. Hence the acronyms *BOP* (base out and plus) and *BIM* (base in and minus).

Vertical Heterophorias.   Nothing has been said in this chapter about the treatment of patients with vertical heterophorias and inadequate adaptive (fusional) ranges. The same treatment principles apply for them; the same four treatment options should be considered. If vision therapy is the treatment of choice, see Table 14.1 for suggested instrument.

□ Compensatory Treatment

When vergence facility is deficient to the degree that it causes patient discomfort and impairs day-to-day visual performance, there is need for treatment. Remediation is the preferred treatment in most cases, *but not always*. The patient who is hard to teach, who does not profit from the "lessons" contained within the remedial activities, the patient who is insufficiently motivated ("I just don't have the time"), and the patient whose deficit is intractable, for some reason, are all candidates for compensatory treatment (see flow diagram in Figure 9.2).

There is no good reason to deny compensatory prism from such patients. Compensatory prisms are generally effective and although they may only mask the problem rather than eliminate it, their value should not be underestimated.

Plus and minus spherical lenses are also useful at times: plus for the esophoric patient with substandard negative fusional convergence ability and a normal or high AC/A ratio; minus for the exophoric patient with substandard positive fusional convergence ability and a normal or high AC/A ratio. The former, of course, usually requires a bifocal because of the blur that the extra plus power is apt to produce at farpoint. Minus spheres may also have to be dispensed in bifocal form, depending upon whether they are to be used for nearpoint, farpoint, or constantly.

Consideration should also be given to the use of moderate power plus lenses for nearpoint activities with those patients who display inadequate positive fusional convergence ability and a low AC/A ratio. True enough, the plus lenses will not enhance positive fusional convergence, but the magnification provided by a pair of +0.75D lenses can be truly helpful without placing very much extra burden on the vergence function.

INTERMITTENT STRABISMUS

The remediation of intermittent strabismus (as the condition is defined on page 378) differs little from the treatment of vergence infacilty, except that the patient with intermittent strabismus will probably require some extra support in order to get started in the therapy sequence. The sequence itself will remain more or less the same. For example, in addition to taking into account the preferences demonstrated by the patient in regard to far versus near fixation, and base-out versus base-in adaptation, it may also be necessary to employ compensatory (sphere/ prism) lenses as a source of additional support at the start-up of the treatment program. In other words, the patient with intermittent esotropia will probably get off to a better start if she is given extra plus spheres (in bifocal form) for near. (See case report 6.) She may also need some base-out prism as well. Conversely, patients with intermittent exotropia often have less difficulty getting started in a procedure if they are supplied with minus lenses and/or base-in prism. If this type of support appears to be called for, it should be supplied, then withdrawn as the patient demonstrates that it is no longer needed. When that time arrives, the patient's problem will probably be more accurately described as a vergence infacility rather than intermittent strabismus.

DEFICIENT ACCOMMODATION FACILITY

□ Remedial Therapy

See flow diagram in Figure 9.1.

FINAL (LEVEL IV) GOALS

Upon completion of therapy, the patient will be able to clear (and keep single) a row of small vertical letters, executing accommodation jumps of:

At far: $-2.50D$/plano*

At near: $-2.50D/+2.00D$*

Once again, notice that these criteria are much more demanding than those of the screening test described in Chapter 7. Farpoint criterion now calls for a 2.50-diopter and nearpoint for a 4.50-diopter "accommodation jump," as compared with the 2.00-diopter adjustments of the screening test. In addition, the speed requirements are more stringent, and the patient must be able to sustain at the task for a much longer period of time. As with vergence facility, the rationale for this is to *overtrain* the patient—to help her achieve a level of facility where the newly acquired behavior can be performed automatically—without conscious effort.

SUBORDINATE GOALS AND THEIR HIERARCHICAL INTERRELATIONSHIP

Defining subordinate training goals for accommodation facility is much the same as defining them for vergence facility. Once more, they are determined arbitrarily. Three levels are identified below, organized in a descending order of difficulty. Also, notice that here again, for the same reason as cited above, there are two strands: one for farpoint, the other for nearpoint.

Level III: At far: The patient is able to execute accommodation jumps of two diopters (from plano to $-2.00D$, then back again), completing at least 60 cycles within 5 minutes.

At near: The patient is able to execute accommodation jumps of 4.00 diopters (from $+1.50D$ to $-2.50D$, then back again), completing at least 60 cycles within 5 minutes.

---

*Sixty cycles within 5 minutes; a cycle = at far, start with no lenses; then introduce the minus lenses, then back to no lenses; at near, start with the plus lenses, then replace these with the minus lenses, then back to the plus lenses.

Level II: At far: The patient is able to execute accommodation jumps of 1 diopter (from plano to −1.00D, then back again), completing at least 60 cycles within 5 minutes.

At near: The patient is able to execute accommodation jumps of 2.5 diopters (from +1.00D to −1.50D, then back again), completing at least 60 cycles within 5 minutes.

Level I: At far: The patient is able to execute accommodation jumps of one-half diopter (from plano to −0.50D, then back again), completing at least 60 cycles within 5 minutes.

At near: The patient is able to execute accommodation jumps of 1.50 diopters (from +0.50D to −1.00, then back again), completing at least 60 cycles within 5 minutes.

PLACEMENT TEST

Begin placement testing at level I. If the patient demonstrates mastery of those goals, test for level II goals, and so on, until failure is demonstrated. The patient is "placed"—i.e., is to begin vision therapy—in the level in which she failed. (See case reports on pp. 507–510 for illustrations of this principle.)

During placement testing, pay special attention to relative differences in performance the patient may display as a function of *fixation distance*. Some patients have much more difficulty exercising accommodation facility at distance than at near; others, vice versa. If there is a marked difference, therapy should begin at the fixation distance that presents the fewest difficulties. If no major difference is observed, then start where it is most convenient.

PROCEDURES

Any task that can be managed out of office and is designed to teach the patient how to activate or inhibit accommodation, independent of vergence, has worth (7,8,9,10,11,12). In fact, it is altogether possible that remediating vergence facility deficits will simultaneously remediate inept accommodation facility or vice versa. In many ways, the two are but different versions of the same basic function.

In its simplest form, the treatment could involve providing the patient with the plus and minus spherical lenses he has difficulty adapting to within the stated time constraints and prescribe their use on daily basis. As he masters these, stronger powers may be prescribed.

Figure 14.8 depicts such a procedure, prepared as an instruction sheet for the patient. Notice that, from the outset, it stresses rapid adaptations to plus and minus lenses. Notice also that each task has its own goal and that these may be made more or less difficult by amending the procedure (in the Special Instructions section) in accord with the patient's entering abilities and the treatment goals. For example, a patient who has difficulty in activating accommodation independent

Accommodation Facility at Near

Binocular Plus and Minus Lenses

EQUIPMENT
1. Vectogram 9 or any other target that provides monocular and binocular feedback (e.g., red-green or polarized bar reader)
2. Compatible filter glasses
3. The following pairs of plus (+) and minus (−) lenses:

+_____   −_____
+_____   −_____
+_____   −_____
+ 2.00 D   − 3.00 D

EQUIPMENT SETUP
1. See special instructions at the end of this procedure.
2. Start with the +_____ D and −_____ D training glasses.
3. Seat yourself under a good light, holding the near-point target in one hand, about 16 inches away from your eyes, and the training glasses in the other hand.
4. Put on the filter glasses.

ACTIVITIES
1. Look at the vectogram without using the training lenses. The print should appear single and clear. Make sure that none of the rows of letters are missing—specifically, rows 4 and 6; this would indicate that one eye is not working. Now look at the print through the +_____ D lenses. If the print is not as clear as it was or if it doubles, blink a few times. If this does not help, move the card closer or farther away from you. When the print does clear (and become single), return the card to the 16-inch holding position and continue.

When the print is clear through the plus training lenses designated above, replace them with the opposing pair of minus training lenses: −_____ D. Refocus the letters. If you have trouble doing this, change the holding distance, as described above. Always make sure to read or spell out some of the material so that you are certain of its clarity. Do not simply look. Continue alternating the lenses from the plus pair, to the minus pair, to the plus pair, and so forth, striving for rapid adaptation as you do.

Figure 14.8   Accommodation facility training procedure (from Rosner J, Rosner J. Vision therapy in a primary care practice. New York: Professional Press, 1988). (Continues on next page)

Goal: 36 cycles within 3 minutes. (For one cycle, obtain single and clear print through plus lenses, then through minus lenses, then again through plus lenses.)

2. Replace the training lenses designated in activity 1 with the following: +_____ D and −_____ D. Repeat the exercise described in activity 1 above.

Goal: 60 cycles within 5 minutes using these powers.

3. Work your way through the sequence of lens powers we prescribed in this same manner. Your final pairs of training lenses are +2.00 D and −3.00 D.

Goal: 60 cycles within 5 minutes using the lens powers designated to activity 3.

SPECIAL
INSTRUCTIONS

When you do this procedure, follow the special instructions checked below.
☐ Wear your glasses.
☐ Use the training prism we supplied *until* you are able to achieve the goal of activity 3. Then go back to activity 1 and work through all the activities again, this time without the prism.
☐ Use the training prism we supplied *after* you have achieved the goal of activity 3 without it. Wear it as you once more work your way through all the activities, starting with activity 1.
☐ Repeat activities 1 through 3 while holding the print _____ inches from your eyes.

Figure 14.3   (Continued)

of vergence (i.e., adapting efficiently to minus spheres) is likely to have relatively less difficulty if she wears some base-out (compensating) prism at the same time; the innervational link between convergence and accommodation will provide additional support. Later, as she progresses, the prism will be withdrawn and ultimately, perhaps, a base-in (anticompensating) prism may be introduced to make the task even more demanding. A similar link exists, of course, between base-in and base-out prism and the inhibition of accommodation.

SUPPLEMENTARY PROCEDURES

Combine the accommodation facility training procedures described above with the various vergence facility training procedures described earlier in this chapter.

□ Some Final Remarks Regarding Vergence and Accommodation Facility Treatment

Vergence and accommodation facility are significant skills, especially for the school-child who is required to engage in visually demanding tasks on a regular basis. They are easy to treat; they should not be ignored.

□ Compensatory Treatment

If the patient does not appear to be a good candidate for vision therapy, consider prescribing compensatory lenses to reduce some of the stress she faces when engaging in demanding nearpoint visual activities (e.g., additional plus power for near work; in bifocal form, if necessary). This will enable her to perform more comfortably despite the functional deficit, even though it is not designed to eliminate the problem. How much lens power? That will vary with the case, but as a rule-of-thumb, use enough power to put into balance the relationship between the patient's positive ("minus-to-blur") and negative ("plus-to-blur") relative accommodation.

□ Reassurance Therapy

The effect of "leaving well enough alone" in the management of accommodation infacility may not be detrimental, but neither is it very helpful. The condition rarely deteriorates into a worse condition, but neither is it likely that the patient's symptoms will disappear. Hence, this is not the treatment of choice.

PRACTICAL SUGGESTIONS

14-1. There are a number of sources for vision therapy procedures. (See, for example, the catalogs of Bernell Mfg. Corp., P.O. Box 4637, South Bend, IN 46634; Mast Development Co., 2212 E. 12th St, Davenport, IA 52803.) These are all more alike than different. If they are effective—and many are—they provide various ways (instruments/procedures) in which the patient will learn how to activate or inhibit vergence or accommodation, while keeping the other stable; how to appreciate physiological diplopia; and so on. The clinician should examine these devices and procedures and select those that seem to fit his/her needs the best.

14-2. In recent years, a number of computer-assisted vision therapy programs have been developed and are now being marketed. (For example, Rapid Research, 11940 W. 70th Way, Arvado, CO 80004.) In our opinion, they have both good and negative features. On the plus side, they are, by definition, programmed— designed to proceed in a step-by-step manner to a goal. (Obviously, this is not a positive feature unless they have been programmed properly.) In addition, the computer is a passive instrument; it will give the patient as many tries as she wishes—and do so without becoming irritable. Also, computers are often motivating; some children who would complain about daily activities with a stereoscope will interact with the computer in an enthusiastic manner.

On the negative side, the therapy programs we have seen tend to be "padded"; that is, they seem to delay patient progress by introducing steps in the treatment regimen that are not integral to effective treatment. As such, they lengthen treatment time, raise costs, and increase the possibility of the patient losing interest in the therapy before reaching the goal for which the treatment was initiated. In addition, they force the patient to limit therapy sessions to the optometrist's office or to obtain a compatible computer for home use.

In balance, they are worth considering.

─── ■ ──

REFERENCES

1. Daum KM. Characteristics of exodeviations: I. Characteristics of three classes. AJOPO 1986; 63(4):237–43.
2. Rosner J, Rosner J. Vision therapy in a primary care practice. New York: Professional Press, 1988.
3. Schrock R, Heinsen A. Schur-mark out-of-office training program. Meadville, Pa.: Keystone View Co., 1966.
4. Cashill G, Durran L. Handbook of orthoptic principles. 3rd ed. Edinburgh: Churchill Livingstone, 1974.
5. Griffin JR. Binocular anomalies. Chicago: Professional Press, 1976.
6. Gibson HW. Textbook of orthoptics. London: Hatton Press, 1955.
7. Bobier WR, Sivak JG. Orthoptic treatment of subjects showing slow accommodative response. AJOPO 1983; 60(11):678–87.
8. Mannen DL, Bannon MJ, Septon RD. Effects of base-out training on proximal convergence. AJOPO 1981; 58(12):1187–93.
9. Grisham JD. Treatment of binocular dysfunction in Schor CM, Ciuffreda KJ. Vergence eye movements: basic and clinical aspects. Boston: Butterworths, 1983.
10. Suchoff IB, Petito GT. The efficacy of visual therapy: accommodative disorders and non-strabismic anomalies of binocular vision. JAOA 1986; 57(2):119–25.

11. Daum KM. A comparison of the results of tonic and phasic vergence training. AJOPO 1983; 60(9):769–75.
12. Scheiman M, Gallaway M, Ciner E. Divergence insufficiency: characteristics, diagnosis, and treatment. AJOPO 1986; 63(6):425–31.
13. Daum KM, Rutstein RP, Eskridge JB. Efficacy of computerized vergence therapy. AJOPO 1987; 64(2):83–89.
14. Cooper J, Citron M. Microcomputer produced analglyphs for evaluation and therapy of binocular anomalies. JAOA 1983; 54(9):785–88.

15

Delayed Development

□

This chapter is organized into two parts. The first concentrates on the child whose performance on the Denver Developmental Screening Test (DDST) is inadequate; the second on the youngster who, at age 5 or above, reveals substandard visual and/or auditory analysis skills.

Each part is then organized into two subsections: one for the optometrist who prefers to limit her postexamination involvement to reporting screening test outcomes and making appropriate referrals; the other for the optometrist who elects to assume greater responsibilities, such as managing remedial treatment programs and offering selective guidance to parents and teachers.

Throughout, the central theme is that such children can be helped with remedial and/or compensatory treatment, and that all optometrists have a contribution to make to the effort—a contribution that will vary in accord with the optometrist's personal interests and the availability of competent multidisciplinary services within their respective communities.

■

INADEQUATE DDST PERFORMANCE

Upon encountering a child whose performance on the DDST is inadequate, the optometrist is obliged to inform the parent and recommend an action. What she recommends, and the urgency with which she does it, is governed by the nature of the deficits uncovered by the DDST.

As a rule of thumb, if the problem is observed in the:

Personal-social sector. Refer the child/parent to someone qualified to assess and treat emotional development problems: a clinical psychologist, perhaps, or someone with similar background and experience.

Fine-motor adaptive sector. Refer the child/parent to a child development specialist, or manage the case personally. More will be said about this shortly.

Language sector (including children who display a speech deficit). Refer the child/ parent to a speech and language specialist; i.e., someone whose clinical specialty goes beyond audiology; someone who is trained in the treatment of language disorders.

Gross motor sector. Refer the child/parent to a pediatric neurologist (if there are signs to substantiate taking a position of serious concern), or (if medical factors are ruled out) to an agency that provides motor training in a recreation context, such as a local community center.

□ More about Fine Motor-Adaptive Deficits

The point was made in Chapter 8 that the DDST items of the fine motor-adaptive sector are not dissimilar to items that appear on many visual perceptual skills tests: probes of the child's ability to identify the task-pertinent, concrete features of spatially organized patterns. Hence, inadequate performance in that sector represents substandard visual analysis skills development, a clinical problem that falls within the scope of the optometrist. This is particularly so in those cases where there is an associated ametropia. It is not difficult to appreciate the connection between reduced visual acuity due to uncorrected high hyperopia, for example, and delayed development of visual analysis skills (1,2). In a very real sense, the infant engaged in a preferential looking assessment of visual acuity is exercising basic visual analysis skills. If he lacks acuity, it will be apparent in his visual analysis skills development.

There is, however, a qualifying consideration. If the child's development appears to lag generally, across most or all sectors, then long-term, multidisciplinary treatment will probably be needed. Such a child and his parents will be served best by a referral to a child development clinician who, most often, will be found on the professional staff of a community-sponsored child development clinic. This does not rule out optometric participation. It merely shifts pivotal responsibility to someone who is accustomed to coordinating multidisciplinary treatment programs.

If, on the other hand, the child's general development appears to be progressing normally, and his shortcomings in the fine motor-adaptive items are his only observable difficulty, then there is no reason why the optometrist should not manage the remedial effort. Such children usually do not need extended and diverse treatments. Often, all they need is gentle but direct instruction in how to deal with visual analysis tasks.

□ Remedial Therapy

See flow diagram in Figure 9.1.

DESIGN THE REGIMEN

The activities described in this section are intended for use with young children (up to about age five) whose visual analysis skills are deficient, but not to an alarming degree (3). The activities are not so structured as those presented in previous sections. They are written in the form of suggestions to a parent or a nursery-school teacher; descriptions of activities that most children enjoy and often engage in spontaneously; activities that facilitate the development of spatial analysis skills (see Figure 15.1).

Placement Tests

There are neither formal placement tests nor formal goals, although it is helpful to advise the parents that they should (a) select activities that challenge but do not frustrate, and (b) take note of the child's progress, moving on to more difficult activities in accord with that progress.

The child's progress should be evaluated about once a month, using tasks similar to those that initially revealed the deficit; block design and geometric design reproductions, for example. (Care should be taken to select tasks that are not specifically taught in the homebased activities, and caution the parent to avoid the temptation.)

The average 3- and 4-year-old who will profit significantly from these activities will display at least some of the benefits within a month or so. If improvement is not observed within that time, it may be due to inadequate implementation or an unforeseen complication. In either event, the treatment recommendations should be reconsidered (see J in Figure 9.1 flow diagram).

☐ Compensatory Treatment

Extensive compensatory therapy (see flow diagram in Figure 9.2) is rarely necessary with this type of child. However, if there is a need for some parental guidance while the remedial effort is underway, the following suggestions will be helpful. Advise the parents that when they are attempting to instruct the child, they should:

1. Organize the task for the child. Divide it up into small, accomplishable steps, and present them one at a time.
2. Point out the organization to the child; e.g., *"First* you do this." Then, when the first step is accomplished: *"Now,* you do this," and so on; *but do not overexplain.*
3. Correct the child's errors at once. That does not mean punish. Rather, it means that when the child makes an error, show him the correct version and, if possible, an easy way to remember it.
4. Practice the task until he can accomplish it without assistance, but do not prolong any single session to the limits of (child or parent) patience.

Suppose, for example, that the child is learning to print his name.

1. Start with the first letter.
2. Identify it as the *first* letter and that, as such, it is positioned on "this" (point to the left) side.

Visual Analysis Skills Training Procedures

To parent:

We suggest that you engage your child in the following activities. They are designed to help him/her acquire certain classroom-related skills. (Feel free to modify the activities in any way that might make them more interesting and enjoyable. Your general goal with these activities is to sensitize the child to details—certain key characteristics—that cause "things" (visual and acoustical patterns) to be similar yet different. (As long as your modifications do not get in the way of that goal, they are perfectly acceptable.)

Sorting tasks. There is a vast array of materials that may be used for this activity. Whatever you use, have the child organize the materials according to a characteristic that you identify. Have him do the following:

a. Sort buttons according to size. In every household there is usually a box full of buttons. Have the child sort these into containers, a specific size in a specific container.

b. Sort buttons according to color.

c. Sort buttons according to color *and* size. If you have enough buttons, this adds an extra dimension. Thus one container will hold all the black buttons of a certain size, for example, and another container all the white buttons of the same size. This is a good place to teach the concept that things can be the same one way, yet different another way. Proceed with care. This can be a confusing concept. Do not stress it. Simply point it out periodically. He will catch on in time.

d. Sort playing cards according to suit or numerical designation or both.

e. Sort screws, nails, nuts, bolts, washers, and other hardware items according to size.

f. Sort paint chips (cards showing various colors—these are usually obtainable from a paint store) according to color. Homemade chips can be made with crayons.

g. Sort food cans according to size or according to the pictures on the labels.

h. Sort samples of fabric according to texture; for example, all smooth fabrics in one pile, all rough fabrics in another.

i. Sort shapes. You will probably have to prepare this yourself, but it is quite easy. Cut paper into a variety of shapes—circles, squares, and triangles—and have the child sort these according to shape, size, color. Add more shapes when he appears to be ready for more complex tasks. (You may also have him cut out the shapes himself.)

j. Sort silverware according to size or function or both.

k. Sort books according to size or color of cover.

l. Sort strands of yarn according to color or length or both.

Figure 15.1   Visual analysis activities suitable for preschool children (from Rosner J. Helping children overcome learning difficulties. New York: Walker Publishing Co., Inc., 1979). (Continues on next page)

m. Sort photographs of people according to their sex, their family relationships, or their ages.

n. Sort cards showing capital letters. You may have to make these yourself, but it is easy to do. All you need is a pencil and some paper. Cut the paper (or have the child do it) into playing-card size and print a capital letter on each. Start off with only two or three different letters and add to the assortment as he shows competency. For example, "Put all the *A*'s in one pile, all the *B*'s in another."

o. Sort bottles according to weight. Purchase a number of medicine bottles from your local drug store and wrap adhesive tape around them so that the contents cannot be seen, or use empty tin cans or soft-drink bottles. Then pour sand (or salt or sugar or dried beans) into each container, so that even though they are equal size, some are of one weight and others are either lighter or heavier.

This list could be extended, but I think you must have the idea by now. Any task is useful if it involves sorting objects that are similar in one way and vary in another—and if the child can figure it out.

Matching tasks. In all these activities you construct a pattern, and the child constructs one just like it, positioning his alongside yours. If he encounters difficulty matching your pattern, have him place his *on top* of yours rather than alongside. To add further interest and to foster better visual memory, play "Flash" with him. To do this, hide your pattern from the child's view with a sheet of cardboard. Tell him to get ready, then flash your pattern for a brief period (count to 10, or 5, or 1, or whatever works), then cover it again. The child is to match your pattern from memory. Start with simple patterns. Increase their complexity as he displays the ability to deal with them.

a. Match playing cards. Line up one, two, or more playing cards and have the child match your pattern. (These need not be lined up; they can be arranged as a triangle, or what have you, so long as the child can manage the task.)

b. Match silverware. Line up a spoon, a fork, and a knife, and have the child match your pattern.

c. Match a button pattern.

d. Match a color pattern, using crayons or other colored articles.

e. Match a hardware pattern made up of screws, bolts, nuts, washers, and so on.

f. Match letters. Construct your pattern with cards on which letters have been printed. Give similar cards to the child and have him match the pattern.

g. Match shapes. Parquetry blocks are particularly useful here. You can purchase these in most toy and variety stores. They include three basic shapes (square, triangle, diamond). Arrange them in patterns and

Figure 15.1 (Continued)

have the child match the patterns. Caution: Do not use complex patterns until the child shows that he can match simple ones.

h. Match glassware (drinking glasses) of different shapes and sizes.

i. Match pipe-cleaner patterns.

j. Match toothpick patterns.

As you undoubtedly see by now, virtually any material can be used for this activity. Simply construct a pattern and have the child copy it. You can vary this by switching roles; have the child construct the pattern and you match it. He, of course, must then check your work for accuracy. Make an occasional error. He will enjoy finding them, and looking for them will sharpen his skills.

Organizing tasks. In these activities the child is given materials and asked to organize them according to some attribute. Show him how; give him a model to follow. Then, in time, withdraw your model and encourage him to figure it out for himself. For example, have him

a. Organize buttons according to size. Give the child a number of buttons, one of each size. He is to arrange them in a row, from smallest to largest. If necessary, start out with only three buttons and add to the task as he grasps the concept.

b. Organize playing cards according to their numerical designation.

c. Organize bolts, screws, washers, or other hardware items according to size, from smallest to largest.

d. Organize shoes according to size. For example, Dad's, Mom's, big sister's, baby's.

e. Organize shapes according to size—squares, circles, triangles, and others.

f. Organize colors according to hue, for example, from light blue to dark blue.

g. Organize pictures according to time sequence. Show the child three pictures that are sequentially related; for example, drawings from a comic strip that shows (1) the sunrise and a rooster crowing; (2) a child awakening; (3) a child playing. Then have him arrange them in a logical sequence. (Other examples: pictures of articles of clothing to be arranged in the order in which he puts them on when getting dressed or in the order in which he removes them when getting undressed; pictures of food items—appetizers, main course items, desserts—to be arranged according to the sequence in which they are customarily eaten.)

h. Organize wood blocks according to thickness, ranging from thin to thick, like a staircase.

i. Measure objects, rooms, or people, and organize them according to size. He can measure with a ruler, a length of rope, a footstep.

Figure 15.1   (Continues on next page)

Again it is apparent that the number of activities involving the organizing of information is virtually unlimited. The general skill you are trying to foster here is the ability to order information.

Classification tasks. This is an extension of what has already been described. In these activities the child is shown a picture and asked to classify it. For example, have him

a. Classify food. Show him pictures cut out of magazines and have him classify them according to whether they are (1) good tasting or bad tasting; (2) breakfast food or dinner food; (3) eaten hot or cold; (4) appetizer, main course, or dessert; (5) eaten cooked or raw.
b. Classify household objects. Use pictures or real objects and have him classify them according to whether they are (1) hard to move or easy to move, that is, heavy or light; (2) for sitting on or lying on; (3) livingroom pieces, bedroom pieces, or kitchen pieces; (4) constructed of metal, wood, or plastic; (5) rough or smooth in texture.
c. Classify clothing. Show him pictures and have him classify them according to whether they are (1) for boys or girls; (2) for winter or summer wear; (3) rough or smooth; (4) heavy or light; (5) worn above the waist or below the waist.
d. Classify sports equipment. Show him pictures and have him classify them according to whether they are (1) used indoors or outdoors or both; (2) used in summer or winter; (3) heavyweight or lightweight; (4) thrown, kicked, or batted in some way (for example, a golf ball, a tennis ball, a football).

Find hidden shapes. Here the child is to learn the concept that large patterns contain collections of identifiable smaller patterns. For example, have him

a. Find all the hidden circles. Show him pictures of automobiles, household objects, and other things, and have him find all of the hidden circles—for example, the *wheels* of an automobile; the *bottom* of a pot. You need not use pictures; real objects will do. Also, this may be extended to hidden squares, triangles, and so on.
b. Find all the hidden numerals in a room—in calendars, clock dials, radio and television dials.
c. Find all the hidden flowers in the house—in carpet and towel designs, hanging paintings, kitchenware.
d. Find the hidden letters—on book covers, newspapers, mailboxes, street signs, billboards. (This procedure can be modified to focus the child on specific letters; for example, "Find all the *A*'s you can," or "Find the letters of your name."

Painting, drawing, and other graphic tasks. The purpose here is to give the child the opportunity to see and reproduce details—and have

---

Figure 15.1 (Continued)

some fun doing it. This should range from coloring books and follow-the-dots, to weaving and finger painting. As I mentioned earlier, do not be afraid to use coloring books. I do not think it will limit his artistic development. Every creative artist worthy of the designation knows his craft and the potentials of his media. He knows these things as a result of disciplined training or disciplined self-instruction. Coloring books will not make your child into an artist, but neither will they prevent him from being one.

Block play and other construction activities. There are a great variety of construction toys on the market. They are all useful, so long as they do not impose unreasonable demands on the child. Start with simple ones, then progress to the more complex ones as he shows that he is able. You need not be limited to commercial toys. Popsicle or paste sticks and straws are all good construction materials that can be glued together. For that matter, so is construction paper, which may be cut into various shapes and assembled into a number of designs.

"How Do You Get There?" Have him tell you how to get from one place to another. For example, from the kitchen to the living room, from home to school, to grandmother's house, and so forth. Teach him to read simple road maps, tracing the route between two points. Then, when he can, have him tell you how to get from *here* to *there* by consulting the map. As a variation, you describe a specific route but do not designate the destination: have him do that.

Predict a line. This works well on the chalkboard. Start off by marking two X's on the board. Position the X's so that they are about 12 inches apart and at about the same height. Give the child a stick of chalk and ask him to "pretend there is a straight line on the board connecting the two X's." Then ask him to mark one or two X's *on that imaginary line.* In other words, he is to demonstrate the capacity to project an imaginary line between two points on a chalkboard.

Once he has drawn his X's, check his performance by drawing a straight line (use a straight edge) between the two X's and discuss with the child the accuracy of his performance.

When the child understands the concept, alter the task by varying the relative location of the X's, so that they are farther apart and at different heights.

Experiment with positions and keep him interested. This is a particularly useful activity for children who display persistent visual perceptual skills dysfunction.

As another variation, draw a short, straight, horizontal line at one edge of the chalkboard and have the child mark an X at the opposite edge of the board in the location where he thinks your line would terminate if it were extended. Once he has done this, extend the line in accord with its beginning segment and see how close the child was to

Figure 15.1   (Continues on next page)

being on target. Continue this, changing the line's orientation—vertical, oblique, from right to left, and so on—with the child's task remaining the same: to imagine where the line would end up once drawn to completion.

Matching sizes. Draw a line on the chalkboard. Then have the child draw a second line, making it the same length as yours. Check him for accuracy. At first his line may be positioned adjacent and parallel to yours. When he is ready—that is, when he can accomplish this initial task fairly well—have him draw his copy farther away from yours and not parallel. You may also replace the line with a geometrical shape such as a square, rectangle, triangle, and so on, but only after the child has displayed accomplishment at the basic level.

Memory games with cards. Concentration is a good activity. Do you recall it? All you do is arrange a full deck (less than that, if you think it advisable) facedown, in 13 rows—4 cards in each row. (This arrangement can be changed to suit your own taste.) The first player chooses two cards at random, looks at them, shows them to all players, and, unless they are a matched pair, returns them, again facedown, to their original positions. If they are a matched pair, he keeps them and chooses another pair. He keeps on choosing until he misses. The second player then chooses one card, turns it faceup, and tries to choose a second one that matches it. Obviously if the first card is a match to either of the two shown by the first player, it is helpful for him to remember where that card is. The game ends when all cards have been paired. The player with the most cards wins.

Memory games without cards. There are many of these, and they are adaptable. This one can be played at the dining room table after dinner. Everyone should participate. All players study the table, generally laden with dishes, utensils, and condiments. Then the first player closes his eyes while someone else removes one object from the table. The question to the first player then is, "What's missing?" As the game proceeds, the challenge lessens (and the table gets cleared!). *Note:* start off with a limited assortment of objects. There is no need to make the game too difficult. "What's Missing?" can be played anywhere, with any assortment of objects: playing cards, household objects, candy, or whatever is handy. It can also be modified to "Which One Was Moved?" or "Which One Was Just Added?" and so forth.

Figure 15.1   (Continued)

3. If he reverses a letter (e.g., *b* for *d*), correct it with a *very brief* explanation. See p. 468 for suggestions regarding remediation of letter reversals. Certainly, there is no need to punish him for the error, but just as certainly there is no benefit in allowing it to pass uncorrected.

4. Practice the letter and add the next one continuing until he can print his name without significant conscious effort.

——■——————————————————————————————————

PERCEPTUAL SKILLS DYSFUNCTION

This section commences with the remediation of visual and auditory analysis skills deficits in school-aged children and is followed by a discussion of school-based compensatory instruction: when to recommend it and the general principles that should underlie those recommendations.

The discussion regarding visual analysis skills remediation is longer and more detailed than is the one concerning auditory analysis skills, for two reasons. One, auditory analysis skills have not been investigated as long nor as thoroughly; hence, less is known about them. Second, most optometrists choose to refer such patients to speech and language therapists or remedial reading specialists—not an unreasonable decision. What is included here regarding auditory analysis skills, then, is more for background information than for direct application.

The school-age child who does not perform satisfactorily on one of the visual or auditory analysis skills tests cited in Chapter 8 will reveal his deficit in many ways, some fairly obvious, some not. His problem has been defined as an inadequate awareness of the task-pertinent concrete features of visual or spoken patterns; i.e., an inability to identify *what* to pay attention to rather than an inability to pay attention. It is conceivable that the child also has the latter problem, either because it is difficult to pay attention to stimuli that appear to lack order (How long can one pay attention to an unfamiliar language text or speech?) or because he is coping with a process skills deficit (e.g., a lack of adequate accommodation or vergence facility) along with his perceptual skills dysfuction. The result: he will not remember enough of what he is taught. He will be hard to teach. He will not make satisfactory progress in the standard classroom. The result of that: the gap between what he should know and does know will widen (3).

The examples used in Chapter 8 simulated an arithmetic lesson and a reading lesson, and properly so. Making satisfactory progress in these two basic school subjects is dependent upon many factors, but two fundamental ones are: (a) the ability to remember "facts"—and "to remember" means to be able to recall at once, without the need to figure it out; (b) the ability to recognize the relationships between already-learned (memorized) facts and those yet to be learned. To recognize, for example, how knowing the answer to the problem $2 + 2 = ?$ contributes to the solution and easy retention of the answer to $2 + 3 = ?$ or, at a higher level, how knowing the answer to $6 \times 6 = ?$ contributes to remembering the answer to $6 \times 7 = ?$, or, in reading, to recognize how being able to read *cat* contributes to the recognition and easy retention of such words as *scat* and *scatter*.

Perceptual skills deficits are revealed in other ways as well. As noted in Chapter 8, in the primary grades, the child with deficient visual perceptual skills is likely to (a) be uncertain in identifying some of the lower case letters, such as the *b* and *d*, (b) produce sloppy ("messy") paperwork, (c) have difficulty completing tasks ("He forgets what he was to do"), and (d) be generally disorganized. In the intermediate and secondary grades, it will manifest as an extension of those basic deficits, except that by this age, school difficulties will be compounded by the knowledge deficits that have accumulated over the years, and by the psychological effects of chronic school failure.

Because of this, treatment of deficient analysis skills produces best results with younger children: i.e., up to about the third grade level, before the "race" is too far gone (see Chapter 8). With the older child, compensatory methods should be stressed. Ideally, of course, treatment should comprise a mix of remedial and compensatory methods. But that statement must be counterbalanced with the acknowledgment that no treatment will be effective unless the child is motivated. This is not possible unless he makes at least some classroom gains fairly quickly. This becomes increasingly more difficult as the child grows older. It is a true dilemma.

□ Historical Overview

Over the past few centuries, man has been fascinated with the prospect of fostering intellectual development through environmental forces. Itard (4) described his experience with "The Wild Boy of Aveyron" in 1807. A few decades after that, also in France, Seguin (5) hypothesized on remediating children of low intelligence (children who would today be called "retarded") with a "physiological method" that emphasized visually directed motor skills training. At the turn of this century, Maria Montessori (6), an Italian physician, spawned the notion of "stimulating the senses" of the young children who attended what today would be called day-care centers in the poorer sections of Rome.

In the late 1940s, Gesell and his coworkers reintroduced the notion of guiding development (7). One of Gessell's coauthors was Getman, an optometrist who since that time has devoted much effort to disseminating the concepts of what he and his colleagues call "developmental vision" (8).

From that time, events proliferated rapidly. The era of heightened concern over school achievement began, in earnest, in the United States during the post-World War II era and the term *learning disability* entered the scene to describe the child with an enigmatic learning difficulty, the child who obviously was not impaired cognitively, yet encountered great difficulty in reading and/or arithmetic. (But not without a struggle. The condition has also been called *minimal brain dysfunction, neurological handicap, dyslexia, specific language disability, specific learning disorder,* and more. These now appear to be obsolete, but not yet completely forgotten [9,10].)

As noted in Chapter 8, many investigators have offered explanations of the problem and proposed remedial treatment methods. Prominent among these: Ayres (11), Kephart (12), Eisenberg (13), Cott (14), Feingold (15), Levinson and Frank (16), Pavlidis (17), Stein (18), Geiger (19), and Irlen (20). Their treatment methods varied from a strong emphasis on motor training (gross, fine, extraocular, etc.) to the control of behavior through medication, to megavitamin therapy, to special diets that avoided artificial food colorings to the use of antivertigo drugs on the presumption that the children suffered from vestibular dysfunction, to eye movement exercises, to patching one eye, to wearing colored lenses.

All have argued rationally, all cite their successes; all have their believers and their supporters. None has yet published convincing data.

Education slowly assumed its obligation by recognizing that, regardless of cause, such children need to be taught in nonstandard ways (see footnote on p. 313 for a description of "standard instruction"). It was not enough to step aside and wait for the various health-care disciplines to "cure" the child. At best, a cure meant improved information processing skills, a child who was easier to teach. But even then, the effects of his unsuccessful school years remained like the scar that follows the cut, and the only way that it could be removed was through the "plastic surgery" of special instruction that helped the child overcome his knowledge deficit (21).

The era of partnership appears to have arrived. Educators now see their role more clearly and so do the health-care professionals. Each group has a part to play. The child who fails to make satisfactory progress may be approached in either one or both of two ways: (a) Attempt to change the child. Improve his ability to profit from standard instruction. (b) Attempt to alter instruction so as to accommodate the child (22). The first is referred to below as *remedial*, the second as *compensatory*.

□ Remedial Therapy

See flow diagram in Figure 9.1.

VISUAL ANALYSIS SKILLS

The goal of such a program is to teach the child a systematic method for identifying the task-pertinent, concrete features of spatially organized patterns, *thereby* enabling him to recognize how new information may link up with previously acquired knowledge on the basis of attribute similarities and differences, thereby giving him insights into invention and/or application of effective mnemonic strategies, *thereby* making him easier to teach.

There are many books that describe remedial treatment regimens and, indeed, there are many commercially produced programs.* They vary in their effectiveness, of course, but not all that much at the conceptual level. A few attempt to teach basic visual analysis skills directly. Most engage the child in activities where (presumably) he will be motivated to learn the basic analysis skills so as to be able to do what the activities require. The distinction between the two is noteworthy. The first is analogous to teaching someone how to read, the mechanics of the act. The second is similar to presenting the nonreader with interesting easy-to-read books on the assumption that he will be inspired to read, and will thereby become a reader. The former method is more effective with the type of child being discussed here.

At the operational level, most remedial therapy programs fall within one of the following four categories:

1. *Hand-eye coordination tasks.* Tracing, coloring, connect-the-dots, scissors cutting, lacing, and so on. Ordinarily, these are used with young children (see the remedial activities for preschool children in Figure 15.1). Their *main value:* successful performance depends upon following a sequential, step-by-step series of actions in order to generate a product, a work habit worth fostering. Their *main drawback:* they do not teach analysis skills, only a subordinate ability.

2. *Discrimination tasks.* Sorting, matching, identifying similarities and differences, embedded figure puzzles, and so on. These are useful with all ages; they may be constructed so as to be very easy (see the preschool remedial activities in Figure 15.1) or very difficult (e.g., locating a specific character on a page of Chinese text). *Their main value:* successful performance depends upon correct feature analysis, with the level of difficulty depending upon the number and nature of the features and the number and nature of the distractors in the display. *Their main drawback:* they do not teach analysis skills; they attempt to inspire them.

3. *Replication tasks.* Copying block, mosaic, pegboard, matchstick, etc., designs. The level of difficulty may be influenced by the complexity of the design, the time allowed to copy it, the time allowed to study it before (and if) it is removed from sight, and so on. *Their main value:* successful performance depends upon correct feature analysis; i.e., identifying the task-pertinent concrete features of the designs to be copied. It is possible to teach this skill directly, within this context. *Their main drawback:* once again, the activities may not overtly teach the child *how* to identify such features as quantity, magnitude, and relationships, depending instead upon the child discovering a method for doing this by engaging in activities that require their application.

4. *Problem-solving tasks that involve analysis process.* Jigsaw puzzles, classifying objects according to one or more attribute, defining size and position relationships (e.g., completing the patterns: ↑ ↑ ↑ ?; | / ╱ ?), mapping out blank space (e.g., figuring out how many steps will be required to walk across a

---

*See, for example, the catalogs of Developmental Learning Material (DLM), Allen, TX, and Walker Educational Book Corp., New York, NY.

Figure 15.2
9-pin geoboard.

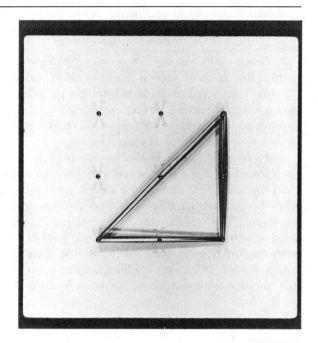

room or, at a more complex level, drawing a reasonably accurate floor plan of a classroom). *Their main value:* successful performance requires analysis skills and reasoning; i.e., applying the knowledge gained through analysis in order to solve a new problem. (This is not unlike applying a known number fact to the solution of an unfamiliar calculation.) *Their main drawback:* once again, the underlying abilities may not be taught explicitly.

Prototype Program
The program described below illustrates how a single device may be used for all types of tasks (3). The device: a geoboard that may be purchased* or homemade with nuts and bolts attached to perforated plywood.** Three configurations are used: 5-pin, 9-pin, and 25-pin. Figure 15.2 shows a 9-pin, commercially produced geoboard.

1. *Hand-eye coordination tasks.* Stack metal washers on each pin or stack them only on designated pins. Stretch rubber bands between certain pins perhaps only those that hold washers; etc.
2. *Discrimination tasks.* Compare the designs on two geoboards and decide whether they are the same or different (e.g., one 5-pin geoboard and one 9-pin

*Walker Educational Book Corp., DLM; Cuisenaire Corp.
**See *Helping Children Overcome Learning Difficulties*, 2nd ed., by J. Rosner (New York: Walker Pub. Co., Inc., 1979).

geoboard; or two 9-pin geoboards, one containing fewer washers than the other; or two similar geoboards that contain matching [or nonmatching] rubber band designs; etc.).

3. *Replication tasks*. (a) Two matching geoboards, one containing a rubber band pattern that is to be copied onto the other and then, when the child is able, (b) child copies drawn geoboard designs on geoboard with rubber bands (i.e., drawn lines connecting certain dots indicate rubber bands connecting those respective pins: see Figure 15.3). Then, (c) child copies geoboard designs onto a map of dots; i.e., the reverse of preceding step.

4. *Problem-solving tasks that involve analysis*. At this stage, the geoboard may be replaced by a compatible maps of dots. A number of activities are possible: child copies designs drawn on a 25-dot (geoboard) map onto a second map from which certain dots have been deleted. He is instructed how to "pretend the dots are there." The specific aim, of course, is to teach him how to map out spatial relationships on the basis of an incomplete set of reference points. As he learns, more dots are deleted until, finally, all that remains is the blank space within the square border, still a very useful reference point.

The similarity between these activities and the TVAS is apparent (see Chapter 8).

Placement Test

In fact, the TVAS may be used as a placement test for this program (1). It identifies the level at which the child encounters difficulty and portrays what goals he has yet to master before reaching the level of visual analysis skills that all children should achieve, naturally, by about the age of 10.

Once placed, the child follows a prescribed sequence that parallels the sequence portrayed in the TVAS. In other words, he is taught to "pass" the TVAS, not by familiarizing him with its specific designs but, rather, by teaching him the analysis process that is needed to pass the TVAS. It has been shown that not only will the child show improvement on the TVAS, he will also show improvement on any of the other standardized visual analysis skills tests listed in Chapter 8. And, most important, he will also reveal the effects in related school activities such as arithmetic—if he has not slipped so far behind that "catching up" is impossible regardless of the improved visual analysis skills (22).

Additional instructive activities are possible with this device (23). For example:

1. Spatial manipulation. Teach the child how to alter perspective; i.e., construct the designs as if they were viewed from the opposite direction.

2. Variation of parts, retention of the whole. Teach the child how to construct the same design using a different internal structure; i.e., by reorganizing the distribution of the subcomponent parts.

3. Variation of size, retention of form. Teach the child how to construct shapes that differ in total size but not in the quantity and interrelationships of the component parts (e.g., a square remains a square, regardless of its size).

Figure 15.3
Constructing a pattern
on a 25-pin geoboard.

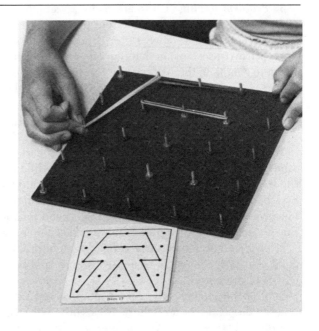

It is apparent that the potential for apparatus and procedure variations is great, but it is also important to remember that the variations should subserve the same ultimate goal: to teach the child how to identify the task-pertinent concrete features of a spatially organized array; how to figure out what to pay attention to in order to do what he is expected to do.

In fact, the optometrist has access to some optical devices that could be used very effectively to foster the development of competent visual analysis skills: prisms, spheres, and stereograms.

Prisms. Prisms may be used for three levels of activity:

1. *Discrimination.* Demonstrate the effects of a prism to the child; i.e., the shift of the image in the direction of the apex. Demonstrate also that if both eyes are kept open when a prism is placed before one eye, diplopia results, which may or may not be overcome by a fusional vergence. Once he understands these two optical effects, engage him in activities where he is asked to (a) select the "different" prism from a group of three unmarked prisms (e.g., one = 2 prism diopters; the other two = 4 prism diopters each); (b) select the two prisms that are the same.

At the beginning, large prism power differences may be provided. Later, use smaller differences. Also vary the direction of the prism base.

2. *Replication.* Child looks through an unmarked prism, as described above; then he selects another prism that matches the effect from a box of unmarked prisms. This may be extended to a two-prism, two-direction task (e.g., a 3 base down combined with a 3 base out).

3. *Problem solving.* There are many possibilities. For example: (a) given a set of unmarked prisms, each a different power, have the child order them in accord with their respective powers (i.e., from the weakest to the strongest); (b) given three prisms in succession that represent a pattern, have the child select the fourth prism to complete the pattern (e.g., sequence: 2 base up, 2 base left, 2 base down . . . ?. . . . ; or 4 base left, 4 base right, 2 base left, . . . ? . . .).

Spheres. These may be used in ways similar to those described for the prism.

1. *Discrimination.* Given a set of three unmarked spherical lenses, two of the same power, the third a different power, the child identifies the *different* lens on the basis of its optical effect (e.g., +2.00D, +2.00D, −1.00D). Obviously, this may be varied in many ways, with the task difficulty increased as performance improves. (Note: here again there is no need for the child to become expert at this level. It is but a step in the sequence, not an end in itself.)

2. *Replication.* Given three unmarked spherical lenses of different powers, the child selects three matching lenses from a trial case on the basis of the optical effects of the lenses.

3. *Problem solving.* Given a set of unmarked spherical lenses, each a different power, the child orders these in accord with their respective powers (e.g., +1.00, +2.00, +3.00). Another version: Given a set of three unmarked spherical lenses that represent a pattern, the child selects the fourth lens to complete the pattern (e.g., +1.00, −1.00, +1.00, . . . ? . . .).

Stereograms. The variable disparity anaglyph or vectogram devices work well here. Once again, all three levels may be implemented:

1. *Discrimination.* Upon being shown three pairs of vectograms, two representing the same disparity, the third a different disparity, the child identifies the "different" one (e.g., three minivectograms, set up to present [a] 2 p.d., base out; [b] 2 p.d., base out; [c] 2 p.d., base in).

2. *Replication.* Given a pair of vectograms positioned to represent, say, 4 base out, the child sets up a matching condition with his vectograms (i.e., he determines the disparity of his stereograms based on where the image appears to be and its size, not on the instrument's scale).

3. *Problem solving.* Given three pairs of vectograms, each providing a different disparity condition, have the child order them in accord with the relative size and position of the perceived images (e.g., 6 base out, 4 base out, 2 base out). Given three pairs of vectograms that represent a pattern, the child sets up the fourth pair (e.g., 2 base in; 2 base in; 2 base out;. . . . ? . . .).

Summary
The limiting factor is the scope of one's imagination. The world is full of objects that share certain concrete attributes and differ in others. Most of these may be used at all the levels defined above. And all will be useful. Some will be more

useful than others, however, because some stress identification of the spatial attributes that count most in school: quantity, magnitude, relationships.

In that regard, some may wonder at the light treatment given here to motor training activities (e.g., walking rail, balance board). These were very popular in the 1950s and 1960s but have since faded out of the picture. They faded not because they are useless but, rather, because they are not as useful as some of the other devices. *Their main value:* they provide a means for variation in the training of visual analysis skills. There is no reason why activities have to be limited to small spaces (e.g., 10-inch square geoboards). Most playing fields are organized spaces, having bases (in baseball), yardlines (in football), and so forth. These provide reference points. These may be used as "maxi" geoboards and should be, if the child enjoys it. *Their main drawback:* the implication that it is the motor coordination that is critical. There are no data to support this notion. Its origin is easy to trace: children with neurological deficits often display motor dysfunction and substandard perceptual skills. Hence the reasoning: train the motor function.

This ignores two basic facts. One, the relationship is not cause and effect. Training motor skills will not remediate the neurological deficit. Second, many well-coordinated children lack adequate visual analysis skills.

AUDITORY ANALYSIS SKILLS

There are fewer auditory programs, but what does exist resembles, in concept, the visual analysis skills programs just described. Once more, they tend to fall within one of the same four categories (3).

Vocal-Ear Coordination.　Mimicking speech patterns. Generally, this falls within the province of the speech and language therapist and, like the aforementioned hand-eye coordination tasks, stresses the skills needed to produce a sequence of sounds accurately and in correct order.

Discrimination Tasks.　Identification of precise similarities and differences in spoken words. Typically, these subdivide into beginning sounds, final sounds, and medial sounds.

Replication Tasks.　Listening to and repeating clusters of sounds that do not constitute meaningful words (e.g., "Repeat 'flib' or 'linderplan' "). The complexity of the clusters (length, sound sequence) may be varied. In all cases, the child is taught to listen, analyze, and repeat. (Foreign language recordings are very useful in this activity.)

Problem-solving Tasks.　(a) Reorder sound sequences (e.g., "Say the word *cat* backwards"); (b) delete a single sound from a sequence (e.g., "Say *coat;* now say it again, but don't say /k/"); (c) substitute sounds (e.g., "Say *fit;* now again, but instead of /f/, say /m/"); (d) complete patterns such as "boy," "toy," "ban," "?".

Placement Tests

The connection between these activities and the TAAS is apparent (see Chapter 8). Indeed, the TAAS may be used as a placement test for a remedial program. That program is not described here, in accord with the previously acknowledged, generally accepted attitude that it is best managed by persons trained in the remediation of reading problems that are connected with speech and language problems. In fact, of course, there is no good reason why the optometrist should not manage such cases, particularly in communities where speech and language specialists are unavailable (1).

WHERE SHOULD THE REMEDIAL PROGRAM BE CONDUCTED?

A properly managed perceptual skills remediation program requires the same kind of structure as any of the other remedial programs described in this book. In many ways, it is easier to administer a perceptual skills remedial program than one that concentrates on binocular function; the materials and procedures are less technical. For the same reason, however, it also generates certain difficulties because it involves the child in activities that are perceived as relatively uncomplicated. Failure to deal with them successfully is therefore viewed as a personal failure rather than a deficit that reflects no personal blame, such as strabismus. This may heat up the emotional climate considerably, especially if a parent is the out-of-office supervisor.

Not always, however. In many instances, a parent is an excellent home-therapist. But, when a choice exists, it is best if the perceptual skills deficits are treated in school. It is, after all, an educational problem. Treatment, therefore, should be centered in an educational setting.

Shifting the responsibility to the school yields benefits: (a) The parent and child are spared the emotional conflicts that often erupt when the parent attempts to teach the child a difficult (for him) behavior. (b) The child's teacher gains insights into some of the youngster's basic deficits and how they affect his school performance. This often enhances the teacher's ability to design more effective lessons.

There was a time when convincing schools to accept responsibility for implementing a remedial perceptual skills program was very difficult. This has changed; U.S. Public Law 94–142, mandates school involvement in such enterprises, and, although how the law is interpreted varies across the nation, it is a rare school district that does not now provide some special services and might provide more if petitioned appropriately. The optometrist has a strong petitioning potential.

□ Compensatory Treatment

The child in the fourth grade and beyond, who has been dealing with inept visual and/or auditory analysis skills since her early years, needs compensatory treatment (see flow diagram in Figure 9.2) taught in a way that takes her deficits into account, in a way that accommodates the deficits (24). This does not rule out perceptual skills remediation, but it does argue for a sensible ordering of priorities. The child and those who work with her have a finite amount of available energy, patience, and time. These should be expended as efficiently as possible, and the most efficient approach with this age group is through compensatory instruction.

Because compensatory instruction is really special education, the optometrist shies away from direct involvement. This is reasonable. She is not, after all, an educator.

But, another perspective is possible. If the patient were a low-vision case, with best corrected visual acuity limited to no better than 20/100, then the optometrist would have no reservations about requesting—insisting, if necessary—that the child be given special education support. The same circumstances exist with the child who has a perceptual skills disorder. In identifying the problem and pre-scribing a compensatory instructional approach, the optometrist is not usurping the educator's role. She is merely using her professional authority on behalf of her patient, and legitimately so.

The recommendations need not be accompanied by anything more than a report of the outcome of the tests that revealed the deficit, although it is not overstepping legitimate boundaries to explain perceptual skills behaviorally and to suggest some of the principles that make compensatory methods effective.

In order to to this, the optometrist is obliged to be somewhat familiar with the instructional environment and process. (True, all have attended school, but that is insufficient.) The information that follows is to serve that purpose. It is intended to enhance the optometrist's ability to communicate effectively on his patient's behalf. It is not intended to, nor will it, transform the optometrist into an educator.

Standard instruction comprises many components. For discussion purposes, these remarks will be limited to three major ones: *teacher, instructional program,* and *instructional environment.* One or more of these should be modified to ac-commodate the child with perceptual skills deficiencies (3).

TEACHER

The teacher is a central factor. A "good" teacher can use average materials and procedures and generate superior achievement. A "poor" teacher can use the same materials and procedures with opposite results. Some teachers are "good" with all types of children, regardless of whether they are easy to teach or the opposite. Some teachers are "good" only with the easy to teach, and so on.

When a choice exists, teachers of children with perceptual skills deficits should be (1): (a) *Knowledgeable;* i.e., know the business of teaching very well. A distin-guishing characteristic of hard-to-teach children is that they fail to recognize what to pay attention to and what to ignore unless someone tells them, and then reminds them. Not all teachers have yet achieved the level where they, themselves, can identify just what it is that the children are to pay specific attention to in a lesson. (b) *Pleasantly pedantic.* Not all children need slow, careful, step-by-step instruc-tion. Many, in fact, do not need it and abhor it when it is provided. The children under discussion here do need it and their teacher should be temperamentally suited to the role. (c) *Professionally secure*. The child with visual analysis skills deficits does not show regular gains in the classroom. There are times when the situation appears hopeless, that she will "never learn." Then, a sudden spurt. The teacher who is not secure will not be consistent in method. Many methods will be tried. The result: insufficient depth, ambiguity, and no academic gains.

INSTRUCTIONAL PROGRAM (25)

The vast majority of schools purchase their instructional materials from publishers. Ordinarily, these materials are organized into programs that cover a subject over a number of grade levels. A school may purchase a math program, for example, or a reading program that is introduced in kindergarten or first grade and is designed to be used through the sixth grade.

All reading and arithmetic programs tend to be the same in respect to *what* they are designed ultimately to teach. They may differ markedly, however, in *how* and *when* it is taught: i.e., the sequence in which subskills are introduced and the methods employed to teach them.

All programs work reasonably well with easy-to-teach children. That is not the case with the child who is hard to teach because of perceptual skills deficits. She needs a specific type of instruction, an approach that accommodates her deficits.

READING

Although there are a great number of hybrid variations, reading programs tend to follow one of three approaches: *whole word, linguistic,* and *phonic*. The major difference among the three is the size of the unit presented to the child for retention.

Whole Word Programs

From the outset, these introduce the child to reading stories. The stories are made up of familiar words, but the words do not have much in common in respect to their phonic or visual makeup. The "Look, look, oh look . . ." instructional sequence is representative. Words are repeated often and illustrations are usually present on each page, this to help the child become facile at recognizing the words rapidly. The words are usually well established in the average 6-year-old's speaking vocabulary. In addition, they are words that are easy to represent visually, allowing for pertinent picture clues.

The memory burden that this imposes on some children is enormous, especially the child with substandard auditory analysis skills. By definition, she lacks the ability to isolate the separate sounds that, when linked with the letters that comprise the printed word, facilitate retention. She fails to "see" the pertinent similarities and differences in the sounds and letters of *me* and *mother*, of *lit* and *little* and *brittle*, and so on, that would allow her to link new information to facts already learned. She is burdened with the need to invent an alternative strategy

that will enable her to remember all of her reading words, and there simply is
no reasonably effective alternative (26).

Linguistic Programs

These, too, stress whole word recognition, but the words that are used to introduce
the child to reading are chosen because they contain pertinent, reasonably obvious,
similarities and differences. Instead of having to remember such diverse words
as *run*, *mother*, *jump*, *look*, and *something*, the child starts with such words as
fit and *fat*, followed closely by *bat*, *sit*, and *sat*. Thus, remembering one word of
the group helps the child recall the others as well. Auditory analysis skills are
needed for this method, too, but they need not be so well developed. The key
phonic attributes of the words are very apparent.

The approach has a flaw, of course. The program cannot get very far along
before irregularly spelled words have to be introduced and, with this, ambiguity
of the type that confuses the child with auditory analysis skills deficits.

Phonics

Here the linkup between letters and sounds is made evident from the beginning.
The child is taught that individual letters have their distinctive sounds. She is
then taught how to blend these into words. This is very helpful to the child with
inept auditory analysis skills because it does for her what she cannot do for herself:
Analyze spoken words into separate sounds. It also has two obvious major faults.
First, it is extremely difficult to blend words made up of more than a few sounds;
the child forgets the initial sounds while working on the fourth and fifth ones.
Second, many letters have more than one sound (e.g., the *a* in cat, cake, saw,
said, above). This, combined with the irregular spellings of the English language,
require that something beyond a strict phonic approach be used fairly early in
the program.

Which Type of Reading Program Is Best?

What, then, should be recommended for the child with auditory analysis deficits?
In general terms:

1. The more impaired the child's auditory analysis skills, the greater her need,
initially, for a program that is based on phonics.

2. As she masters phonics principles, a linguistic approach should be introduced, and the child *should be shown* how those words may be remembered on
the basis of their shared phonic and spelling similarities and differences. For
example, how *bit*, *bat*, *sit*, and *sat* may be remembered as a related group rather
than as separate units; how remembering any one of them facilitates recall of the
others.

3. As linguistic units are mastered, the standard whole-word approach should
be introduced, and the child *should be shown* how groups of words may be
remembered on the basis of their shared linguistic-unit similarities and differences.

For example, how the words *sand, stand, standard,* and *withstand* are easier to remember on the basis of the linguistic unit *and*.

ARITHMETIC

Although there are many variations, arithmetic programs tend to follow one of two approaches: some emphasize *math concepts;* others, *math facts*. In the former, the child is taught that arithmetic is based on concepts that may be proven by counting. The rest is "simply" a matter of application, and, with practice, arithmetic fluency is attainable. This resembles, in many ways, the phonics approach to reading instruction.

In the other type of approach, number facts are taught as units to be remembered, with instruction regarding the underlying concepts introduced afterward. This is much like the whole word reading instruction approach.

The child with a visual analysis skills deficit will experience difficulty with both methods. Initially, the *concept* approach will seem to be effective, but it will be because she can solve simple problems by counting without understanding the concept. Counting cannot satisfy demands, however, when the child is confronted with such problems as $8473 \times 96 = ?$ or $65 \sqrt{759397} = ?$

On the other hand, a *number facts* approach will not work effectively because there are too many number facts. Unlike reading, an "educated guess" based on partial clues produces disastrous results in arithmetic.

Which Type of Arithmetic Program Is Best?
Like reading, a combination approach is essential. In general terms:

1. The child with visual analysis skills deficits should be introduced to arithmetic through a counting (concept) approach.

2. Relationships must be stressed; e.g., that $3 + 3 = 6$ and $3 + 4 = 7$, though separate problems, are related. The former is neatly contained within the latter, just as the word *and* is embedded in **stand** and *standard*. As such, no number fact is independent of other number facts.

SUMMARY

All of this reduces to a set of general guidelines that help in designing compensatory instruction for children with perceptual skills deficits. Teachers already know these, but occasionally overlook them in their anxiety to teach the child who is hard to teach. It does not hurt for the optometrist to remind them, diplomatically, that in accommodating the child's deficiencies in the classroom (see case report regarding patients 3,8,9,13), *the goal* is to make it possible for the child to learn—remember what she is taught—despite a persistent deficit in the ability to identify the concrete attributes of spatial and spoken patterns (3). To facilitate this:

COMPENSATORY INSTRUCTION GUIDELINES

1. Limit the amount of new information presented in any single lesson.

2. Present new information in a simple, organized way that highlights what is especially pertinent to such an extent that it is readily apparent to the child.

3. Make certain that the child really does have the factual knowledge that she will need to profit from the lesson. Assume nothing. Just because a student seemed to know something at an earlier time does not guarantee that she retains it. Find out.

4. Make clear the system that links up the new information with the information she already knows. The system should be made as explicit and basic as is necessary; and when there are exceptions to the system, these too should be made obvious. Do not assume that the student will be able to figure out an effective system from what appears to be appropriate examples. A system, probably; an effective system, no. The former happens frequently, meaning that the teacher may also have to help the child unlearn some "bad habits."

5. Encourage the student to use all her senses—not just her eyes and ears— to examine the concrete aspects of the task at hand. This forces her attention to those attributes that may escape her because of her perceptual skills deficits (e.g., virtually every adult reader will recognize the word *embarrass* on sight; fewer are able to spell it correctly).

6. Provide enough repeated experiences to establish the information securely in the student's long-term memory. Construct for her the associations and larger "chunks" that she fails to identify on her own, and have her practice until she can identify these instantaneously and virtually automatically—"on sight." In other words, have her practice until she no longer needs to use a system in order to "figure it out," but simply "knows it," has the information at her fingertips (e.g., as in learning how to drive a car or ascertain a refractive error with a retinoscope). In essence, this means that breaking things down for her into subunits is not enough. The relationship of the unit within the larger entity has to be made explicit.

INSTRUCTIONAL ENVIRONMENT

This refers to such diverse conditions as number of school days in an academic year, number of hours per day devoted to a specific subject, teacher-student ratio, heterogeneity of class makeup, physical space, social climate of school and the community, and so on.

Most of this goes well beyond the optometrist's concern, but there are some recommendations she can make that will benefit her patient with perceptual skills dysfunction. They all tend to emphasize the child's need for explicit, unambiguous, direct instruction; in other words, as much of the teacher's attention as possible. For example:

1. The child should be in a small class (e.g., student-teacher ratio of 8:1), at least when receiving instruction in those areas of greatest difficulty.

2. The class should be homogeneously teachable. It is unreasonable to expect a teacher to prepare different lessons for each child. It is far more efficient to group children so that the same approach is appropriate for all—at least during the times they are receiving instruction in their areas of greatest difficulty.

3. If necessary, additional tutorial assistance should be provided, but the tutor's approach should match, not conflict with, the classroom teacher's approach. Ambiguity must be avoided.

THE OPTOMETRIST'S ROLE BEYOND MAKING DIAGNOSIS AND RECOMMENDATIONS

This is a debatable topic. No single answer is correct. The optometrist's role depends at least in part on the services available at the child's school and the community at large. Certainly, the optometrist should not be cast in the role of team captain unless she functions as part of the education "team." The child's major problem is inadequate school achievement. The principal treatment site should be the school.

But, the optometrist does have a role to play, if only as a child advocate. Some day all schools will have well-developed, compensatory instruction capabilities for all their students. That day has not yet arrived. It behooves the optometrist to monitor her patient's progress, intervening whenever and wherever it appears to be desirable in order to obtain for the child the type of services she needs. It is not a comfortable role, but if often is an essential one.

■

PRACTICAL SUGGESTIONS

Parents and teachers are often puzzled by children with perceptual skills dysfunction, children who display adequately developed cognitive abilities in some aspects of their school work and severely impaired abilities in other areas. They often relate some of these idiosyncratic behaviors to vision and, therefore, direct their questions to the optometrist. Listed below are a number of these.

15-1. Q: What should be done to help the child who tends to read certain words in reverse, such as *was* and *saw?*

A: The general rule: Provide the child with a system for helping him overcome his problem. For example, as he reads aloud, have him move his finger across the lines of print, from left to right, in accord with his eyes and voice. Stress the importance of looking first at the first letter of the word, then at those that follow.

Another method: With a felt-tip pen, draw a vertical line down the left edge of each page the child is to read and make sure that he understands that he is *always* to start reading the words from *that side* of the page.

15-2. Q: What will help the child who frequently loses her place while reading?

A: Once more, use of the finger as a pointer is helpful. Many teachers will prefer a ruler, or some other device, to be held beneath the sentence in lieu of the finger. Their antipathy toward pointing with a finger usually derives from the observation that poor readers tend to use their finger as a pointer. This may be true, but it hardly supports the cause-and-effect inference. After all, a person with a broken leg is apt to use a crutch; eliminating the latter will not cure the former. Urge the teacher to encourage the child to use her finger as a pointer until she no longer needs it; until she can "pretend" it is there. (This assumes that the child's visual process skills—vergence and accommodation facility—are adequate.)

15-3. Q: What will help the child who has difficulty copying from the chalkboard?

A: In most cases, this is caused by substandard reading ability rather than a hand-eye incoordination. The greater the child's reading deficit, the more likely it is that he will encounter problems in copying. (An illustrating experiment is to copy the three visual patterns shown in Figure 8.15. Which of the three offers the greatest challenge? Obviously, the one that is not legible.) The answer, therefore: help the child become a better reader. The copying abilities will then improve without special intervention.

15-4. Q: Should the child be retained in her current grade for another year?

A: This, too, evokes high anxiety from the optometrist. It is a difficult question, worthy of a wise, knowledgeable answer. Ordinarily, the optometrist should limit her response to the observations that promoting the child to a higher grade when she lacks the knowledge expected of children in that grade is not beneficial. On the other hand, retention without a modification of how the child is taught is like urging a drowning swimmer to keep trying even though there is no shore in sight. The solution: retain, but take advantage of the opportunity by providing the necessary remedial/compensatory treatments.

15-5. Q: Is it possible for an illiterate adult to learn to read?

A: Yes, unless the individual is lacking in basic cognitive skills. Illiterate adults can (and do) learn to read, if properly instructed (28). The key question they have to face is whether they are willing and able to devote the time and energy that learning to read requires, regardless of age.

15-6. Q: Does the child have a learning disability?

A: There is a legal definition for learning disability, but it is long and relatively nonspecific. And, worse yet, it implies that a learning disability is a "disease," rather than simply a descriptor for the child whose learning problem is limited to the classroom. The best answer to this question appears to be: ignore the labels (including dyslexia) and deal with the problem.

15-7. Q: What is the cause of the child's problem?

A: Implicit in this question is the parent's anxiety that it is "their" fault. This is unfortunate, but reasonable, given the pervasive influence of psychological environmental factors on children during their formative years. The best, and indeed most honest response: probably not. In most cases, both parent and child are served best by persuading the parent that (a) the cause is unknown (unless, of course, it is known, which is rare) and (b) identifying the cause is no longer the key to the solution; effort now should be devoted to helping the child overcome his problem, whatever the original cause.

15-8. Q: The child is taking a behavioral-control drug (e.g., Ritalin). Should she continue?

A: Clearly, this is beyond the optometrist's scope. But, she should urge the parent to pose that question to the prescribing physician. In most cases, the answer is based on pragmatics. If it seems to help, why not? But no drug should be taken over a prolonged period without some assessment of its direct effects and side effects.

15-9. Q: The child's eye movements are erratic when he reads. Should he have eye-movement training?

A: This is a prevalent notion, based upon valid observations. Poor readers do display erratic eye movements. But, it is not the cause; it is the effect. There is evidence that the eye movements of poor readers are not worse than those of good readers when engaged in a task that does not involve reading (29).

15-10. Q: My youngster is having some difficulty in kindergarten. He is a "bright child," but he is "immature." I think I baby him too much. Also, his birthday is in August. That means that he will be among the youngest in his class—keeping in mind that in this community, the date for entry into school is September 1. In other words, had he been born a week or two later—in September—he would not have been allowed to enter kindergarten until next year. What should we do? Should he repeat kindergarten, enter first grade, be tested, what?

A: This question, heard frequently by optometrists, is difficult for us to answer with authority. It requires a judgment of the child's academic readiness rather than his vision. And, in fact, there is no absolutely correct answer; but some answers are better than others. As a rule of thumb, the best single predictor of the child's readiness for grade 1 is the quality of his performance in kindergarten. Clearly, that is in the educator's domain. From the optometrist's point of view, the important variables are (a) the status of the child's visual and auditory analysis skills and (b) his general development. The first of these is fairly easy to determine. The second is more complex, but it too can be judged on the basis of such factors as the child's DDST profile: If he manifests "delays," then by all means suggest something other than going on to grade 1. Regarding his birthdate: If he is significantly closer to his sixth than his seventh birthday upon entering grade 1, it probably is wise to suggest a year's delay; there is no inherent advantage in being the youngest and most immature child in the class. Besides, what is the hurry?

15-11. Q: Shouldn't we find out if the child is a "visual" or an "auditory learner" and then teach her accordingly?

A: No. This idea is hard to put to rest; it sounds reasonable, but it does not work. In simple terms, the (erroneous) hypothesis is: Some children have good visual analysis skills and poor auditory skills. Therefore, they should be taught to read with a "sight" (whole word) method—a method that avoids explication of phonetic principles.

The fact is that learning to read cannot be reduced to modality preference constructs. Regardless of whether the child is deaf, blind, or has normal sight and hearing, reading is the process of mapping language onto symbols. With most (sighted/hearing) children therefore, it is the process of mapping oral language onto graphic symbols. In order to be able to do this, the child must be familiar with the oral language, the graphic symbols, and how the two are linked.

The 6-year-old child with appropriately developed auditory and visual perceptual skills will probably learn to read with any standard reading program, be it sight or phonics based, or something in between. The same is true of the child with visual perceptual skills dysfunction, so long as her auditory analysis skills are adequate and her visual deficits are not so great as to impair her ability to learn to recognize the letters without confusion.

The child with auditory perceptual skills dysfunction presents a different challenge. By definition, she lacks the ability to isolate the separate sounds ("phonemes" in the jargon of reading teachers) in the context of spoken words. Hence, she will not make satisfactory progress in a "sight" reading program because it is not designed to make the separate phonemes apparent to her. She will not recognize the "system"; she certainly will not be able to memorize enough words by rote. She needs a reading program that *emphasizes* phonetic principles—a "phonics" program that makes clear to her what she cannot discover for herself because of her lack of auditory analysis skills.

Thus, the question is not: "Visual learner or auditory learner?" Rather, it is: "How important is it to teach the child phonetic principles?" with the child's TAAS score serving as the determinant.

15-12. Q: Where/how does spelling fit into this discussion? Is spelling affected by deficient visual or auditory perceptual skills? If so, which of the two is the most important?

A: Spelling is affected by both abilities—visual *and* auditory analysis skills—in different ways. The poor speller typically lacks one or both of the following: (a) the ability to analyze spoken words into their phonemic elements, i.e., adequate auditory analysis skills; (b) the ability to invent mnemonics for remembering the correct letter sequences in those parts of words that are not spelled phonetically. Therefore, to help the poor speller the teacher should attempt to improve the child's auditory analysis skills, if needed, and then go on to teach the child useful mnemonics; or inspire him to invent effective ones on his own. (Note: A fundamental rule when teaching a mnemonic to a child: Keep it short and simple— memorable; base it on something the child already knows well and can therefore build upon. Hence, there is no need to teach a mnemonic for remembering how to spell an entire word; rather, teach a mnemonic for remembering that part of the word that is spelled irregularly, i.e., nonphonetically; for example, "i before e except after c;" or have the child "say" the word to himself in a way that accentuates the spelling irregularity; e.g., pronounce the /k/ sound on "knife," the /h/ sound in "ghost," and so on.)

15-13. Q: How do these principles apply to helping a child who has difficulty with reading comprehension?

A: First of all, it is essential to make sure that the child understands the meaning of the words she is attempting to read and comprehend. If she is lacking in this, all other attempts at remediation will fail. Once this potential problem has been ruled out, consider her comprehension problem to be the product of poor organization skills. Show the child how to organize information: categorize events or objects discussed and shown in stories and pictures, encouraging her to invent alternative organizations and then to judge the relative effectiveness of each.

15-14. Q: Many children with substandard visual analysis skills also have poor handwriting. Will a child's handwriting improve if he is given visual analysis skills training?

A: Yes, handwriting is likely to improve as a result of visual analysis skills training. However, there are faster, more direct ways of improving a child's handwriting; specifically, teach him the "rules" of penmanship, the mechanics that he did not learn when they were originally taught—if, indeed, they were taught. Teaching him those rules, and having him practice them, is bound to improve his handwriting. Simplistic? Yes. Effective? Absolutely.

15-15. Q: At what age should I worry about my child's tendency to reverse letters; i.e., to print the "b" for the "d," etc? And what should I do when that time comes?

A: It is not uncommon for kindergarten (and younger) children to reverse letters; hence, it is not cause for worry at that level. However, there is no reason to allow even the young child to learn a bad habit, if it can be avoided without difficulty. Hence, rather than worry, it is often helpful at the outset to teach the child a dependable mnemonic for distinguishing confusable letters, such as the "b" and "d". One way that usually works: Find a related letter that the child does not confuse—the capital "B," perhaps. If she does not confuse its orientation, then it is but a small step to teach her that the lower case "b" is "hidden" in the capital "B." Refrain from the temptation to show how the "b" differs from the "d." Ignore the "d." Once the child has securely learned the "b", the "d" will not present a problem; it will simply be the "other one"—the one that is not the "b."

15-16. Q: My second-grade child is having trouble with arithmetic; he does satisfactorily in reading. What could explain this?

A: Learning arithmetic is, in some ways, similar to learning to read in that the child has to learn to map language onto symbols. The difference: There are two languages in arithmetic: a verbal one (the spoken words that pertain to arithmetic; e.g., "more," "less," "same as," "one," "two," "three," etc.), and a nonverbal one (the recognition of such spatial attributes as quantity, magnitude, and relationships; in other words, visual analysis skills). The child should be familiar with both (verbal and nonverbal) languages when he begins formal instruction in arithmetic. If he is not, he has only two ways of meeting classroom standards—and neither works very well. One, memorize the answers to all arithmetic problems—an impossibility. Two, solve arithmetic problems by employing a counting algorithm—a reasonable condition as long as the numbers involved are relatively small; hardly sensible when larger numbers are introduced. (In other words, it is one thing to solve, by counting, the problem $3 + 4 = ?$ It is another to solve the problem '$7 \times 9 = ?$' in this way.)

15-17. Q: What about mixed hand-eye dominance; does that cause learning problems?

A: No, it does not appear to cause learning problems. Granted, over the years this notion has surfaced many times, only to be rejected when studied scientifically (27). There is no apparent validity to the proposal that the child who "sights" with her left eye and prints with her right hand is more at risk to school learning problems than the child who is "right eye dominant," and right handed.

15-18. Q: To what extent does hand preference (dominance) influence a child's school performance?

A: There is a lot yet to be learned about the influence of hemispheric (sensory and motor) dominance on cognitive functioning. At present, the honest and most practical approach is to acknowledge that although there are relatively more left-handed children in "learning disability" populations, there are also many left-handed children who do very well in school. In that same vein, a great many children who have difficulty in school are right handed. Hence, hand preference, in itself, does not seem to be a significant factor.

15-19. Q: My first grader is ambidextrous; that is, sometimes he uses his right hand for printing, sometimes his left. Do you think that his printing reversals are connected with this in some way? And, if so, should I do something about it?

A: Yes, if by "ambidextrous" you mean that he has not yet established a preferred hand for printing, etc. (Usually, it is more accurate to describe such children as "nondextrous.") Hand preference develops; very few children settle on being right or left handed until they are about four. Sometimes they eat, draw, throw, etc., with their right hand, sometimes with their left. But this should all be resolved by the time they reach their fifth birthday. Children who are late in establishing consistent handedness are demonstrating a developmental lag—one that will affect their ability to remember spatial relationships. Obviously, the child who does not remember spatial relationships will display confusion when it comes to remembering which is the "b" and which the "d," etc. In other words, it is highly likely that the child who does not develop a consistent hand preference at the expected age will also reveal a (related) lag in visual perceptual skills.

What to do about it? Many kindergarten teachers advocate selecting a preferred hand for such children by determining empirically which hand is already the most adept and requiring the child to limit all printing, coloring, drawing, and other one-handed activities to that hand. This has not been found to create any "deeper" problems for the child; in fact, most often it seems to resolve a problem.

15-20. Q: My kindergarten child is having difficulty learning the names of the colors. Her teacher wonders if she is color blind. Is that her problem?

A: We will test her color vision, although the test is somewhat demanding; it may be confusing for her. Most children do not manifest a color vision anomaly. Rather, they simply have difficulty remembering which color is which.

You may investigate this in a number of ways. The simplest: show the child a colored wooden cube (blue, for example) along with three additional cubes—one red, one yellow, one blue (or whatever combination you please)—and ask her to find the cube among the three additional cubes that is the same color as "this (the blue) one."

To teach the names of the colors, have the parents initiate an organized program:

Once it has been established that the child can match colors (as described above), have her engage in some activities that require her to discriminate colors in various ways: e.g., "find the cube that is a different color," "sort these cubes into two (or three, or four) piles, with all of this color (e.g., yellow) together, all of this color (e.g., red) together, etc."

Designate a given week as being devoted to a specific color; e.g., "This week is *red* week. Every day this week you will have to wear something red and find as many red things as you can. Next week we will work on a different color— green; for now, let's work on red."

15-21. Q: My 6-year-old is enrolled in a bilingual program; we are recent immigrants and we do not speak English at home. Is such a program good for him?

A: The program is probably good for him. Remember, the definition of reading is "mapping language onto symbols." If the child does not know the spoken language, he can hardly be expected to learn how to map it onto symbols. Such children are best served by first having the time and experiences needed to learn the spoken language, then learning how to read it.

15-22. Q: Are visual and auditory perceptual skills totally dependent upon development; i.e., can they be influenced by specific instructional experiences? For example, would my child do better on a copying test if I prepared her with some instruction in how to copy circles, squares, and so on?

A: Visual and auditory perceptual skills can often be stimulated by appropriate activities; in other words, instruction frequently helps. But, such instruction should not be devoted to tutoring in how to copy specific geometric designs. It is true that most preschool children could be taught literally how to draw a square, or a triangle, but this would not foster general development. It would simply help them score better on tests that used those forms. It would be analogous to teaching a preschooler the square root of 16, or a myope the 20/15 letters on the Snellen visual acuity chart. With sufficient practice, most would be able to respond correctly—but that could hardly be evidence of acquisition of a general ability.

REFERENCES

1. Rosner J, Rosner J. Differences in the perceptual skills development of young myopes and hyperopes. AJOPO 1985; 62(8):501–504.
2. Rosner J, Rosner J. Some observations of the relationship between the visual perceptual skills development of young hyperopes and age of first lens correction. Clin & Exper Optom 1986; 69(5):166–68.
3. Rosner J. Helping children overcome learning difficulties. 2nd ed. New York: Walker Publishing Co., 1979.
4. Itard J. Rapporte fait a son excellente le ministere de l'interieur: sur les noubeaux develouppement et l'eteat acteral du sauvage de L'Aveyron. 1807.
5. Seguin E. Idiocy and its treatment by the physiological method. New York: Columbia University Press. 1866.
6. Montessori M. The Montessori method. New York.: F.A. Stokes Co., 1912.
7. Gesell A et al. Vision—its development in infant and child. New York: Paul B. Hoeber, 1949.
8. Getman GN. How to develop you child's intelligence. Luverne, Minn.: published privately, 1962.
9. Clements SD. Minimal brain dysfunction in children. Washington, D.C.: Pub. Health Serv. Publication #1415, 1966.
10. Chalfant JC, Scheffelin MA. Central processing dysfunction in children: a review of the research. Washington, D.C.: H.E.W., 1969 (NINDS Monograph #9).
11. Ayres AJ. Learning disabilities and the vestibular system. J Learn Dis 1978; 11(1):30.
12. Kephart NC. The slow learner in the classroom. Columbus, Ohio: C. S. Merrill, 1960.
13. Eisenberg L. Principles of drug therapy in child psychiatry with special reference to stimulant drugs. Am J Orthopsychiatr 1971; 41:371.
14. Cott A. Orthomolecular approach to the treatment of learning disabilities. Schizophrenia 1971; 3:95.
15. Feingold B. Why your child is hyperactive. New York: Random House, 1975.
16. Frank J, Levinson H. Dysmetric dyslexia and dyspraxia. Synopsis of a continuing research project. Acad Therapy 1975-76; 11(2):133.
17. Pavlidis GT. Do eye movements hold the key to dyslexia? Neuropsychologia 1981; 19:57–64.
18. Stein J, Fowler S. Effect of monocular occlusion on visuomotor perception and reading in dyslexic children. Lancet 1985; July 13:69–73.
19. Geiger G, Lettwin JY. Peripheral vision in persons with dyslexia. N Engl J Med 1987; 316:1238–43.
20. Irlen H. Successful treatment of learning disabilities. Unpublished paper presented at American Psychological Association, August 1983.
21. Ross AO. Psychological aspects of learning disabilities and reading disorders. New York: McGraw-Hill Book Co., 1976.
22. Rosner J. Testing for teaching in an adaptive educational environment. In: Hively W, Reynolds M, eds. Domain-referenced testing in special education. Reston, Va.: Council for Exceptional Children, 1975.
23. Rosner J. Two developmental training devices. San Rafael, Calif.: Academic Therapy Publication, 1971.

24. Rosner J. Teaching hard-to-teach children to read: a rationale for compensatory education. In: Resnick L, Weaver P, eds. Theory and practice of early reading. Vol. 2. Hillsdale, N.J.: LEA, 1979.
25. Rosner J. Adapting primary grade reading instruction to individual differences in perceptual skills. Reading World 1975; 14(4).
26. Barr R. The effect of instruction on pupil reading strategies. Reading Res Quart 1974–75; 10(4):555.
27. Robbins MP. A study of the validity of Delacato's theory of neurological organization. Exceptional Children 1966; 32:517.
28. Robinson MH. "Kenneth Johnson": a progress report on a search for literacy. Bull Orton Society 1969; 19:134.
29. Adler-Grinberg D, Stark L. Eye movements, scanpaths, and dyslexia. AJOPO 1978, 55(8):557–570.

16

Case Reports

☐

Ordinarily, case reports are published to document novel clinical conditions and/
or sets of circumstances. That is not our purpose. The case reports contained in
this chapter do not describe unusual, never before reported types of conditions.
On the contrary, they were selected because they are representative of a variety
of typical pediatric patients. In most instances, each of the reports describes a
different condition; however, some of them are representative of the same condition but differ in the age of the patient or some other circumstance that necessitates a different approach to clinical assessment and management.

We do not suggest that the treatments we prescribed in these cases are the
only or the best. On another day, with another patient, we might have prescribed
something a bit different. But, we do believe that what we prescribed was appropriately derived from the available information.

We publish these cases as a means of illustrating the integrative processes that
drive good clinical pediatric practice. The competent clinician knows the signs
and symptoms of the various conditions presenting in his/her practice. The competent clinician knows which tests to administer and how to administer them so
as to obtain differential information. The competent clinician knows which types
of treatments are most appropriate for different conditions. And, in addition to
all this—and probably most important of all—the competent clinician knows how
to synthesize all of this information, accurately and rapidly, and communicate
with the patient: to advise them as effectively as possible. Our major purpose in
presenting these case reports is to illustrate the deductive, synthesis, and communication processes as they apply to the different conditions and circumstances
that arise with young patients and their parents.

Each case report is organized in a similar fashion. Each begins with a short
overview of the case, then a presentation of the salient clinical data obtained at
the first visit, then our diagnosis and treatment recommendations, followed by a
summary of treatment outcomes. Each report ends with a section devoted to
"general comments," and a listing of "questions worthy of discussion," in which
alternative viewpoints are posed.

■
_____

PATIENT 1: ANDREW
(NORMAL FIVE-MONTH-OLD)

The chief purpose of this report is to illustrate how clinical assessment methods change in relation to the patient's age. It describes the management of an apparently normal youngster whose parents initially sought consultation solely because of the prevalence of amblyopia in the family. Patient was 5 months old at his first visit; 5 1/2 years old at his last (fifth) visit.

☐ Visit #1 (June 1980)

SALIENT CLINICAL DATA

Age: 5 months (Date of birth [DOB]: January 1980).

Chief concern: Parents report no evidence of any ocular or visual abnormality. Their sole reason for this visit is that both the child's father and his paternal grandfather manifest unilateral amblyopia, attributable (purportedly) to anisometropia, and they do not want to risk neglecting a similar condition in their child.

Relevant history/initial impressions: Andrew appears to be a healthy, contented, well cared for youngster. He is responsive to his environment. Pregnancy was full term; birthweight = 7 pounds, 8 ounces. APGAR = 9, 10. His postnatal development and health have been normal to date.

Visual Acuity: 20/200+ each eye; measured with preferential looking cards held at 0.5 meter. No evidence of specific resistance to occlusion of either eye.

Ocular health: No evidence of pathology or structural abnormalities as observed by external and opthalmoscopic examination. Motilities unrestricted, both eyes.

Refractive status (dynamic retinoscopy): O.D., +2.00 −0.75 cx 180; O.S., +1.75 −0.50 cx 180.

Binocular status (unaided): At distance = apparent alignment by direct observation; more formal testing not possible. At near = Hirschberg test indicates normal binocular alignment.

Developmental status: No evidence of a lag in any sector of the DDST; passed all items intersected by age line.

DIAGNOSIS

Moderate hyperopic astigmatism, O.U. No other noteable conditions. No evidence of acuity or binocular deficit that could be linked with amblyopia.

RECOMMENDATIONS

Reassurance. Parents advised that their youngster's eyes appear to be healthy, normally formed, and functioning as expected for his age; that we observe no evidence of amblyopia, nor any reason to anticipate it occurring in the foreseeable future. We also reassure them that Andrew's moderate refractive error is well within normal limits for his age, that compensatory lenses are not justified at this time. When satisfied that their anxieties have been adequately addressed, we close the visit with the suggestion that they return with Andrew for a follow-up examination in about a year and that, in the interim, they feel free to contact us if a question arises or if they observe something that concerns them.

□ Visit #2 (June 1981)

SALIENT CLINICAL DATA

Age: 17 months.

Chief concern: None. This appointment was made on the basis of our previous recommendation.

Relevant history/initial impressions: Parents report no events or observations during the past year that caused them to be concerned about Andrew's eyes. He has obviously thrived. He now walks unaided, inspects objects in his view with keen interest, and jabbers in a way that, though unintelligible, reflects the cadence of normal speech.

Visual Acuity: Reasonably adequate, as determined with a candy-bead procedure (i.e., Andrew was able to discriminate a 1-mm candy bead from a distance of 3 meters). No resistance to occlusion of either eye.

Ocular health: No evidence of pathology or structural abnormalities as observed by external and ophthalmoscopic examination.

Refractive status (dynamic retinoscopy): O.D., +1.50 −0.50 cx 180; O.S., +1.25 −0.50 cx 180.

Binocular status (unaided): Cover test at distance = orthophoria; at near = 2 pd exophoria. Stereopsis at distance = not measurable; at near = at least 600 seconds arc, as measured with a two-item, forced-choice, modified Frisby stereotest (see p. 254).

Hirschberg test also indicates normal binocular alignment in all positions of gaze.

Developmental status: No evidence of a lag in any sector of the DDST.

DIAGNOSIS

Moderate hyperopic astigmatism. No other noteable conditions. No evidence of acuity or binocular deficit that could be linked with amblyopia.

RECOMMENDATIONS

Parents advised that Andrew's eyes continue to appear healthy, normally formed, and functioning as expected for his age. We also suggest that they return with Andrew for routine reexamination in about a year.

☐ Visit #3 (January 1983)

SALIENT CLINICAL DATA

Age: 3 years.

Chief concern: None. This appointment was made on the basis of our previous recommendation.

Relevant history/initial impressions: Parents report no events or observations since their last visit that caused them concern. Andrew obviously continues to thrive. He now demonstrates relative independence; he separates from his parents with comfort, is curious about his environment, and responds appropriately to our queries. His speech seems to be reasonably articulate and his language appropriate for his age.

Visual Acuity (Sheridan Gardiner test): O.D., 20/30; O.S., 20/30.

Ocular health: No evidence of pathology or structural abnormalities as observed by external, slit lamp, and ophthalmoscopic examination.

Refractive status (static retinoscopy): O.D., $+1.25 -0.25$ cx 180; O.S., $+1.25 -0.25$ cx 180.

Binocular status (unaided): Cover test at distance = orthophoria; at near = 2 pd exophoria. Stereopsis at distance = at least 2 minutes arc (A.O. vecto); at near = 40 seconds arc (Titmus stereotest); RDE at 1.5 meters = pass.

Developmental status: No evidence of a lag in any sector of DDST.

DIAGNOSIS

Moderate hyperopic astigmatism. No other noteable conditions.

RECOMMENDATIONS

Reassurance. Parents advised that their son's eyes continue to appear healthy, normally formed, and functioning as expected for his age, and that they return with Andrew for routine reexamination in about a year.

☐ Visit #4 (June 1984)

SALIENT CLINICAL DATA

Age: 4½ years.

Chief concern: None. This appointment was made on the basis of our previous recommendation.

Relevant history/initial impressions: Parents report no events or observations since their last visit that caused them concern. Andrew now communicates effectively and freely both verbally and nonverbally. He is enrolled in a neighborhood preschool where he spends four half-days per week. According to his teacher (as reported by his parents), he is doing well.

Visual Acuity (Tumbling E test): O.D., 20/25; O.S., 20/25.

Ocular health: No evidence of pathology or structural abnormalities as observed by external, slit lamp, and ophthalmoscopic examination.

Refractive status (static retinoscopy): O.D., +1.00; O.S., +1.00.

Binocular status (unaided): Cover test at distance = orthophoria; at near = 3 pd exophoria. Stereopsis at distance = 1 minute arc (A.O. vecto); at near = 20 seconds arc (Randot stereotest); RDE at 1.5 meters = pass.

Developmental status: No evidence of a lag in any sector of DDST.

DIAGNOSIS

Moderate hyperopia, O.U. No other noteable conditions.

RECOMMENDATIONS

Reassurance. Parents once again advised that their son's eyes appear healthy, normally formed, and functioning as expected for his age. We suggest that they return for routine reexamination in about a year.

□ Visit #5 (June 1985)

SALIENT CLINICAL DATA

Age: 5 ½ years.

Chief concern: None. This appointment was made on the basis of our previous recommendation.

Relevant history/initial impressions: Parents report no events or observations since their last visit that caused them concern. Andrew attended prekindergarten this past year and progressed as expected.

Visual Acuity (Snellen letters): O.D., 20/20; O.S., 20/20.

Ocular health: No evidence of pathology or structural abnormalities as observed by external, slit lamp, and ophthalmoscopic examination.

Refractive status (static retinoscopy): O.D., +1.00 D sphere; O.S., +1.00 D sphere.

Binocular status (unaided): Cover test at distance = orthophoria; at near =3 pd exophoria. Stereopsis at distance = 1 minute arc (A.O. vecto); at near = 20 seconds arc (Randot stereotest); RDE at 1.5 meters = pass.

Vergence facility (unaided): At distance: pass; at near: pass.

Accommodative facility (unaided): at distance: pass; at near: pass.

Developmental status: DDST = no evidence of a lag in any sector; TVAS = 5 (within expected limits for his age/grade); TAAS = 2 (within expected limits for his age/grade).

DIAGNOSIS

Moderate hyperopia, O.U. No other noteable conditions.

RECOMMENDATIONS

Reassurance. Parents advised that Andrew's eyes continue to appear healthy, normally formed, and functioning as expected for his age. His perceptual skills development also appears to be age-appropriate; he is "ready" to enter kindergarten insofar as these aptitudes are concerned. His hyperopia remains clinically insignificant; it may be safely ignored for at least the next year. We suggest that they return for routine reexamination in about a year.

□ General Comments

Andrew's case follows a very typical path; seen initially during his first year of life, primarily because his parents were alert to the possibility of a vision problem and wished to address it early if it did manifest; seen at subsequent visits on the basis of our recommendations. Notice that although we followed the same structure at each visit (chief concern, relevant history, visual acuity, health status, refractive status, binocular status, adaptability, and developmental status), our testing methods changed. For example, we initially tested visual acuity with preferential looking cards, then with candy beads, then with the Sheridan-Gardiner test, then with tumbling E's, and finally with Snellen letters. Similarly, our assessment of the child's binocular status began with the Hirschberg test, then with the modified, two-item Frisby, then with the Titmus stereotest, and finally with the RDE at 1.5 meters. Had we not been able to adapt our testing methods to the child's behavioral and cognitive abilities, we would not have been able to conduct adequate evaluations; as such, we would have not been able to offer his parents adequate valid and reliable advice.

□ Questions Worth Discussing

1. What other tests would have served us equally well in examining this youngster at his first, second, third, fourth, and fifth visits? That is, are there other methods we could have used to measure visual acuity, binocular status, etc., at any those visits?
2. Did we omit any important measures during any of the visits? If so, which? And why are they important; why should we not have omitted them?
3. Would you have prescribed compensatory lenses at any of the visits? If so, what powers, and why? What benefit(s) would they have provided? What undesirable consequences might they have caused or prevented.

4. Should Andrew's visits have been spaced closer together. Farther apart? Why?

5. Is there sufficient information in this report to enable you to predict if Andrew is likely to become more or less hyperopic? Myopic? Astigmatic? if yes, what would you predict? If no, what additional information, if any, would enable you to make such a prediction?

■
___

PATIENT 2: ALICE (NORMAL PRESCHOOLER—ANXIOUS PARENT)

The chief purpose of this report is to illustrate one approach to the clinical management of a healthy, normal preschooler whose mother is concerned about her child's readiness for kindergarten. It describes the clinical picture of a 4-year-old who is behaving in the manner typical of a 4-year-old, but whose parent—anxious about her daughter's cognitive development—is not familiar with just how well 4-year-olds should be able to draw human figures. It also includes a copy of the report we sent to the child's pediatrician at the request of Alice's mother (see Figure 16.1).

□ Visit #1 (November 1984)

SALIENT CLINICAL DATA

Age: 4 years, 11 months (DOB: December 1979).

School: Neighborhood preschool.

Chief concern: Child's mother has read an article that stressed the desirability of an early eye examination and emphasized the importance of assessing visual perceptual skills. This, in combination with the fact that Mrs. Smith did not believe her child's preschool "paper work" (drawing skills, etc.) was as neat as it should be, prompted her to seek advice from her pediatrician who, in turn, referred the child to us.

Relevant history/initial impressions: Alice's health and developmental histories are uneventful. She appears to be a very bright, socially adept, attractive youngster. She separates easily from her mother and responds readily to our initial requests and questions.

Unaided distance visual acuity: O.D., 20/20 (Tumbling E's); O.S., 20/20.

Ocular health: No evidence of pathology or structural abnormalities.

Refractive status: O.U.: +0.75 D spheres.

Binocular status (unaided): Cover test: at distance = orthophoria; at near = 4 pd exophoria. Stereoacuity: passed RDE at 1.5 meters. Vergence/accommodation facility: not tested.

Developmental status: DDST: Passed all items intersected by age line. Gesell Copy Forms: Satisfactorily copied circle, plus sign, square, and triangle; encountered difficulty with the other forms (divided rectangle; diamonds); i.e., performed at about a 5-year-old level. TAAS: score = 1 (appropriate for age/grade).

DIAGNOSIS

The child displays no significant visual/ocular deviations. Perceptual skills development appears to be progressing at a normal rate. This, in conjunction with the fact that Alice's birthdate prevents her from entering kindergarten until she is well past her fifth birthday, allows us to predict that she will be "ready" for school—at least to the extent that this is predicted by the instruments cited above.

RECOMMENDATIONS

Reassurance. Re-examine child in one year. Send report to her pediatrician and preschool (see Figure 16.1 below).

☐ Follow-up Data

Alice returned for routine re-examination the following November. At that time, she was attending public school kindergarten and doing well. Our assessment revealed nothing significantly different from the previous year other than normal growth and development.

Alice's last visit occurred when she was about midway through the first grade. She continued to enjoy good ocular health, 20/20 visual acuity, emmetropia, normal binocular abilities, and an appropriate developmental status. Her school performance was reported to be very satisfactory.

☐ General Comments

Alice's case is not unusual. She is a "product of our times," the child of a well-meaning, concerned parent who is ambitious for her child—who wants her child to be able to excel in school so that she can reap the benefits of all that a good education will offer her. The optometrist's obligation in such cases: Be aware of what normal development would predict for a child of this age, compare the patient's performance with this set of standards, and counsel the parent accordingly. In Alice's case, the optometrist's function was simply that of offering assurance and teaching the mother that although her child's development will have important effects on how well she will be able to adapt to the demands that society places upon her, it is innately guided, and should be respected so long as it is progressing normally. Treatment might not be all that simple in other cases. Not all children are as intact as Alice; some really do lag in one or more aspect of their

Report re: Alice Smith
Age: 4 years, 2 months
School: Neighborhood Preschool
Date of visit: November 22, 19..

Alice was referred to this office because of her mother's concern regarding the child's visual development. Mrs. Smith had read an article that pointed out the importance of early eye examinations and, along with that, had decided that her daughter's drawings seemed to be "immature." Alice's general health is and always has been excellent. She is a personable youngster, participating in the examination in a communicative, cooperative manner.

Alice has never had an eye examination prior to this visit. Her eyes appeared to be healthy and normally formed. Her visual acuity is normal (20/20, each eye). Refraction revealed a very moderate hyperopia (farsightedness), not enough to cause any concern.

I also assessed the child's general development, using the Denver Developmental Screening Test (DDST), the Gesell Copy Form Test, and the Test of Auditory Analysis Skills. Nothing unusual was observed in any of these. Alice's responses to the items in the Personal-Social, Fine Motor-Adaptive, and Language sectors of the DDST indicate that she is developing at a normal rate. The second of these (Fine Motor-Adaptive) pertains to visual perceptual skills development; a normal finding here indicates that her mother's concerns regarding the child's drawings are probably not well founded. (Indeed, after inspecting one of Alice's drawings, it is apparent that she draws the way a 4-year-old usually draws.) I also screened the child's auditory analysis skills. Once again, no deviation from the normal was noted.

In summary then, Alice's development, including her visual and auditory analysis skills, appears to be normal. No treatment of any sort is recommended. She should be re-examined at regular (yearly) intervals.

Joy Rosner, O.D.

Figure 16.1 Report regarding Alice Smith.

development, and the sooner that lag is identified, the earlier intervention can begin.

□ Questions Worth Discussing

1. Are there other tests we should have administered at Alice's first visit? If so what, and why?

2. Would you have prescribed lenses for this child, based on the data we obtained at her first visit?

3. Would you have offered the same advice that we did at that first visit? If not, what would you have recommended, and why?

4. Would it have been possible to help Alice acquire better pencil-paper skills? If so, should this have been suggested as a means of (a) calming her mother's anxieties and (b) improving the child's general classroom behavior?

5. What is the long-term prospect for Alice, in respect to her ability to make satisfactory progress in school?

6. What is the long-term prospect for Alice, in respect to her refractive status? Is she apt to become more hyperopic? Astigmatic? Myopic?

■

PATIENT 3: CARL
(IMMATURE PRESCHOOLER)

The chief purpose of this report is to illustrate one approach to the clinical management of a kindergarten-aged child who has not developed basic visual and auditory analysis aptitudes at the expected rate. It describes a situation in which a key ingredient in the treatment (for an "August birthday" boy) is delayed entry into first grade.

☐ Visit #1 (June 1982)

SALIENT CLINICAL DATA

Age: 5 years, 10 months (DOB: August 1976).

School: Neighborhood school (kindergarten).

Chief concern: Carl is scheduled to enter first grade next September. His kindergarten teacher has expressed concern about his "readiness" and has discussed with his mother the advisability of delaying entry for an additional year.

Relevant history/initial impressions: Carl appears to be a healthy, outgoing child. He displays little hesitancy at separating from his mother. He is curious about the environment—too curious, in fact; he tends to handle things that were not meant to be handled and, in general, is more active than is typical of his age group under these conditions.

Carl's health and developmental histories are uneventful. Pregnancy was full-term; birthweight = 7 pounds, 2 ounces. APGAR = 8, 9. He walked and talked at expected ages. He has not had any significant health problems. He attended a neighborhood preschool prior to being enrolled in kindergarten. His preschool teacher never expressed concern regarding his development, although she frequently commented on his "busyness," his tendency to be more active than most of the other children, and his lack of interest in puzzles, crayons, and other activities of this sort. She attributed this to his being a "real boy." Carl's kindergarten teacher, however, viewed these same characteristics with some concern. In her opinion, Carl was not ready for first grade; specifically, she noted his "short attention span, his poor fine-motor skills (as revealed in block play, coloring, etc.), and his relatively limited ability to retain oral instructions." Carl was brought to our office upon her recommendation.

Unaided distance visual acuity: O.D., 20/40; O.S., 20/40 (Tumbling E's). Upon administering this test, we were uncertain as to whether Carl's visual acuity was truly 20/40 or whether he was simply confused by the perceptual demands of the directional E test. We therefore also administered the Lighthouse Flash Card test and obtained the following results: O.D., 20/20; O.S., 20/20.

Ocular health: No evidence of pathology or structural abnormalities.

Refractive status: O.U., +0.50 D spheres.

Binocular status (unaided): Cover test at distance = orthophoria; at near = orthophoria. Stereoacuity at distance = unreliable measure (child confused by test); at near = 60 seconds arc (Titmus); RDE at 1.5 meters = pass. Vergence/accommodation facility: not tested; child not able to participate appropriately.

Developmental status: DDST: Passed all items intersected by age line except for one in the Fine-motor Adaptive sector: Copy a square. TVAS: Score = 1 (unsatisfactory for age/grade). TAAS: Score = 3 (appropriate for age/grade).

DIAGNOSIS

Significant lag in visual perceptual skills development. All else normal.

RECOMMENDATIONS

Carl's visual perceptual skills deficit, in conjunction with the fact that his August birthdate guarantees that he will be among the youngest in his class if he enters first grade this September, inspired us to discuss seriously with his mother the advisability of delaying that first grade entry for an additional year. We also suggest that during this year, two treatment approaches be taken, one designed to be remedial, the other compensatory. In essence, the two are completely compatible. In regard to remediation, Carl should engage in a program designed to teach him the basic spatial analysis strategies he presently lacks, but should have. As this is being carried out, Carl should be taught in a way that takes his inefficient analysis abilities into account: tasks should be laid out in a step-by-step fashion, with limits and rules made evident, clear, and unambiguous. Obviously, these compensatory approaches may be withdrawn as the child develops his own ability to organize tasks. Until that time, however, they are necessary if he is to be spared the frustation of being unable to accomplish what he has been asked to perform.

Parents discuss our recommendations with Carl's pediatrician and his kindergarten teacher, and accept them. We dispense a visual analysis skills training program to his parents, explain its principles and goals to his kindergarten teacher, and heartily endorse the idea that he repeat his kindergarten year with this same teacher. She is obviously well informed as well as interested and sensitive to Carl's particular needs. We also suggest that we monitor Carl's progress on a bimonthly basis.

☐ Follow-up Data

ONE YEAR LATER

Carl has had a productive year. His parents and kindergarten teacher complied fully with the treatment recommendations. He has made significant gains in visual analysis skills development; TVAS score is now 9, well within expected range for a youngster just completing kindergarten. In addition, and obviously just as important, he has acquired better control over his behavior. He enters a new setting in a more organized fashion; he looks around before he goes into action, he responds to signals in that setting that suggest he should or should not be doing what he is doing. He approaches a multi-component, sequential task in an orderly fashion, deciding first where to begin, then what to do, then what, and so on.

Are these gains derived from his TVAS program and/or from the compensatory assistance provided by his parents and teacher? That question is not answerable. He may have made these gains without treatment, simply on the basis of growth and development; or he may not have made them. In any case, he has made them, and more to the point, had he entered first grade last year, without the basic organizational skills he can now display, it is highly likely that he would not have made satisfactory progress. This would have led to frustration and failure, which would have led to additional and more complex problems.

We have no doubt that the most important ingredient in the management of this case was delayed entry into first grade; but we also believe that the treatment provided during that interim year contributed to his improvement.

TWO YEARS LATER

Carl has just completed first grade. He had a successful year. He is not "scholarly," but he performed satisfactorily in all aspects of the first grade program. His visual/ocular status remains unchanged. We are inclined to ignore the moderate hyperopia he manifests (O.U.: +0.75D), at least for the time being. We will reassess him on a regular (annual) basis.

☐ General Comments

Carl's situation is one that is often encountered by optometrists who include developmental assessment in their examinations: an August-born child whose developmental schedule is slightly behind what is expected. Many 5-year-olds, a large proportion of them males, fall into this category. Had Carl entered first grade this September, just after his sixth birthday, he would have been among the very youngest (chronologically) in the class—his classmates would have ranged in age from just past their sixth birthday to just shy of being 7 years old; a large spread when one is only six and already lagging a bit. Hence, our recommendation to hold off a year before entering school. Granted, there were other treatment options. We could have instituted a high-intensity, full-scale program to bring the child's visual analysis skills up to a better level, we could have advised that he begin first grade, but be provided with special classroom conditions that accommodated his perceptual skills deficit, we could have advised both, and so on. Our reason for selecting the treatment we recommended: We considered it the kindest as well as most effective, given the child's status, his parents' reasonable attitude regarding the delayed entry into first grade, and probably some other factors that we cannot articulate (clinical intuition?) but that influenced our decision.

□ Questions Worth Discussing

1. What comes to mind when we refer to "some other factors that we cannot articulate (clinical intuition?)" in the above section? In other words, what other factors would you take into consideration when attempting to decide whether to recommend active remedial treatment in conjunction with standard promotion to first grade versus a 1-year delayed entry?

2. What do you think would have happened had Carl entered first grade just after his sixth birthday? Would he have failed? Is he likely to have developed certain maladaptive (antisocial) behaviors? Anything else?

3. Would Carl's situation have been different if his delayed development had been identified and treated at an earlier age—when he was 3 or 4 years old? If so, what treatment approach would you have taken at that time?

4. Do you think that Carl's present school performance is attributable to the vision therapy administered after that first visit, the delayed entry into first grade, both, or something else altogether?

5. Should we have prescribed the +0.50 D spheres indicated by our refraction?

6. Carl's teacher was concerned about his fine-motor skills. Is that something different than visual analysis skills? If yes, explain the difference.

7. How do you explain the fact that Carl's auditory analysis skills were at an appropriate level while his visual analysis skills were not? Does this indicate an unusual situation?

8. Should we have conducted other tests during our initial examination before we determined diagnosis and recommendations?

PATIENT 4: DENNIS (CONGENITAL ESOTROPIA)

The chief purpose of this report is to illustrate one approach to the clinical management of congenital esotropia as manifested in a very young child. It describes the clinical picture of a 9-month-old who has been esotropic since at least age 1 month.

☐ Visit #1 (August 1982)

SALIENT CLINICAL DATA

Age: 9 months (DOB: November 1981).

Chief concern: Parents report that child's right eye is always turned in. First noticed at age 1 month. Parents sought advice from their pediatrician at that time. He advised them to do nothing for a while; that many children grow out of such conditions. Child has not grown out of it.

Relevant history/initial impressions: Dennis appears to be a healthy, happy baby. He is alert to his surroundings and responds appropriately to social conditions. Pregnancy was full term; birthweight = 7 pounds. APGAR = 8. His development and health have been normal to date.

Unaided distance visual acuity: Unobtainable.

Unaided near visual acuity: Unobtainable, except for child's reaction to unilateral occlusion. Occlusion of the right eye generates very little reaction; occlusion of the left eye produces the opposite effect. (Preferential looking procedure was attempted; child would not attend to stimuli.)

Ocular health: No evidence of pathology or structural abnormalities, other than a very signficiant (>45 prism diopter), constant, right esotropia. Motilities: very limited abduction of right eye past the midline; left eye displays full motilities.

Refractive status: O.D., +1.25 −0.75 cx 015 (cyloplegic); O.S., +0.75 −0.25 cx 165.

Binocular status (unaided): at distance = about 45 pd constant, right esotropia; at near = about 45 pd constant, right esotropia; at near when measured through +3.00 D, O.U.: unchanged.

Developmental status: No lags in any sector of DDST.

DIAGNOSIS

Constant, congenital right esotropia; right amblyopia, probably secondary to the strabismus. Limited abduction, O.D. No evidence of an innervational dysfunction factor; i.e., angle of deviation the same at distance and near; plus lenses had no effect on the magnitude of deviation at nearpoint.

RECOMMENDATIONS

Parents advised that their youngster's visual condition is not one that typically responds to vision therapy—that, in all likelihood, surgical treatment will be necessary, not to provide normal binocular vision but, rather, to improve the child's appearance and, perhaps, to facilitate the acquisition of certain gross binocular abilities.

We do suggest, however, that a surgical consultation would be premature at this time. Certain steps should be taken first: To commence, constant unilateral occlusion, following the schedule depicted in Chapter 12; i.e., patch on "good" (O.S.) eye 2 days, then on "amblyopic" (O.D.) eye for 1 day, etc. Child to be monitored weekly. Compensatory lenses not warranted.

☐ Follow-up Data

Dennis's parents followed the patching regimen for 6 weeks; we saw the child weekly. Effects of treatment were evident in three ways: one, the child's reaction to occlusion of left eye no longer differed significantly from his reaction to occlusion of his right eye; second, his right eye demonstrated full abduction capacity; third, he began to manifest an alternating fixation pattern. Hence, by inference, we believed that his visual acuities were now approximately equal in the two eyes and that any danger of secondary contractures of the right medial rectus had been markedly reduced.

The child's refractive status remained unchanged. We continued to be unable to identify any innervational factor as contributing to the child's binocular status. Hence, our diagnosis remained as stated above.

We advised Dennis's parents that a surgical consultation was now justified and gave them the name of a pediatric ophthalmologist whose opinions and skills we respected. We also forewarned them—on the basis of previous experiences with this surgeon—that even if surgery was recommended, it was very likely that there would also be the recommendation of glasses to be worn for a few months before surgery took place. (Glasses, in this instance, would be primarily to place neutralizing prisms before the child's eyes in the hopes/anticipation of stimulating *some* fusional ability [albeit peripheral] in advance of the surgery. This approach, practiced by some, is not yet validated; those who advocate it to do so because they believe that it might enhance the child's potential for obtaining peripheral fusion; those who do not recommend it probably believe otherwise. We are inclined to side with the proponents but are not able to provide any evidence to support that inclination.)

TWO YEARS AFTER FIRST VISIT

Dennis is now almost 3 years old. His parents did follow our advice (as defined above); the surgeon did recommend surgery, to be preceded by 3 months of wearing 45 diopters of base-out prism. Surgery took place when the child was about 14 months old and was successful, in terms of cosmesis. Dennis now manifests a 12-pd, constant, right esotropia in addition to a small hyper component that varies in accord with the direction of gaze. His eye's "look straight." He is able to appreciate stereopsis with the stereofly but not with any more demanding stimulus. His refractive status remains about the same as it was at his first visit. He does not wear glasses, and his unaided visual acuity is O.D.: 15/30 +; O.S.: 20/30 +, as measured with the Allen Picture Card test.

His parents are very pleased with the outcomes of the child's treatment. Prognosis for further improvement through vision therapy is very poor; there is no reason to believe that this child has—or ever had—the neurophysiological prerequisites for binocular vision. On the plus side: He looks "normal" (even though he will probably manifest a monofixation syndrome when old enough to respond reliably to the necessary tests), and with the exception of being excluded from such vocations as commercial airline pilot, he probably will not be hampered by his visual status.

☐ General Comments

Patients with conditions like those manifested by Dennis are exceptionally common in a primary-care optometric practice. Unfortunately, they rarely, if ever, respond to any remedial treatment beyond what is described above. They display no evidence of an accommodative component being related to their binocular problem and no potential for normal binocular vision, even when their strabismus is neutralized with prisms and both fovea are stimulated simultaneously. It may be that in some cases that strabismus really does derive from an innervational dysfunction, but at this point such comments are more "wishful thinking" than scientific fact. For the present, therefore, the most effective treatment for such children is one that focuses on cosmesis rather than binocular function. Hence, a surgical consultation when the child is about 18 months old is usually appropriate. Surgery, if successful, will not provide the child with normal binocular vision, but it will provide him with a more normal appearance—and that is no small consideration in our culture.

☐ Questions Worth Discussing

1. Are there other tests we should have administered at that first visit? If so what, and why?

2. Would you have made the same recommendations as we did at that first visit? If not, what would you have recommended, and why? (i.e., would you have recommended glasses? bifocals?)

3. Do you think Dennis's visual status would be different today had we put off referral for a surgical consultation and, instead, had prescribed as much plus lens power as possible and used unilateral occlusion to prevent maladaptation?

4. Do you think that the use of neutralizing prisms in advance of surgery is beneficial? Why?

5. Do you think that Dennis would have developed amblyopia in one eye if we had not prescribed unilateral occlusion during his first year of life? Do you think he would have remained a unilateral strabismic, or would the alternating fixation pattern have developed on its own?

6. What reasons are there to recommend surgery by age 18 months? What are the possible consequences if surgery is delayed until later—until the patient is 8 years old, say?

■
_____

PATIENT 5: SAM
(CONGENITAL ESOTROPIA)

The chief purpose of this report is to illustrate one approach to the clinical management of congenital constant esotropia when the patient is of school age. It describes the clinical picture of a 6-year-old who first manifested strabismus at the age of 4 months.

□ Visit #1 (April 1985)

SALIENT CLINICAL DATA

Age: 6 years, 4 months (DOB: December 1978)

Chief concern: One of the child's eyes is "always turned in. Sometimes it is the right eye, sometimes the left."

Relevant history/initial impressions: Eye turn was first noticed at about age 4 months. The parents were advised by their pediatrician at that time to obtain ophthalmological consultation, but they decided to wait; the eye turn was not all that noticeable to them, and they had heard of children who grew out of such conditions. They did obtain a consult when Sam was about age 3, but the doctor who saw him at that time did not impress them as sufficiently knowledgeable. They therefore decided to put off any decisions "for a while." They are now concerned; the condition persists and the youngster is about to enter first grade. Sam is and has been a healthy, happy youngster. Pregnancy was full term; birth-weight = 8 pounds, 2 ounces. APGAR = 8, 9. He accomplished all of the developmental milestones "on schedule." He seems to communicate effectively.

Unaided distance visual acuity: OD, 20/20− (Snellen letters); OS, 20/20−.

Ocular health: No evidence of pathology or structural abnormalities, other than a constant, alternating, comitant esotropia. Motilities are full in all directions of gaze, both eyes.

Refractive status: O.D., +1.00 −0.50 cx 090 20/20; O.S., +0.75 −0.25 cx 090 20/20 (cycloplegic).

Binocular status (both aided and unaided): Cover test: at distance = 25 pd constant, comitant alternating esotropia; at near = 22 pd constant, comitant alternating esotropia. When measured through +3.00 D, O.U.: unchanged.

Stereopsis (measured through 25 pd base-out): at distance = none (fails A.O. vectographic test); at near = none (fails Titmus stereo fly). Worth Dot test (measured through 25-pd base-out): at distance = alternating supression; no evidence of second-degree fusion; at near = alternating supression; no evidence of second-degree fusion.

Developmental status: TVAS = 8 (pass; acceptable for child about to enter grade 1). TAAS = 3 (pass).

DIAGNOSIS

Constant, comitant, congenital alternating esotropia. No evidence of an innervational dysfunction factor; i.e., angle of deviation the same at distance and near; plus lenses had no effect on the magnitude of deviation at nearpoint. Compensatory prisms had no effect on the patient's ability to perceive second- or third-degree fusion.

RECOMMENDATIONS

Parents advised that their youngster's visual condition is not amenable to treatment with eye glasses or vision therapy—"exercises." We therefore suggest that they obtain surgical consultation, but stress that such treatment would not "cure" the condition. If successful, the child's eyes would simply "look better," not "work together better."

□ Follow-up Data

Sam's parents accepted our recommendation and obtained a surgical consultation. Surgery was recommended for cosmesis. Parents accepted the recommendation.

ONE YEAR AFTER FIRST VISIT

Surgery was reasonably successful, in terms of cosmesis. Sam now manifests a 10-pd, constant, alternating esotropia. His refractive status remains about the same as it was at his first visit. He does not wear glasses, but neither does he experience any ocular discomfort. His unaided visual acuity is 20/20, each eye. His eyes "look straight"; his parents are pleased.

□ General Comments

The prevalence of congenital strabismus in the United States is approximately 1.5 percent. There is some debate about whether a distinction should be made between children who manifest the strabismus at birth (congenital) versus those who are not identified until later on in their first year of life (infantile); but for our purposes, there is no need to belabor the point. In both instances, the accepted view today is that the condition does not emerge from a functional disorder (abnormal accommodation-convergence linkup), nor from a neuromotor impairment. Rather, it seems to be related to some deficit in the CNS and, as such, does not respond to lens or prism therapy; only surgery will bring about improvement, and even then, if the surgery is successful, the improvement will be purely cosmetic. In effect, such children simply do not develop sufficient binocular cells in visual cortex; hence they are deprived of any potential for developing normal binocular vision.

A different argument could be made. There is some evidence that a number of so-called congenital esotropias are really undetected accommodative esotropias. Rethy and Gal, for example (see reference 10, Chapter 11), reported remarkable success in treating over 1000 strabismic patients with lenses and occlusion only; but they stress the fact that they sometimes did not achieve success for many years—often not until the patient was 8, 9, or 10 years of age. Their observations, in addition to the commonly observed phenomenon of accommodative esotropia occurring in postoperative strabismics, may very well indicate that surgery is performed more often and too early than it should be. However, all of this is speculation. The optometrist is compelled to offer an opinion and advice when such patients present. Society does not admire esotropia. Parents are unhappy when it occurs in their children. Surgical treatment in this country is well accepted, not only by ophthalmologists, but by pediatricians and other health-care professionals. The optometrist who takes a strong position against surgical intervention for congenital strabismus will probably find himself swimming upstream, and without much company.

□ Questions Worth Discussing

1. Would Sam have had a better opportunity for binocular function if treatment had been initiated earlier? If so, at what age? What treatment?

2. Should we have administered any other tests at that first visit in order to make a more valid diagnosis?

3. Why did we not test for anomalous retinal correspondence?

4. Why did we not test for eccentric fixation?

5. Should we have tried vision therapy? If so, where should we have started; i.e., with what basic goals in mind?

6. Should we recommend postoperative vision therapy? If so, where should we start—with what basic goals in mind?

7. What is your opinion of the Rethy and Gal paper? Would you be willing to follow their recommendations if a child in your immediate family manifested what appeared to be congenital esotropia?

■
_____

PATIENT 6: MICHAEL (INTERMITTENT ESOTROPIA: CONVERGENCE EXCESS)

The chief purpose of this report is to illustrate one approach to the clinical management of convergence excess (intermittent esotropia manifesting only upon nearpoint fixation) in a preschool-aged child. It describes the clinical picture at first visit, when the child was 3 year old, and the changes that occurred in the condition and its treatment over the following 5 years.

☐ Visit #1 (August 1981)

SALIENT CLINICAL DATA

Age: 3 years, 7 months (DOB: January 1978).

Chief concern: Parents report that the child's right eye turns "in" at times, most often when he is looking at something close to his face.

Relevant history/initial impressions: Eye turn first noticed when child was about 18 months old. Parents mentioned it to their pediatrician at that time, but he was not able to elicit it and decided that they were probably being a bit overanxious about their only child. Michael is and has been a healthy, happy youngster. Pregnancy was full-term; birthweight = 6 pounds, 10 ounces. APGAR = 9, 10. He accomplished all of the major developmental milestones "on schedule." He seems to communicate effectively.

Unaided distance visual acuity: O.D., 20/30; O.S., 20/30 (Allen cards).

Ocular health: No evidence of pathology or structural abnormalities. Motilities unhindered in all directions of gaze, both eyes.

Refractive status: O.D., +2.00 20/30; O.S., +2.00 20/30 (cyloplegic).

Binocular status (unaided): Cover test: At distance = orthophoria; at near = 6 pd esophoria; when measured through +3.00 D; O.U. at near: unchanged. Near point convergence: 30 cm. When target is held closer than 30 cm and patient fixates on a target that stimulates accommodation, right esotropia (50 pd) is elicited. When retested through +3.00 D spheres, O.U., squint does not manifest. Stereopsis: At distance = inconclusive (child confused by test); At near = 100 seconds arc (Titmus animals).

Developmental status: No delays displayed on DDST; passed all items intersected by age line.

DIAGNOSIS

Intermittent right esotropia, elicited only when high levels of fixation and accommodation are required.

RECOMMENDATIONS

Parents advised that their youngster's visual condition appears to be functional in origin; that is, it is not due to a disease or a muscle weakness but, rather, to an inappropriate link-up between the eye's "pointing" and "focusing" muscles when the child looks at something held very close to his eyes (see p. 354). In our opinion, vision therapy is not the treatment of choice at this time. Michael is much too young to profit from such a sophisticated educational approach. Rather, we suggest bifocal lenses, to be worn full time. We caution them that the glasses will not "cure" the condition, but will prevent maladaptations—the acquisition of "bad visual habits." We also assure them that the condition is not progressive, that Michael's eye will not cross permanently, and that in time, therapy in conjunction with lenses should alleviate the condition. They accept the recommendation.

□ Follow-up Data

SIX MONTHS AFTER VISIT #1

Michael obtained his glasses (O.U.: +2.00/+2.50 add) and wore them without complaint. Condition unchanged.

THREE YEARS AFTER VISIT #1

Michael is now in first grade and is doing well. We have examined him every 6 months since his initial visit. The only change in his binocular status observed during those 3 years is that it is now more difficult to evoke the strabismus with nearpoint fixation. Everything else is as it was, except that his perceptual skills development has progressed at an expected rate.

FIVE YEARS AFTER VISIT #1

Michael is in third grade. He does very well in school. Examination reveals some reduction in hyperopia (Rx: O.U.: +1.25 D spheres). With these lenses in place, we are not able to evoke the strabismus, regardless of fixation target and distance. Without glasses, the child does display some binocular instability when fixating at an object closer than about 25 cm. His (unaided) nearpoint phoria is 8 pd esophoria; when remeasured through +3.00 D spheres, it reduces to orthophoria. On the strength of this, we advise his parents that treatment should remain the same, that we believe Michael will give up lenses in time, but that for the present, they are desirable, not because of the strabismus but because of the esophoria and the discomfort it might provoke if ignored. We have not altogether rejected the possibility of vision therapy; we may very well institute a program someday, but we fail to see any advantage for it at the present.

□ General Comments

This case illustrates clearly the importance of assessing binocular alignment not only at standard farpoint and nearpoint distances, but also at other distances and directions of gaze. This case also provides an example of the importance of taking parents' observations seriously, even when the condition does not manifest during a single office visit. Our method of managing the case was hardly innovative. We simply took advantage of the link-up between accommodation and convergence, and the availability of the optical device know as the bifocal. With this device, we were able to eliminate virtually all episodes of esotropia. Thus, we were able to allay parental anxiety as well as avoid any maladaptions that Michael might have developed from the strabismus itself. We did not institute vision therapy for two reasons: (1) the binocular condition was well controlled by lenses; (2) because the child was significantly hyperopic, he would need to wear lenses even if vision therapy were successful. As such, we saw no real advantage to vision therapy at this time. Perhaps, as he matures, we will recommend it—particularly if he continues the trend of reduced hyperopia. On the other hand, as is often the case, the convergence excess may completely disappear as he matures.

□ Questions Worth Discussing

1. How can we explain the fact that, at Michael's first visit, +3.00 D spheres did not change his nearpoint phoria yet did eliminate his esotropia when fixating at an object closer than 30 cm?

2. What rationale do you think we employed in deciding to prescribe Michael's nearpoint add? Would you have prescribed a different lens power? If so, what? For that matter, would you have prescribed a bifocal?

3. Should we have instituted vision therapy before this? Why? What detrimental effects have we risked?

4. What other tests should we have done at that first visit?

5. What clinical evidence made it possible to be reasonably certain that Michael's strabismus was intermittent?

PATIENT 7: SCOTT (SIGNIFICANT HYPEROPIA AND ACCOMMODATIVE ESOTROPIA)

The chief purpose of this report is to illustrate one approach to the clinical management of high hyperopia and accommodative esotropia as manifested in a preschool-aged child. It describes the clinical picture of a 3-year-old who began to manifest intermittent esotropia at about age two. (For a report of a similar condition occurring in a 7-year-old, see report regarding Patient 8: Ann.)

□ Visit #1 (March 1986)

SALIENT CLINICAL DATA

Age: 3 years, 1 month (DOB: February 1983).

Chief concern: Child's left eye tends to "cross;" i.e., turn inward. Condition first noticed about 1 year ago. The eye doctor he was taken to at that time recommended surgery. Parents were apprehensive about treatment and sought a second opinion. Second opinion contradicted the first; recommended against surgery and advised the parents to do nothing for a while, explaining that child might very well "grow out of" the problem. Parents much more accepting of the second opinion but are now once again becoming anxious because, rather than disappearing, the problem (esotropia) appears be getting worse—occurring more often than before.

Relevant history: Scott's prenatal, perinatal, and postnatal histories are free of unusual circumstances. His development has been normal. He has always seemed to see clearly—his parents have always been sensitive to the child's eyes because his mother is somewhat myopic (O.U.: −1.75 −0.75 cx 180) and his father has significant hyperopia (O.U.: +6.50). In fact, his father thinks he had a crossed eye when he was younger, but is not certain. His eyes now appear to be aligned.

Unaided distance visual acuity: O.D., 10/30; O.S., 10/20 (Lighthouse cards).

Ocular health: No evidence of pathology or structural abnormalities; motilities unrestricted.

Refractive status: O.D., +3.00 D sphere 10/20; O.S., +2.50 D sphere 10/15 (cycloplegic).

Binocular status: Cover test, unaided: at distance = 10 esophoria; at near = 30 esophoria (which quickly decompensates to an esotropia). Aided: at distance = 2 esophoria, at near = 18 esophoria. Stereoacuity (aided) at distance = 3 minutes arc (A.O.); at near = 100 seconds arc (Randot).

Developmental status: No delays in any sector, but some hint of a lag in the Fine motor-Adaptive sector.

DIAGNOSIS

Significant hyperopia in combination with a higher than normal AC/A ratio. Moderate amblyopia, O.D., secondary to accommodative esotropia.

RECOMMENDATIONS

Glasses, to be worn full time (Rx O.D., +3.00 D sphere; O.S., +2.50 D sphere; add O.U., +3.00 D). The need for bifocal lenses was explained to Scott's parents following the terminology used in Chapter 9; see p. 354. We also explain that Scott might continue to manifest some moderate amblyopia in his right eye and that we might prescribe vision therapy, but that for at least these first few months that would not be necessary. In addition, we express some mild concern over the child's visual perceptual skills development, based upon what has recently been reported about the connection between hyperopia and visual perceptual skills, and the fact that Scott was lagging just a bit in the Fine-motor Adaptive Sector of the DDST, the sector that addresses early levels of visual analysis skills development. We schedule a follow-up visit in 3 months.

□ Follow-up Data

Scott returned on schedule. He has been wearing his glasses without complaint. His parents are not exceptionally pleased about his need for glasses but are happy about the fact that his eyes do not cross as long as he wears his glasses. They did note that his eyes continue to cross when he is without his glasses. (They had expected the glasses to be a cure, obviously a flaw in our explanation.)

Our assessment indicates that the visual acuity of Scott's left eye is 20/20 (aided), and his right eye just a trifle less (20/25). Cover test reveals othophoria at distance (when he uses the upper portion of his lenses), and just about the same at near (when he uses the segs). His stereoacuity has also improved. At distance it is (aided) 2 minutes arc; at near (through seg), 50 seconds arc.

We reassure Scott's parents, and urge them to accept the fact that he, like his father, is farsighted and will probably need to wear glasses (or contact lenses) all his life. (We also reminded them that there are worse fates.) We encourage them to expose the child to various activities that will foster the development of spatial analysis skills; e.g., construction toys, sorting, matching, classification tasks, workbooks of various sorts. They are scheduled to return in about 6 months. If, at that time, Scott's visual analysis skills continue to lag, we will recommend a more structured approach to eliminating the problem.

□ General Comments

This type of case is not uncommon in a primary-care optometrist practice, and it is one that the primary-care optometrist is well prepared to manage effectively. The key ingredients are high hyperopia accompanied by esotropia that begins to manifest at about age 2 years, when the child is introduced to more nearpoint activities than ever before. An accurate, cycloplegic refraction, and a careful, clear explanation of the condition and the role that lenses play: bifocals, perhaps; perhaps not; depending upon the child's binocular status at near, measured through his distance lens Rx.

□ Questions Worth Discussing

1. Are there other tests we should have administered at Scott's first visit? If so what, and why?

2. Would you have recommended bifocal lenses? Why? If not, what would you have recommended, and why?

3. Why, in your opinion, did we prescribe a +3.00D add? How do you make such a determination?

4. Scott's parents are very likely to ask: "Will he always have to wear glasses; will the vision therapy eliminate or, at least, reduce his need for lenses?" What would you reply?

5. Do our findings (at the follow-up visit) indicate that Scott may have a small-angle strabismus? Why?

6. What do you think would have happened in this case if Scott's parents had delayed seeking professional help until after he entered first grade?

■

PATIENT 8: ANN (SIGNIFICANT HYPEROPIA, CONSTANT ESOTROPIA, AND VISUAL PERCEPTUAL SKILLS DYSFUNCTION)

The chief purpose of this report is to illustrate one approach to the clinical management of high hyperopia that is related to esotropia and to visual perceptual skills dysfunction. It describes the clinical picture of a 7-year-old who began to manifest intermittent esotropia at about age two, constant esotropia about six months later, never wore glasses, and is now in first grade and experiencing significant learning difficulties.

□ Visit #1 (February 1986)

SALIENT CLINICAL DATA

Age: 7 years, 1 months (DOB: January 1979).

Chief concern: Child failed her school vision screening tests. In addition, she is not performing well in her classroom work. She is midway through the first grade and has been described by her teachers as being distractible and inattentive. In addition, her paper work (printing/coloring) is very sloppy.

Relevant history/general impressions: This is Ann's first eye examination, even though her mother reported that "Ann's one eye (the left) seems to cross once in a while" and has since she was about 2 years old. The eye turn did not manifest very often at first, but became constant after about 6 months. Oddly, the parents still do not view the esotropia as something serious. They are more concerned about her learning problems. Ann is now midway through the first grade and has fallen well behind her classmates. Her school difficulties began early—immediately after she started kindergarten. (She had not attended any preschool.) Ann's prenatal, perinatal, and postnatal histories are free of unusual circumstances and events. Her development has been normal, although she has "always seemed to do better at talking than in fine motor coordination activities. She has never been interested in sitting quietly with a book or a puzzle. She much prefers playing outdoors."

Unaided distance visual acuity: O.D., 20/80; O.S., 20/30 (Snellen letters).

Ocular health: No evidence of pathology or structural abnormalities. Unrestricted motilities.

Refractive status: Without cycloplegic: O.D., +4.00 D sphere 20/50+; O.S., +3.25 D sphere 20/25. With cycloplegic: O.D., +6.00 D sphere 20/80; O.S., +5.00 D sphere 20/50.

Binocular status: Cover test (unaided): at distance = 19 esotropia, O.D.; at near = 28 esotropia, O.D. Cover test (aided): at distance = 4 esophoria; at near = 10 esophoria. Stereoacuity (aided) at distance = 4 minutes arc (A.O.); at near = 200 seconds arc (Randot).

Developmental status: TVAS = 6 (unsatisfactory); TAAS = 9 (satisfactory).

DIAGNOSIS

Significant hyperopia, constant right esotropia related to a higher than normal AC/A ratio, moderate amblyopia (O.D.), and substandard visual perceptual skills.

RECOMMENDATIONS

Glasses, to be worn full time (Rx O.D. +4.00D sphere; O.S.: +3.25 D sphere; add: +2.00 D, O.U.). The need for bifocals was explained to Ann's parents following the terminology used in Chapter 9; see p. 354. We also advised them that Ann would continue to manifest moderate amblyopia in her right eye unless vision therapy was successfully implemented. We set aside discussion of the child's visual perceptual skills deficits until her next visit, which we scheduled 1 month hence. (Note: We considered prescribing the lens powers determined by the cycloplegic refraction [single vision], but opted instead for the bifocals because Ann's parents did not strike us as being able to deal with what would be needed as a follow-up: [a] administering a cycloplegic agent on a daily basis until the child's acuity [with lenses] achieved an asymptotic level and/or [b] insisting that the child wear her new glasses despite their initial blurring effect.)

☐ Follow-up Data

The parents' report at first follow-up visit was favorable. They stated that Ann did not resist wearing her glasses, although neither did she seem to be uncomfortable when not wearing them. They also reported that there seemed to be an increase in the incidence of her esotropia "when she takes her glasses off."

Ann's corrected visual acuity at that first follow-up visit was unchanged from what was recorded during the initial examination. We also confirmed our earlier observation of the effect of the lenses on her strabismus. With her lenses in place, she was more often an esophore than an esotrope. In other words, her binocular status appeared to have changed from constant to intermittent strabismus. We hesitated, at first, to call it that (rather than small-angle strabismus) because of the reduced stereoacuity, but we ultimately reasoned that this (the reduced stereoacuity) was more likely to be attributable to refractive amblyopia than to bifoveal misalignment. In order to treat the amblyopia and the child's visual perceptual skills problem simultaneously, we prescribed a variety of therapy activities that involved red/green filter lenses and a red crayon. Of particular value were various geoboard (pattern copying) activities.

Ann's parents were surprisingly diligent in supervising her vision therapy program, and the outcomes were very satisfying. During the course of the year following her first visit, she was able to adapt to a full single vision prescription and demonstrate good visual acuity (O.D. = 20/30; O.S. = 20/20). In addition, her visual perceptual skills improved significantly, as did her school work, although not enough to enable her to move on to second grade. She is repeating first grade and is doing very well. Her teacher believes that she will have no further school difficulties.

☐ General Comments

Ann responded exceptionally well to the treatment. Why? Because apparently she was binocular long enough (during her first 2 years of life) to develop the neurophysiological capacity for binocular vision. This, once developed, does not irreversibly erode. As a result, her visual acuity and her binocular status improved, even though lenses were not applied until 5 years later. Ann also acquired more competent visual analysis skills. This does not always happen when lens application has been delayed as long as it was in this case. Why it happened in this case and not in others is inexplicable as of now.

☐ Questions Worth Discussing

1. Are there other tests we should have administered at that first visit? If so what, and why?

2. Would you have made the same recommendations as we did at that first visit (i.e., bifocal lenses)? If not, what would you have recommended, and why?

3. How do you interpret her parent's remarks (in the Follow-up section) about the increase in esotropia "especially when she takes her glasses off?" Do you think their observation was correct? And, if so, how do you explain this increase in frequency?

4. Do you think we should attempt to improve further the acuity of Ann's right eye? If so, describe the vision therapy regimen you would recommend.

5. Do you think the visual acuity will improve beyond its present level (20/30+) if we do not prescribe a program of remediation?

6. Is it possible that Ann manifests a small-angle strabismus? What information do you need to answer this question?

7. Do you think Ann's visual status would be different today had she obtained her first glasses when the strabismus was first observed? If so, speculate as to what the lens prescription would have been at that earlier date? The same as what we measured? Stronger? Less strong?

■
_____

PATIENT 9: ROBERT (SIGNIFICANT HYPEROPIA, VISUAL ANALYSIS SKILLS DYSFUNCTION, LEARNING DISABILITY, AND SCHOOL-BASED REMEDIATION)

The chief purpose of this report is to illustrate one approach to the clinical management of visual perceptual skills dysfunction that appears to be related to hyperopia. It describes the clinical picture of a hyperopic, 7-year-old, second-grade boy who obtained his first glasses about a year ago, and who displayed a significant lag in the development of visual perceptual skills. (For a description of a similar situation occurring in a child who also manifested esotropia, see report of Patient Ann.)

□ Visit #1 (October 1981)

SALIENT CLINICAL DATA

Age: 7 years, 3 months (DOB: July 1974).

School: Neighborhood elementary; grade 2.

Chief concern: Child displays a tendency to print certain letters backward (e.g., b/d). He is making satisfactory progress in reading, but not in arithmetic. His paper work is not appropriate for a second-grader. This same problem existed in first grade but was attributed then to "immaturity" and a need for glasses.

Relevant history/initial impressions: Robert's health is and has been good; his developmental history, uneventful. He has worn his glasses constantly and without complaint since they were prescribed (by another optometrist) about a year ago. He appears to be a pleasant, inquisitive, talkative child.

Unaided distance visual acuity: O.D., 20/50; O.S., 20/50 (Snellen letters).

Present lens Rx: O.D., +4.25 D sphere 20/20−; O.S. +4.25 D sphere 20/20−.

Ocular health: No evidence of pathology or structural abnormalities.

Refractive status: O.U., +4.50 D sphere 20/20−.

Binocular status: Cover test (unaided): at distance = 5 esophoria; at near = 11 esophoria. Cover test (aided): at distance = orthophoria; at near = 2 exophoria. Stereoacuity (aided): at distance = 1 minute arc (A.O.); at near = 30 seconds arc (Randot). Vergence facility at distance and near: satisfactory. Accommodation facility at distance and near: satisfactory.

Developmental status: TVAS score = 7 (unsatisfactory). TAAS score = 11 (satisfactory).

DIAGNOSIS

A significant lag in visual perceptual skills development accompanied by (and probably related to) hyperopia. Very moderate bilateral amblyopia, probably due to late acquisition of compensatory lenses.

RECOMMENDATIONS

Visual perceptual skills remedial therapy in conjunction with appropriate compensatory instructional conditions in his classroom. Continued use of present lenses; no need for a change at this time. Send reports to his pediatrician and his school (see Figure 16.2 for a copy of this report).

Report re: Robert Jones
Age: 7 years, 3 months
School: Neighborhood Elementary School; Grade 2
Date of visit: October 10, 19..

Bob was referred to this office because of his tendency to print certain letters backward (e.g., b/d). He is reported to be making satisfactory progress in reading, but not in arithmetic. In addition, his paper work is not appropriate for a second-grader. Bob's mother stated that these same difficulties existed in first grade but, at that time, were attributed to "immaturity" and an (unsuspected, until then) need for glasses. These were obtained. Bob wears them without complaint. His general health is and always has been good, his developmental history is free of unusual circumstances. Bob appears to be a very pleasant child; he participated in the evaluation in a cooperative manner.

As noted above, Bob has worn glasses for about one year; he is significantly farsighted. My examination corroborated this. I observed no evidence of disease or structural abnormality. His present lenses are correct; there is no need for a change in prescription at this time; he should wear them full-time. With his glasses on, Bob sees clearly (about 20/20, each eye) and his eyes function efficiently; that is, they coordinate without undue effort. That is not the case when he is not

Figure 16.2 Report regarding Robert Jones. (Continues on next page)

wearing his glasses; then his two eye coordination is far below the satisfactory level.

I also evaluated the boy's perceptual skills. His auditory analysis skills—that is, his ability to detect the separate sounds in spoken speech—is well within normal limits for his age. The same is not true about his visual analysis skills—his ability to detect the separate components and relationships of a spatially organized pattern. His responses to the TVAS (a standardized copying test) were far below what is expected from a second grade child.

In consideration of the above, the following was recommended: As noted, Bob should continue to wear his present glasses. Bob's visual analysis skills deficit requires attention; he should engage in an organized program of remediation that is designed to teach him the basic skills he presently lacks. Such a program usually requires daily (5 days/week) activity under the supervision of an adult—parent or teacher. A proper program, effectively administered, should help him overcome his present deficit in about four months. As improvement is made, it should also be apparent in the quality of his paper work and his ability to retain number facts. In addition, as Bob is doing this, his classroom activities should be structured somewhat more than is common in second grade. That is, he should be told explicitly what aspects of a lesson to pay attention to, how to organize his paper work, and so on, rather than be expected to induce such information on the basis of less than complete directions. He will not require this type of aid for very long, but it will be very useful in the short term.

Ideally, the perceptual skills remediation program should be administered in school. As this is going on, I will arrange to see Bob monthly in this office in order to monitor his progress and make updated reports.

Should suggestions about the skills training program—or any other information—be desired, please do not hesitate to contact me.

Jerome Rosner, O.D.

Figure 16.2   (Continued)

□ Follow-up Data

Our recommendations were accepted. Bob participated daily (for 20 to 30 minutes) in a visual perceptual skills remedial training program in school, under the supervision of a classroom aide. (The school had requested some guidance in this endeavor. We assisted them in selecting an appropriate program and provided some consultation services to the classroom aide as she initiated the treatment. See Chapter 15.) Bob returned to our office once each month; he demonstrated improvement each time. Skills training was halted in April, at which time his TVAS score was 15. His teacher reported remarkable changes in his classroom performance. Bob's paper work had become significantly neater, his capacity to grasp mathematical concepts had improved nicely, and he was, in general, "better organized." She continued to provide the boy with some extra classroom structure (until the end of that school year), more because she did not want him to regress than because he seemed to need it.

Robert is now in the fourth grade. His visual/ocular status remains unchanged; he continues to wear his glasses constantly. His school performance is satisfactory in all subject areas, but his teachers and parents all agree that his "talents" lie in the language arts areas: he would rather talk than do.

□ General Comments

Robert's case is very common, although not all are as hyperopic as he; in fact, a good number are emmetropic. Many children enter first grade with what appears to be adequate cognitive development but substandard visual analysis skills. Such children are often quite articulate—their ability to express themselves in spoken form is well within normal expectations. Their problem is revealed only when they are required to demonstrate spatial (visual) analysis skills—the capacity to analyze spatially organized patterns in terms of such attributes as quantity, magnitude, and interrelationships of the pattern's structural components. In other words, they do not lack "potential"; What they lack is the capacity to address sequentially organized tasks in a way that enables them to work through the tasks successfully, step by step. Do such cases fall within the scope of optometry? Perhaps; perhaps not; it depends upon who defines the scope. Do such cases present with great regularity in an optometric practice? You bet! Almost all of these children have, at one time or another, printed or read a letter or numeral backward. This, in itself, is usually sufficient reason to motivate a school person to refer the patient to an optometrist—and it is probably sufficient reason for the optometrist to be willing to include within her assessment a screening test for visual perceptual skills.

□ Questions Worth Discussing

1. Are there other tests we should have administered at the first visit? If so what, and why?

2. Would you have made the same recommendations as we did at that first visit? If not, what would you have recommended, and why?

3. Do you think Robert's binocular status was correctly defined; i.e., do you think he had normal binocularity? If so, or if not, why?

4. Do cases such as this one fall within the scope of an optometrist? In other words, should optometrists conduct screening tests for visual and auditory analysis skills development? Should optometrists treat cases of perceptual skills dysfunction?

5. Nothing was mentioned in this report about Robert's capacity to discriminate figure from ground, or his visual memory, etc. Are these important oversights? Would the availability of such information have altered your diagnosis and/or treatment? Why? And why do you think we chose to ignore them?

■

PATIENT 10: ARTHUR (INTERMITTENT EXOTROPIA AT DISTANCE FIXATION— DIVERGENCE EXCESS)

The chief purpose of this report is to illustrate one approach to the management of intermittent exotropia when the patient is too young for effective vision therapy. It describes an emmetropic, 3-year-old boy who manifests normal binocular alignment at nearpoint and intermittent exotropia at distance, most often noticed when he is tired or "daydreaming"; e.g., staring out the kitchen window during a lull in the evening meal, gazing at the TV set, etc. (For a report of a similar condition occurring in an 8-year-old, see report regarding Patient 11: Richard.)

☐ Visit #1 (January 1981)

SALIENT CLINICAL DATA

Age: 3 years, 1 month (DOB: December 1977).

Chief concern: Child periodically manifests right exotropia; noticed at least a few times each day, more often when he is tired, or simply staring out the window or at the TV set.

Relevant history/initial impressions: Arthur's parents report first noticing the intermittent strabismus about a year ago, although they admit that it might have been present before then. (He is the fourth in a family of five children; hence, he does not receive a lot of individual attention.) Their pediatrician corroborated their observation and made this referral. In examining some photographs of the child taken when he was younger (these were brought along at our request), we could not detect strabismus; although some of them—those taken in bright sunshine—show him in a very characteristic pose: one eye open; the other shut. Arthur's health and developmental histories are uneventful. He appears to be a pleasant, inquisitive, talkative youngster.

Unaided distance visual acuity: O.D., 20/30; O.S., 20/30 (Allen Picture cards).

Ocular health: No evidence of any pathology or structural abnormalities.

Refractive status (static retinoscopy): O.U., $+0.50 -0.50$ cx 180.

Binocular status (unaided): Cover test at distance = 22 pd intermittent exotropia; at near = orthophoria. Stereoacuity at distance = inconclusive; child's responses were unreliable; at near = passed RDE at 1.5 meters. Cover test at distance through − 3.00 D, O.U. = 2 pd exophoria. Vergence facility, at distance: unable to test; child not compliant. At near: again, child not compliant. Accommodation facility at distance: unable to test; at near: unable to test.

Developmental status: No delays on the DDST; passed all items intersected by the age line.

DIAGNOSIS

Intermittent exotropia at distance fixation only; orthophoria at near fixation (i.e., divergence excess). Very moderate hyperopic astigmatism.

RECOMMENDATIONS

Reassurance. Parents advised that their youngster sees clearly and that he does not need glasses. We also inform them of the child's binocular status (divergence excess) and assure them that his eye muscles are "strong enough," that his problem stems from a lack of coordination between the two eyes. We also tell them that the condition is very amenable to treatment, but that the treatment involves *instruction and learning* rather than a medical/surgical intervention. As such, the treatment is well beyond their youngter's present level of cognitive development. The best course of treatment at this time is to do nothing, to delay vision therapy until he is about 6 or 7 years old. There is no reason to believe that his condition will worsen during this period, but as a safeguard against that, we suggest that he be seen for routine evaluation every 6 months or so. Parents accept our recommendation and arrange for their next office visit, 6 months hence.

□ Follow-up

Arthur was seen twice a year until he was about 7 years old. His basic condition did not change. Neither did our recommendations. Finally, at age seven, vision therapy was instituted and successfully carried out. (For a general idea of that treatment, see the report of Patient 11: Richard. Arthur's regimen was very much like Richard's, give or take a few minor variations.)

□ General Comments

The key point in this case report is the advisability of delaying vision therapy for divergence excess (and other conditions that do not become progressively worse through neglect) until the patient is mature enough to profit from the treatment in a reasonable length of time. True, we could have conjured up a few useful activities that he might have engaged in at age three, but they would not have been effective in eliminating his binocular problem. As such, we would have risked sponsoring two undesirable situations: one, disappointing his parents who, despite our caveats, would have expected to see "some benefit" from the therapy; two, generating "burn-out" in the child (and his parents) who, having engaged in whatever activities we had prescribed for him at age three, would begin to rebel long before he reached the age where the vision therapy could have been optimally effective. (It is somewhat like trying to teach a prekindergarten child to read. Some few, of course, do learn—to some extent. Some others learn a little, but hardly enough to make it worth the effort, compared with how much more effective these same lessons would have been if they had been delayed until the child was a bit more mature. The rest do not learn anything; they acquire the experience of failure and all that accompanies it.)

☐ Questions Worth Discussing

1. Do you agree that Arthur was too young for vision therapy when he first presented? If not, how would you have managed the therapy, keeping in mind the typical behavioral and cognitive capacities of a 3-year-old?

2. Do you agree that Arthur's condition (at his first visit) was not apt to deteriorate if left untreated (i.e., increase in magnitude or frequency)?

3. Would you have prescribed minus lenses at the first (or a subsequent) visit as a means of reducing the frequency of the child's exotropia? (Note the effect of −3.00 D spheres, O.U., upon his phoria at distance.) What benefits would these lenses have provided? What are the possible drawbacks?

4. If you had prescribed minus lenses at that first visit, what lens power would you have designated? What effects would you have expected? Would the lenses have elimated the intermittent exotropia? Would the lenses have stimulated the development of myopia? How and when would you have eliminated them (i.e., in small or large increments; by a certain age, etc.)?

5. Why do children with this type of condition characteristically close one eye in bright sunshine? Speculate freely.

6. Should compensatory lenses (O.U.: +0.50 −0.50 cx 180) have been prescribed at his first visit? What effect would they have had on Arthur's condition?

7. What were the risks involved in delaying vision therapy until the child achieved a more mature state? Could he have developed constant exotropia, amblyopia, etc.?

8. This report fails to state whether Arthur manifested right, left, or alternating intermittent strabismus. Does that affect your capacity to make treatment decisions about this case?

■
_____

PATIENT 11: RICHARD
(INTERMITTENT EXOTROPIA
AT DISTANCE FIXATION—
DIVERGENCE EXCESS)

The chief purpose of this report is to illustrate one approach to the clinical management of intermittent exotropia when it manifests in an emmetropic patient who is old enough to participate effectively in vision therapy. The report describes the clinical picture of an emmetropic 7-year-old who began to manifest intermittent exotropia at about age two, never wore glasses, and is now in first grade. (For a report of a similar condition occurring in a 3-year-old, see report concerning Patient 10: Arthur.)

□ Visit #1 (June 1978)

SALIENT CLINICAL DATA

Age: 8 years, 3 months (DOB: March 1970).

Chief concern: Child periodically manifests right exotropia; noticed two or three times a day, most often when he is seated before the TV but not paying close attention to what is taking place on the screen—in his parent's words, "when he is daydreaming."

Relevant history/initial impressions: Richard appears to be a pleasant, bright youngster. His parents have noted the intermittent strabismus for some time; they believe they first observed it when he was about 3 years old. Their pediatrician reassured them at that time, and because of this and the fact that Richard is always able to straighten his eye once he has been asked to do so, they have not sought further opinion. In examining some photographs of the child (which were brought along at our request), no evidence of overt strabismus was noted, but the child did display the often-seen behavior of shutting one eye in bright sunshine. Every photo taken under those conditions shows him doing that.

Richard's health and developmental histories are uneventful. He is doing well in school, although he has recently begun to be a bit embarrassed about the reaction his eye—when turned—elicits from some of his classmates.

Unaided distance visual acuity: O.D., 20/20; O.S., 20/20 (Snellen letters).

Ocular health: No evidence of pathology or structural abnormalities.

Refractive status: O.U.: Plano.

Binocular status: Cover test at distance = 16 exotropia (intermittent); at near = orthophoria. Stereoacuity at distance = 1 minute arc (A.O.) when eyes are aligned; at near = 20 seconds arc (Randot). Passed RDE at 1.5 meters. Vergence facility at distance: fails screening test; at near: passes base out; fails base in. Accommodation facility at distance: fails (plus lens); at near: fails (plus lens).

Developmental status: TVAS = 14 (satisfactory). TAAS = 11 (satisfactory).

DIAGNOSIS

Intermittent exotropia at distance fixation; orthophoria at near fixation (i.e., divergence excess).

RECOMMENDATIONS

Vision therapy, if the child/parents are sufficiently motivated to devote about 30 minutes per day to the effort and visit this office every 2 weeks for the next 2 months—this to be followed by daily sessions of briefer duration that do not require parental supervision nor frequent visits to this office. We also reassured the parents that their youngter's binocular condition was not "dangerous"; if left unattended, it would not deteriorate into something "worse"; e.g., reduced sight or permanent exotropia.

□ Follow-up Data

Richard and his parents elected to attempt vision therapy. The parent's motivation: it should be done; Richard's motivation: he was embarrassed when his friends in school commented on the exotropia.

We dispensed a regimen that initially called for the daily use of a TV (red/green) stereotrainer and scheduled bi-weekly visits in this office to monitor his progress. This allowed us to exploit and improve the binocular abilities Richard already had available at distance fixation. At first, he worked on trying to take notice of what his eyes "felt like" when they were straight—with knowledge of alignment (feedback) provided by the TV stereotrainer.

Then he was supplied with some loose prisms to stimulate vergence facility at near and farpoint, again using the stereotrainer. A secondary, but important, goal of this initial period of treatment was to sensitize the youngster to physiological diplopia. A "Brock string" was used for this. (For a description of one prototype vision therapy regimen, see Rosner J, Rosner J. *Vision therapy in a primary care practice.* New York: Professional Press, 1988.)

Richard was conscientious in his efforts and made excellent progress. By the end of the first four weeks, he had developed reasonably good vergence facility at all fixation distances and an immediate awareness to physiological diplopia. He continued to manifest intermittent exotropia, but less often. (He was disappointed that, when it did manifest, the amount of exotropia was as much as it always was; he had thought that his progress would be reflected in a reduction of the magnitude of the deviation. We apologized for not forewarning of this—that "improvement" in his case would be documented by reduced frequency, not reduced magnitude.)

We then introduced Richard to nearpoint chiastopic and orthopic fusion techniques, using a pair of hand-held stereo targets. The procedure confused him at first, but he persevered and caught on. After he had practiced these procedures for a few weeks, enhancing vergence facility even further, we added farpoint chiastopic and orthopic fusion to his regimen. (He no longer used the stereotrainer.) In addition, the frequency of exotropia had dropped to the point where it rarely occurred during the course of a normal day—only when he was very tired. And even then, he was immediately aware of its occurrence and devoted the "mental effort" needed to bring the eyes back into alignment. In fact, at this point, Richard had acquired sufficient awareness of his binocular function to be able to manifest exotropia or alignment on request. In other words, he could allow the eye to drift temporally, if so inclined, or keep it in line. (When asked to describe this "awareness," the child replied, "My eyes feel different when they are straight." He was unable to offer anything more specific or concrete.)

Richard was advised to practice vergence facility via chiastopic and orthopic fusion as often as he could during the day—and nothing more. A few months later, he reported almost no episodes of exotropia, unless he chose to exercise it. We then suggested that he continue to practice what he had been doing, but not necessarily as often as before.

We did not see Richard again for about 6 months. At that visit, he and his parents happily reported a "cure"; no exotropia except for one occasion when he had a respiratory infection and an accompanying elevated body temperature. Our assessment corroborated this report. For all practical purposes, the treatment could be stopped. However, we suggested that it was advisable for him to continue to practice what he had learned about once each week—preferably selecting a time of the week when he usually did the same thing; e.g., just before going to church on Sunday morning, just before a favorite TV program, etc.

This was 2 years ago. We have seen Richard twice during that time. The last visit—a few weeks ago—found his status to be unchanged, except for one feature. He could no longer produce the exotropia at will; he had "forgotten" how to disassociate his eyes. We view this as a very favorable sign—an indication that alignment has become his habitual behavior.

□ General Comments

This case follows a prototype course. The patient was young, malleable, intelligent, and motivated. His parents have similar attributes. His binocular status was uncomplicated; he manifested divergence excess and nothing more. He had well-established potential for binocular function; when his eyes looked aligned, they really were aligned. Richard simply needed to alter some "bad habits" that had developed over the years, probably the outcome of a higher than average AC/A and an inability to compensate adequately for this when fixating at distance.

□ Questions Worth Discussing

1. Are there other tests we should have administered at that first visit? If so what, and why?

2. Would you have made the same recommendations as we did at that first visit? If not, what would you have recommended, and why?

3. Do you think Richard's visual status would have been different had he been treated earlier in life? If so, speculate how you would have treated it.

4. Do you agree with the treatment regimen? If not, how would you have altered it? Would Richard have progressed faster if training had started at near rather than at distance?

5. Would you have used minus lenses in this case, as an assist in facilitating binocular performance—at least until the benefits of vision therapy had started to become evident? Would minus lenses, if used, have caused Richard to develop myopia?

6. Why is it that improvement in this case is documented by reduced frequency rather than a reduction in the angle of deviation?

7. Would Richard, having successfully completed his vision therapy program, manifest exotropia if we occluded one of his eyes for a prolonged period of time; e.g., 24 hours?

PATIENT 12: DAVID (SIXTH-GRADE CHILD WITH A LONG-TERM LEARNING DISABILITY)

The chief purpose of this report is to illustrate the pragmatic importance of shifting clinical attention away from remediation (albeit justified) to compensation as the patient grows older and falls further and further behind in school. This report describes the clinical management of a sixth-grade boy who has had significant learning problems since entering school. Over the years, he has had many tests, acquired many diagnoses, and engaged in a variety of treatments, many of which were "successful" in what they sought to treat, but not successful in altering the child's school performance.

□ Visit #1 (January 1965)

SALIENT CLINICAL DATA

Age: 12 years, 8 months (DOB: May 1952).
  School: Neighborhood middle school; grade 6.
  Chief concern: David was referred to this office by his school counselor/psy-

chologist who advised us that the boy has experienced chronic learning difficulties for many years and is now starting to add to his problems by manifesting antisocial behavior, such as disrupting his classes, etc. His reading, writing, arithmetic, and spelling abilities are 2 to 3 years behind what is expected from a healthy, normally intelligent 12-year-old who is midway through the sixth grade.

Relevant history/initial impressions: David's mother reports that her son has had school difficulties since first grade. He has been examined by many different professionals and has had many diagnoses and treatments, none of which has improved his school performance significantly. He once wore glasses—when he was in first grade. Mrs. Green's recollection is that they were "not very strong," and that the "eye doctor did not think they were really necessary, but might help." David does not remember much about them other than that he did not want to wear glasses and was glad to give them up. He states that he sees clearly and that he never experiences visually related pain or discomfort. His general health has always been good, although he was thought to be "at risk" when born. He was born prematurely (birthweight: 3 pounds, 8 ounces) and was kept in the hospital nursery for about 1 month. His APGAR score, at 1 minute, was 6; this subsequently rose to 7 after 15 minutes. His mother did not monitor his development very closely, but her impression is that he was "about on schedule" in motor development, but did lag a bit in learning to speak. David is a short, thin youngster. He did not communicate freely during his visit, although his social behavior was quite acceptable.

Visual acuity (unaided): O.D., 20/20; O.S., 20/20.

Ocular health: No evidence of pathology or structural abnormalities.

Refractive status: O.D., +0.25 D sphere 20/20; O.S., +0.25 D sphere 20/20.

Binocular status (unaided): Cover test at distance = orthophoria; at near = 5 exophoria. Stereoacuity at distance = 1 minute arc (A.O.); at near = 40 seconds arc (Titmus). Vergence facility (unaided) at distance: satisfactory; at near: satisfactory.

Accommodation facility (unaided) at distance: satisfactory; at near: satisfactory.

Developmental status: TVAS score = 13 (unsatisfactory); TAAS score = 11 (unsatisfactory).

DIAGNOSIS

Very moderate hyperopia. Some lag in both visual and auditory analysis skills.

RECOMMENDATIONS

Intensive compensatory education. Send reports to pediatrician and school (see Figure 16.3).

□ FOLLOW-UP

David's parents attempted to persuade his school to provide him with a personalized educational program. The school did not deny their request, but neither could they fulfill it. David needed more help than they could provide; and, to

Report re: David Green
Age: 12 years, 8 months
School: Neighborhood Middle School; Grade 6
Date of visit: January, 19..

David was referred to this office by his school psychologist. The boy has experienced chronic learning difficulties since entering school, and is now starting to add to his problems by manifesting antisocial, disruptive behaviors in school. Mrs. Green, David's mother, reports that her son has had school difficulties since first grade. He has been examined by many different professionals and had many tentative diagnoses and treatments, none of which has been effective. (A complete history is on record, but will not be reported here.) In basic terms, his reading, writing, arithmetic, and spelling abilities are far below what is expected from a normal, healthy 12 year old.

David has had previous eye examinations. Lenses were prescribed once—"for reading." This, when he was about six years old. Glasses were obtained, worn for a short while, then discarded when he was re-assessed by the original examiner. He has not worn glasses since, although his eyes have been examined regularly. Our examination corroborated the last opinion cited above. David's eyes appeared to be healthy and normally formed. Refraction revealed no significant deviation; he is very moderately farsighted. His eyesight is good (20/20, each eye). His binocular coordination is normal.

We also assessed the youngster's perceptual skills. David shows deficits in both visual and auditory analysis skills—not marked deficits, but deficits nonetheless. In our opinion, David's perceptual skills have probably always lagged and, at present, he is starting to "catch up," to acquire these skills, albeit somewhat behind schedule. Carrying that idea further, his school difficulties may therefore be linked, at least in part, with this lag in perceptual skills development—development of basic learning aptitudes that are crucial in standard instructional settings. As a result, by sixth grade, David's knowledge deficits are major, while his perceptual skills deficits are diminishing.

In consideration of the above, I believe that the best way to help David now is to focus directly on his school performance and needs, and treat all other deficits as subordinate to that. In other words, I do not recommend that David engage in a perceptual skills training program at this time, as a means of trying to 'cure' him. Rather, I urge that David be (a) placed in a setting where he will be provided with the opportunity to learn skills that have practical value and that he *can* learn despite his academic deficiencies, and (b) provided with the kind of highly structured, individualized, remedial instructional program that he needs in order to start making *some* progress in reading, arithmetic, spelling, and writing.

Certainly, perceptual skills training is justifiable, but it would be a

Figure 16.3 Report sent regarding David Green.

mistake to address his perceptual skills deficits independently of his educational needs. Once David is convinced that he is capable of learning—and that depends on the amount and quality of his instructional program—he will probably be more responsive to ancillary treatments. Until then, it would simply aggravate his problem to do anything that is not directly related to some easily-observed progress in the classroom. There is only one treatment that can do this: solid, effective, tailor-made instruction—instruction that takes into account his present ability level and builds upon that. There is no reason to believe that David cannot learn; but there is every reason to believe that he will not learn in a standard program. Hence this recommendation.

Please feel free to contact me should additional and/or more specific information be desired.

J. Rosner, O.D.

Figure 16.3   (Continued)

compound the problem, he was not cooperative—he no longer believed that he could succeed in school and he no longer was willing to try.

Following a few sessions with a private tutor, David's parents again met with school personnel and arranged a program for their child that would reduce the stress he was experiencing in the regular classroom.

Upon entering seventh grade, David was allowed to enroll in classes that taught vocational skills. Over time, he displayed an interest and aptitude for electronic equipment. He continued to expand his knowledge in this area during his high school years.

David is now employed by a local computer company. He is competent in his job and socially well-adapted. He can read and calculate at about the sixth grade level—not sufficient to gain him entry into a demanding university program but certainly sufficient for his day-to-day needs.

□ General Comments

The key aspects of this case are (a) the child's age at his first visit in our office, (b) the significant educational lag he displayed at that time, and (c) the fact that his visual/ocular condition was excellent except for a moderate lag in visual and auditory analysis skills development. This combination of circumstances almost invariably leads us to recommend a compensatory instructional program rather than remediation of the perceptual skills deficit. Our reason: The boy has experienced school failure for a long time; he is showing signs of frustration. Engaging him in activities that might, in time, improve his basis analytic aptitudes—thereby making it easier for him to learn—may very well be desirable, but these activities would not provide the child with the school-related information he must have if he is to make satisfactory progress in the sixth grade. If the remediation effort worked, it would be another classic case of "the operation was a success but the patient died." Besides, it is almost certain that David would not commit himself to the remedial program, especially as he recognized that improved visual and auditory analysis skills do not automatically bring about academic success. It is for these reasons that we urged that David be placed in a school setting in which he would not fail, even though it meant acknowledging that he would probably never go beyond a high school education.

□ **Questions Worth Discussing**

1. One could speculate about what earlier intervention might have done for this boy. Assuming that David was a bit slow in developing visual and auditory perceptual skills, could these have been improved when he was in first grade, and if so, would the effects of that improvement have been reflected in his classroom performance? Keep in mind that David's birth history implies significant distress and the possibility of some minimal central nervous system insult.
2. Would David have benefited from a school system that identified and provided for his special educational needs early on—before he had experienced the repeated failures in elementary school.
3. Should David's entry into first grade have been delayed a year or two? Might this have improved his chances for early school success—surely an important factor in subsequent school performance?
4. Was our assessment as thorough as it should have been? That is, should other tests have been administered, and if so, why—how could we have used that information?
5. Describe, in general terms, the nature of the compensatory instruction program that would benefit David? Should we be concerned about whether he is a "visual learner" or an "auditory learner"?

PATIENT 13: CLAIRE (AUDITORY PERCEPTUAL SKILLS DEFICITS)

The purpose of this report is to illustrate how the optometrist may be involved in the management of a child who displays no visual/ocular problems but does manifest substandard auditory analysis skills development. It describes a third-grade child who was referred to us because she has was having difficulty learning to read—a problem that, in our opinion, was closely related to a lag in development of auditory perceptual skills.

□ Visit #1 (February 1982)

SALIENT CLINICAL DATA

Age: 8 years, 7 months (DOB: July 1973).

School: Neighborhood elementary; grade 3

Chief concern: Claire has a persistent reading problem. Purpose of this visit is to rule out any visual and/or perceptual skills factors that might be contributing to that problem. Claire's mother reported that the child has had reading difficulties since first grade—specifically, in "decoding"; in remembering her reading words. The rest of her school work is satisfactory. She has recently been given an extensive battery of psychoeducational tests and found to be of at least average intelligence, with adequate vocabulary and reasoning ability. On the basis of this information, she is to be placed in a Resource Room program at school, so as to provide her with some additional help in reading.

Relevant history/initial impressions: Claire is a healthy child, but does have a history of chronic ear infections during her preschool years. There had once been some question about her hearing, but this was recently tested and found to be normal. She appears to be an attractive, quiet, shy, reasonably intelligent youngster.

Unaided distance visual acuity: O.D., 20/20; O.S., 20/20.

Ocular health: No evidence of pathology or structural abnormalities.

Refractive status: O.D., $+0.50 - 0.25$ cx 180; O.S., $+0.25 - 0.25$ cx 180.

Binocular status (unaided): Cover test (unaided) at distance = orthophoria; at near = 7 exophoria. Stereoacuity (aided) at distance = 1 minute arc (A.O.); at near = 20 seconds arc (Randot). Vergence facility (distance and near): satisfactory. Accommodation facility (distance and near): satisfactory.

Developmental status: TVAS score = 16 (satisfactory); TAAS score = 6 (unsatisfactory).

DIAGNOSIS

Very moderate degree of ametropia that, in our opinion, is not related to child's school difficulties. Significant deficit in auditory analysis skills, which, in contrast, we believe to be closely related to her reading problem.

RECOMMENDATIONS

Auditory perceptual skills remedial therapy in conjunction with appropriate accommodations in her instructional program. Send reports to pediatrician and school (see Figure 16.4).

□ Follow-up Data

Our recommendations (as cited in our report—Figure 16.4) were implemented, although the auditory analysis skills training program had to be home-based.

Report re: Claire Doe
Age: 8 years, 7 months
School: Neighborhood Elementary; Grade 3
Date of visit: February 16, 19..

Claire was referred to us because of her persistent reading problem and a concern that at least some of her difficulties stemmed from visual/perceptual skills factors. Claire has had difficulty with learning to read since first grade. Specifically, her problem seems to be an inability to learn the "decoding" (word recognition) skills that underlie fluent reading. The rest of her school work is satisfactory. Her general health is good, but she does have a history of chronic ear infections during her preschool years. Two of these episodes necessitated the insertion of drainage tubes. There had once been some question about her hearing, but this has been tested and found to be normal. Claire is an attractive, shy, apparently intelligent youngster.

Claire has never had an eye examination previous to this visit. She has always passed the school vision screening test and has never displayed any signs of substandard vision or ocular discomfort. Her eyes appeared to be normally formed and free of disease. Her eyesight is clear—20/20 in each eye. Refraction revealed a trivial amount of hyperopic (farsighted) astigmatism, but not enough to warrant lens use. Her binocular abilities were also within normal limits. In short, whatever the child's reading problem may stem from, it does not appear to be connected to a visual factor.

Claire's visual perceptual skills are normal. She displayed a competent (for 3rd grade) ability to identify the key features of spatially-organized patterns: separate quantities and relationships. In contrast, her auditory analysis skills are substandard; she showed a great deal of difficulty in identifying the separate sounds of spoken words. There is little doubt that this is related to her reading problem.

In consideration of the above, I recommended a two-pronged treatment approach for the child: (1) teach her the auditory analysis skills she presently lacks and needs if she is to make satisfactory progress in a standard reading program; (2) provide her with additional support in reading class until her auditory analysis skills are improved. This latter translates into a greater emphasis on phonics. As noted, Claire's auditory analysis skills deficit means that she is not sufficiently aware of the separate sounds of spoken speech. Emphasizing phonics accommodates that deficit to some extent in that, by definition, "phonics" explicates the link between printed letters and spoken sounds.

An effective auditory analysis program will require about ten minutes per day, five days each week. It is best administered in school, but can be carried out at home under parental supervision if necessary. There are a number of commercially-prepared programs that would help Claire, and I presume that her school already has one or more of these. Should specific suggestions be desired, please do not hesitate to contact

---

Figure 16.4   Report sent regarding Claire Doe.

me. (I should stress here the importance of using a program that focuses on the sounds in words rather than on nonverbal sounds, background noises, etc.)

Once the program has been instituted, I will arrange to see Claire on a monthly basis in order to monitor her progress. Prognosis, in my opinion, is excellent—if she is given the aid she needs *at this stage* of her school career. Further delay would be very detrimental.

Please feel free to contact me if additional and/or more specific information is desired.

Joy Rosner, O.D.

Figure 16.4   (Continued)

Claire's teacher was interested in it but did not have the time or help needed to carry it out on a regular basis. She did, however, see the wisdom in putting more emphasis on phonics as a method for helping Claire recognize the "system" on which reading and spelling are based.

Claire returned to our office about three times between the intial visit and the end of the school year. During that time, her auditory analysis skills improved significantly; TAAS score (in May) = 13 (maximum). More importantly, her reading skills improved—not to the point where she read at the level appropriate for her grade placement, but far better than at the beginning of the treatment period.

At the recommendation of her teacher, Claire's parents employed a competent reading tutor over the summer period. She, too, emphasized phonics, taught Claire how to exploit words she already knew "by sight," to help in reading unfamiliar words; how, for example, rapid recognition of the word "ring" facilitated reading such words as "string," "bring," "ringing," "sing," etc.

Claire is now in the sixth grade. Her visual/ocular status remains unchanged. She has overcome her reading deficit; she now scores at about the average level in school achievement testing.

☐ General Comments

Claire's case is not unusual: a child encountering chronic difficulty learning the basics of reading, yet with at least average cognitive abilities. Such children often present in optometrist's offices and, also often, are not quite so intact visually as was Claire. This presents the optometrist with a dilemma: should the child's school difficulties be attributed to the visual deficits that are observed (e.g., refractive, accommodative, and/or vergence infacility) or should these visual deficits be ignored? In our judgment, neither decision is the correct one. Visual deficits should not be ignored, but neither should they be perceived as the key factor in determining how well a child acquires the basic, "word recognition" skills that underlie reading. Hence, albeit that assessment of auditory analysis skills is beyond the traditionally defined scope of our profession, we argue that they should be investigated, if only because of our basic obligation as primary-care practitioners. How we should then interpret test outcomes is not as clear cut. Some optometrists will limit their involvement to administering the TAAS and reporting results to parents and school. Others, at the opposite end, will mount a full-blown, office-based remedial program, including reading tutoring. Most—including us—will report test findings and make what we believe to be appropriate recommendations.

☐ Questions Worth Discussing

1. Would you have prescribed glasses in this case? If so, why?

2. Would you have administered the TAAS? Or do you believe that optometrists should not intrude into the professional domain of other practitioners? If that is the case, what is your position on assessing blood pressure in your practices? Will you do it, thereby implying that you diagnose and treat hypertension?

3. Claire might very well have grown out of her auditory analysis skills problems; that is, developed those skills on her own, without remediation. If you were assured that this would happen, albeit that you did not know when it would happen, would you have prescribed as we did, of would you have chosen to defer treatment and "let nature take its course"?

■

PATIENT 14: JACK (PSEUDOMYOPIA)

The chief purpose of this report is to illustrate one approach to the clinical management of pseudomyopia. It describes the clinical picture of a 7-year-old who presented with blurred distance vision.

☐ Visit #1 (February 1985)

SALIENT CLINICAL DATA

Age: 12 years, 6 months (DOB: August 1973).

Chief concern: Child failed school vision screening because of reduced visual acuity.

Relevant history/general impressions: This is Jack's first eye examination. His prenatal, perinatal, and postnatal health histories are uneventful. His development has been normal; if anything, he was precocious in development of language skills. He is in second grade, making better than average progress. He is a very good reader, and according to his mother, he likes to read books "for fun."

Unaided distance visual acuity: O.D., 20/50; O.S., 20/50 (Snellen letters).

Ocular health: No evidence of pathology or structural abnormalities. Unrestricted motilities.

Refraction status without cycloplegic: O.D., −0.75 D sphere 20/30+; O.S., −0.75 D sphere 20/30+. With cycloplegic: O.D., +0.50 D sphere 20/25 (under cycloplegia); O.S., +0.50 D sphere 20/25 (under cycloplegia).

Binocular status: Cover test (unaided) at distance = 1 esophoria; at near = 10 esophoria. Cover test (through −0.75D) at distance = 8 esophoria; at near = 18 esophoria. Cover test (through +0.50D) at distance = 2 exophoria; at near = exophoria. Stereoacuity (unaided) at distance = 4 minutes arc (A.O.); at near = 100 seconds arc (Randot). Stereoacuity (−0.75D) at distance = 4 minutes arc (A.O.) (Randot); at near = 200 seconds arc. Sterioacuity (+0.50D) at distance = 3 minutes arc (A.O.) (Randot); at near = 60 seconds arc. Vergence facility tested unaided and with patient wearing −0.75D spheres (O.U.) - In both instances, patient failed to meet passing criteria; could not adapt to minimal amounts of base-in prism. Vergence facility through +0.50D spheres was not tested; patient was too exhausted and under the influence of cycloplegia.

Accommodation facility was tested unaided and with patient wearing −0.75D spheres (O.U.). In both instances, patient failed to meet passing criteria; could not adapt to minimal amounts of minus spheres; manifested diplopia. Accommodative facility through +0.50D spheres was not tested; patient was too exhausted and under the influence of cycloplegia.

Developmental status: TVAS = 12 (satisfactory). TAAS = 13 (better than expected).

DIAGNOSIS

Pseudomyopia in conjunction with ciliary spasm.

RECOMMENDATIONS

Plus lenses for near, to be worn full time until spasm relaxes. Because of need for constant wear, lenses are to be designed in bifocal form. Rx: O.U. Plano/ +1.00 add. Parents advised that this prescription was likely to be changed as the child began to respond to the plus power. Our goal in this case: Patient to demonstrate at least 2.50 diopters of positive relative accommodation. We also advised them that a certain amount of vision therapy might be needed, but that we preferred to delay that decision until the effects of the lenses could be assessed. Parents accepted recommendations.

□ Follow-up Data

Jack wore his glasses as directed, although at the onset he generated some parental anxiety by noting that "they don't help at all." We assessed the clinical situation about 2 weeks after he started to wear the glasses and were able to reassure Jack's parents that "everything was as expected right now." We saw the boy again about a month later. Positive effects were very evident. Unaided visual acuity in each eye was 20/25 +. Manifest refraction: plano. And, most important for Jack's parents, the child reported that he no longer was experiencing difficulty seeing the chalkboard in his classrooms. Following a complete refraction, lens prescription was changed to +0.50/+1.50D add (O.U.). Jack was advised to continue to wear his glasses full time—but that he could look forward to the time when this would no longer be necessary.

Two years elapsed before we felt it safe to allow Jack to reduce wearing time to nearpoint activities only. We did not prescribe any vision therapy during that time.

Jack was last seen a few weeks ago, 5 years after his first visit. He continues to wear his glasses for nearpoint activities, but not as consistently as before. He is symptom free. He shows no signs of pseudomyopia. His visual acuity, binocular status, and adaptability are all normal without glasses. We advised him to continue lens wear as he has been these past few years and allow us to conduct annual examinations. Prognosis is excellent. We anticipate that Jack will wear glasses for near use during his forthcoming college years and beyond—he intends to study law; reading will be an essential aspect of his daily life.

☐ **General Comments**

Pseudomyopia is sometimes difficult to detect. This was not so with Jack. The condition was revealed in his case by (a) an inability to obtain 20/20 acuity with the minus lenses and (b) the high esophoria. Jack responded exceptionally well to the lens therapy. All visual functions returned to a normal status.

☐ **Questions Worth Discussing**

1. Are there other tests we should have administered at that first visit? If so what, and why?

2. Would you have made the same recommendations as we did at that first visit (i.e., bifocal lenses)? If not, what would you have recommended, and why?

3. Do you think dynamic retinoscopy would have done as well as the cycloplegic in revealing the pseudomyopia?

4. Should we have prescribed vision therapy as well as lenses? Why?

5. What do you predict would have occurred had we prescribed the minus (0.75D) lenses measured retinoscopically at the first visit? Would Jack have worn them? Would he have found them helpful? Would it have stimulated the development of myopia?

6. What do you predict would have occurred had we prescribed single vision (convex) lenses for near use only at that first visit?

7. Why should Jack continue to use the lenses so many years after he has returned to a normal status? Or shouldn't he? What are the risks?

8. Why did the ciliary spasm develop in the first place? Would we have been able to detect it at some date prior to Jack's first visit? What would have been the indicators and how early would they have been evident?

INDEX